D1226649

HANDBOOK OF
EMERGENCY TOXICOLOGY

Publication Number 1034

AMERICAN LECTURE SERIES

A Monograph in

The BANNERSTONE DIVISION *of*
AMERICAN LECTURES IN PUBLIC PROTECTION

Edited by

LE MOYNE SNYDER, M.D.
RALPH F. TURNER
RUSSELL S. FISHER, M.D.

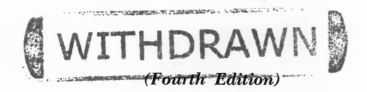

(Fourth Edition)

HANDBOOK OF EMERGENCY TOXICOLOGY

A Guide for the Identification, Diagnosis, and Treatment of Poisoning

By

SIDNEY KAYE, M.Sc., Ph.D.

Professor of Toxicology; Legal-Medicine; and Pharmacology
Chief, Toxicology Section
School of Medicine, University of Puerto Rico

Chief Forensic Toxicologist and Associate Director
Institute of Legal Medicine
University of Puerto Rico

Coordinator, Poison Control Centers
Department of Health
Commonwealth of Puerto Rico

Consulting Toxicologist
United States Army and Navy
United States Veterans Administration Hospital
San Juan, Puerto Rico

Colonel, MSC, AUS (Research and Development), Retired

Consultant Emeritus in Toxicology to the
United States Department of the Army

Formerly, State Toxicologist and
Coordinator, Poison Control Centers, Health Department
Commonwealth of Virginia

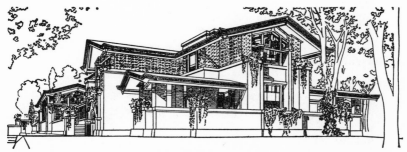

CHARLES C THOMAS • **PUBLISHER**
Springfield • *Illinois* • *U.S.A.*

Published and Distributed Throughout the World by
CHARLES C THOMAS • PUBLISHER
BANNERSTONE HOUSE
301-327 East Lawrence Avenue, Springfield, Illinois, U.S.A.

© *1954, 1961, 1970, 1973, and 1980 by*
CHARLES C THOMAS • PUBLISHER
ISBN 0-398-03960-7
Library of Congress Catalog Card Number: 79-17565

First Edition, 1954
Second Edition, 1961
Third Edition, First Printing, 1970
Third Edition, Second Printing, 1973
Third Edition, Third Printing, 1977
Fourth Edition, 1980

Printed in the United States of America
N-11

Library of Congress Cataloging in Publication Data

Kaye, Sidney, 1912-
    Handbook of emergency toxicology.

    (American lecture series ; publication no. 1034)
    Bibliography: p.
    Includes index.
1. Poisoning. I. Title.
RA1211.K3   1980   615.9'08   79-17565
ISBN   0-398-03960-7

To
Carmen, Cynthia, and Frederic

FOREWORD

THE PAST DECADE has seen remarkable advances in the field of toxicology. Many toxic substances have come into common use, not only as a result of the development of new insecticides and agricultural poisons, but also through the introduction of new therapeutic agents, solvents, and industrial chemicals. It has been difficult if not impossible for the average medical practitioner or medical student to keep abreast of this flood of new poisons, their trade names, common sources of contact, potency, symptoms and treatment of resulting poisonings. When a case of poisoning occurs, little opportunity is afforded for research reading or study; either effective antidotal measures are employed promptly or serious consequences ensue.

During this decade of rapid toxicological development in this country, there has been a dearth of up-to-date books published on the subject, so that one has been forced to turn to clinical and toxicological studies scattered throughout the medical and chemical literature. *Emergency Toxicology* will come as a welcome aid to fill this deficiency. Through his experience in the laboratories of the Chief Medical Examiner of New York City, his services in the St. Louis Police Laboratory, the wartime experience in the toxicology laboratories of the U. S. Army Medical Department, and his duties as Toxicologist to the Chief Medical Examiner of Virginia, the author is preeminently qualified to speak with authority on the subject.

From the viewpoint of the laboratory technician, the analytical procedures given in this book will be most helpful in the identification and determination of toxic agents. Newer methods are given for the identification of poisons by means of their charac-

vii

teristic absorption spectra, and more rapid estimations by means of the photoelectric colorimeter are detailed.

This book is recommended for use by medical practitioners and laboratory investigators, whose prompt action in handling cases of poisoning may result in the saving of life or in minimizing harm from the ingestion of some unidentified toxic substance.

CLARENCE W. MUEHLBERGER, PH.D.

PREFACE TO FOURTH EDITION

IDENTIFICATION AND RAPID DIAGNOSIS of acute poisoning continues to be a serious need. This is especially true in the small hospitals.

When dealing with poisoning cases, time is not available to search the literature. Your nearest poison control center and your own ready references and experience may help to reach a presumptive diagnosis by alerting as to signs and symptoms and by rapid laboratory tests that can be performed.

Supportive and symptomatic treatment in suspected cases of poisoning *should not be delayed* (treat the patient—not the poison). Nevertheless, every effort should be made to identify the toxic agent. A rapid, simple, reliable test to support diagnosis can be very assuring, especially today when specific treatment is available in some cases and can make the difference between survival and death.

In acute emergencies, it is not always possible to send specimens to distant laboratories. Any laboratory regardless of size could be set up to screen or test at least for some of the more common poisonings occurring in your area. As training and experience allows, additional tests may be added as needed.

A simplified general guide is presented to help classify and detect some of the common poisonings by characteristic properties, signs and symptoms, and by screening tests.

All sections have been revised and some were completely rewritten to include new and improved techniques. Each common poison is described according to synonyms, general uses, properties, approximate minimum lethal dose, typical signs and symptoms, suggested general guide for treatment, and rapid presumptive tests for identification.

In most cases, several tests for each poison are described so that each individual laboratory will find at least one or several tests suited to their facilities and immediate needs.

It has been our purpose to update and bring together as much information as possible for a quick reference, to supply a ready guide for dealing with a suspected poisoning. Acetaminophen, methaqualone, paraquat, phencyclidine, and vacor have been added and data of UV spectra, gas chomatography, and thin layer chromatography have been expanded to include other drugs.

Thanks and acknowledgement are due to my staff: José R. Rodriguez, Emma Rodriguez, Carmen Santiago, Lucy Lane, Flor Cabrera, Mildred Collazo, Vanesa Narvaez, and Silvia Martínez.

It has been a pleasure to work with Payne Thomas who has been a stimulating force to produce this 4th Edition. Special thanks is due Hope Wright for her suggestions and diligence in editing the manuscript and galley proofs.

S.K.

PREFACE TO THIRD EDITION

DRUGS AND CHEMICAL PRODUCTS are increasingly being produced and finding their way into our homes and at work. Therefore, poisoning is continuing to be a constant everyday hazard. A rapid diagnosis is essential for proper management. Rapid and more exacting technics have been developed since the second edition.

It has been our purpose to update and bring together as much information as possible for a quick reference, to supply a ready guide for dealing with a suspected poisoning.

Although supportive treatment in suspected cases should not be delayed, every effort should be exerted to identify the toxic agent. There is a great need for more and better toxicology facilities in some of our hospitals.

Rapid presumptive tests for the common poisons such as alcohol (ethyl and methyl), aspirin, salicylates, phenothiazines, barbiturates, arsenic, mercury, carbon monoxide, and bromides are described in detail. These tests are simple, reliable, and easily performed.

In most cases, several tests for each poison are described so that each individual laboratory will find at least one or several tests suited to their facilities and immediate needs.

All sections of this edition have been revised and some completely rewritten. Parathion and morphine, which now have become such major hazards to our society, have been dealt with in more detail. New and improved technics have made necessary additions or revision to previous discussions of barbiturates, Dieldrin, ether, mercury, meprobamate, digitalis, amphetamines, lead, fluorides, phenothiazines, and others; "glue sniffing" and

LSD have been added.   Ultraviolet spectra data for new drugs, near infrared spectrophotometry, gas chromatography, and thin layer chromatography have now been included.

I would like to thank Mr. Payne Thomas and his staff for their constant encouragement and their diligence in converting a manuscript into a handbook.   Thanks also are due to Alma Tudó de Lewis, Eduardo Cardona, Jaime Irizarry, José Rafael Rodríguez, Etanislao Martínez, and Carmen I. Castro de Santiago.   Special thanks to my wife for proofreading and suggestions.

S.K.

PREFACE TO SECOND EDITION

I AM DEEPLY APPRECIATIVE of the cordial reception given to the first edition and hope that the second edition will continue to serve its purpose.

It has been intended to gather together in one small handbook as much information as practical to deal with a suspected common poisoning.

Many new drugs and chemicals have been developed since the first edition, and these multitudes of potential toxic agents now present a perplexing problem in identification and treatment. Fortunately, however, there also have been recent advances in methodology. *Rapid* and more exacting technics have been developed within the past several years employing to greater advantage the ultraviolet range of the spectrophotometer at two different pH's, paper chromatography, microdiffusion, and direct extraction technics, to mention only a few. These new technics and rapid simplified procedures have been included in this revision.

The sections on alcohol, carbon monoxide, and barbiturates have been rewritten and enlarged; also the section on poisonous plants has been greatly expanded, as well as the section on common trade names with their ingredients. New tranquilizers, antihistamines, and hypnotics recently developed are included. Tests for paraldehyde, ethylene glycol, oxalates, amphetamines, morphine, and methemoglobin have been completely revised; others, partially revised or replaced.

Many of the tests have been geared for speed and simplicity to assist the poison control centers to make a rapid evaluation in questions of emergency poisoning. This was specially aimed for the common ones such as ethyl and methyl alcohols, carbon monoxide, barbiturates, arsenic, mercury, and aspirin. Every hospital laboratory of moderate size should be set up to do these rapid determinations.

New concepts of treatment reported in the literature, as well as generalized and specific signs and symptoms associated with the newer potential toxic agents, have been included.

I would like again to thank my many friends and associates for their kind assistance and suggestions. Special thanks, however, are due to Dr. G. T. Mann, Mr. Ramon A. Morano, Mr. Elmer L. Gordon, Dr. H. B. Haag, Dr. C. W. Muehlberger, Dr. H. L. Beddoe, and Mr. C. Reginald Hall for their cooperation.

S.K.

PREFACE TO FIRST EDITION

MANY DEATHS OCCUR ANNUALLY due to accidental, suicidal, homicidal, or industrial poisonings. Some of these deaths could have been avoided with an accurate diagnosis and adequate treatment. Early recognition of the characteristic signs and symptoms of poisons is therefore a very important factor in the prevention of death due to poisoning.

One day, this recognition problem will confront you. Then the question will arise, "Is this ill health, disease, or intoxication caused by a poison or toxic agent and, if so, what can be done to support life?" Before you can answer this question, you must know:

1. Whether signs observed are consistent with the poison or toxic agent in question. Which diseases will exhibit similar signs or symptoms. (Were these ruled out?)

2. Whether poison was demonstrated by analysis of body fluids.

3. If the "alleged" quantity taken approximates toxic levels. Then and only then are you justified in giving specific treatment, which in some cases is not without danger.

S.K.

ACKNOWLEDGMENTS

THE AUTHOR WISHES to express his appreciation to his many friends and colleagues who gave so generously of their time and suggestions. Special thanks are due to Dr. G.T. Mann, Chief Medical Examiner for the Commonwealth of Virginia; Dr. C.W. Muehlberg, State Toxicologist for Michigan; Dr. H.B. Haag, Professor of Pharmacology, Medical College of Virginia; Dr. T.H. Alphin, Chemical Warfare Consultant, Federal Civil Defense Administration, Washington, D.C.; Dr. G.W. Thoma, Assistant Chief Medical Examiner; and Dr. A.E.A. Hudson, Research Consultant, North Carolina State College; Dr. H.G. Kupfer, Professor of Clinical Pathology and Director of Hospital Laboratories, Medical College of Virginia; Dr. L.R. Goldbaum, Chief of Toxicology, Army Medical Center, Washington, D.C.; Drs. R.N. Harger and R. Forney, Toxicologists, Indiana University School of Medicine for their constructive criticisms and many suggestions. And finally, no end of thanks to Mr. Elmer Gordon and Mr. Ramon Morano for their tireless efforts, especially in proofreading.

Suggestions for therapy in this volume have been prepared in kind cooperation with the medical staff of the Department of Legal Medicine, Medical College of Virginia.

S.K.

CONTENTS

SECTION I

SECTION II

Contents

HANDBOOK OF
EMERGENCY TOXICOLOGY

SECTION I

INTRODUCTION

EMERGENCY TOXICOLOGY

*E*mergency Toxicology deals with the problems involved in the rapid presumptive diagnosis and treatment of "alleged" poisoning. Rapid access to some information should be available that could assist the physician in terms of synonyms, common uses, general properties, minimum lethal doses (MLD), nature of injury and signs and symptoms, simple tests or rapid presumptive identification, interpretations and evaluation of these results, suggested guide for antidote and treatment and management.

POISON

By definition, a *poison* is an agent (acting chemically) that may produce an injurious or deadly effect when introduced into the living body; thus, *almost anything* is a potential poison when taken in "sufficient quantity." For practical purposes, however, a poison may be limited to those substances that produce injurious or deadly effect only when taken in quantities of 50 grams (gm) or less. A *potent poison* is one which requires less than 5 gm, and a *very potent poison* is one which requires less than 1 gm to produce these effects.

Poisons and poisonings have been with man since his early days, but never have they been such a problem as today. The problem gets worse with time. New drugs and chemicals are being developed and produced in vast numbers, and as a result (in part) poisonings are on the increase. A quick differential diagnosis is highly desirable to help minimize damage and to ensure that adequate treatment is initiated quickly:

5

Is it a poison? If so, which one?
Was there a bottle? Was a label on it?
Will the poison control center have the brand name cata-
logued?

Many times no bottle is available, or the bottle had no label, or it was the wrong bottle. *Now what?*

In questions of poisoning, diagnosis is not always simple. Every assistance must be solicited: signs and symptoms, speed of onset, intensity, odors, any other leads or clues that may be of some material help in arriving at an early diagnosis. Rapid, simple, sensitive, and reliable tests, especially for the more common poisons, would also help to confirm diagnosis.

Even though you cannot immediately identify the agent, *do not delay treatment.* Symptomatic treatment and supportive measures are given as needed, and in many cases, this is all that is available or that is necessary.

Support all vital functions. Avoid unnecessary drugs; support whenever possible by mechanical rather than by chemical means. Refer to the Physician's Desk Reference (PDR) and to the manufacturer's products package insert for more information.

Simple tests are listed under each specific poison. It may be more fruitful to look first for those poisons more common in your area.

Continue your efforts to try to identify the particular poison so that more definite treatment, if available, may be instituted.

The following, it is hoped, will be of some assistance as a general guide in identifying, evaluating, and treating some of the poisons you may encounter.

LETHAL DOSES

IT IS NOT POSSIBLE to be definite in describing lethal doses because of the many variables and the lack of proper controls. Many animal experiments have been reported, but animals do not always demonstrate the same response as humans to the same toxic agents. Nevertheless, they do make available some knowledge about action and relative toxicities of agents and, although not the ideal method, this constitutes the best one available. Results of these experiments are reported as lethal dose fatal to 50 percent of animals in the experiment (LD/50). Dealing with human toxicities, the minimum lethal dose (MLD) is of more practical value. For the most part, our present available data are those obtained from case histories of poisoning where some indication of quantity and type, and other factors, are "allegedly" known and reported.

The MLDs reported in the literature may vary somewhat, but for the most part they are reasonably close. These variants most likely are due to many factors:

1. History may be misleading; estimated amount taken may be reported in error by witness or patient.
2. Loss of material by vomiting is difficult to estimate.
3. Form in which material is taken is very importnt (whether soluble or not; soluble barium salts are very toxic, but insoluble barium sulfate is not). Bioavailability.
4. Particle size is a factor regulating rate of absorption and speed of action.
5. Whether food was in the stomach at the time (to slow absorption); protein food would act as an antidote for metallic poisons. Presence of other drugs.
6. How poison entered the body—intravenous, intramuscular,

7

lungs, rectum, vagina, mouth or skin.
7. Plus other factors.

The fatal dose varies with the *actual amount absorbed* into the system.   Except for the local irritant action on the gastrointestinal tract, the material that remains in this tract is inert so far as lethal dose is concerned.   The fatal dose also varies with the body weight, age, health, idiosyncrasies, rate of detoxification, and elimination of the drug. It also varies with the amount of material given or taken either in one dose or accumulated over a period of time (acute vs. chronic) .   In spite of all these many variables, there are available some fairly reliable data on the approximate MLD (for a 70 kg person) for many of the common acute poisons:

Arsenic (As_2O_3) —100 mg	Mercuric chloride—0.5 gm
Aconitine—10 mg	Methanol—70 ml
Barbiturates—1 to 5 gm	Nicotine—50 mg
Boric acid—12 gm	Paraldehyde—100 ml
Camphor—2 gm	Parathion—25 mg
Cantharidin—30 mg	Phenols—10 ml
Chloral hydrate—7 gm	Phosphorus (yellow)—O.1 gm
Chlorates (K)—8 gm	Strychnine—50 mg
Formaldehyde—30 ml	Thallium—0.8 gm
Fluorides (Na) 1 gm	Whiskey (100 proof)1 pt–1 qt.

For others, see under specific poisons.

Although this MLD is only approximate, it can be of great assistance to the physician in evaluating the seriousness of a situation and probabilities of injury or fatality.

SYMPTOMS AND SIGNS

SYMPTOMS AND SIGNS are the effects, stated or observed, produced by the action of a particular poison on the physiologic functions of the body. These effects may be characteristic, especially in the absence of other possible causes. The presence of a particular symptom or sign may be enough to direct our attention toward a particular group or type of poisoning and, in like manner, may help to rule out other possibilities. For example, coma may suggest barbiturates and would rule out strychnine. Many diseases, however, produce symptoms similar to those caused by poisons, and special care is urged in the differential diagnosis.

A partial listing of some of these common symptoms and signs follow. However, these symptoms are not infallible because they may or may not be always present. Confirmation of the suspected poison by reliable methods of identification would still be indicated, if possible.

NAUSEA, VOMITING, ABDOMINAL PAIN, OR DIARRHEA

Poisons

acetaminophen
acetanilide
acetic acid
acetone
acids
aconitine
alcohols
alkalies
aminophylline
antimony
arsenic
aspidium
aspirin
benzene
borates
boric acid
bromides
camphor
cantharides
carbamate
carbon disulfide
carbon monoxide
croton oil
DDT (dichlorodiphenyltrichloroethane)
detergents

9

digitalis
3,5-dinitro-o-cresol
emetine
ergot
essential oils
ether
ethyl alcohol
ethylene glycol
fluorides
food poisoning
formaldehyde
halogens
heavy metal salts
hexachlorophene
ipecac
kerosene
methaqualone
methyl alcohol
morphine
moth balls
muscarine
naphthalene
nicotine
oxalates
oxalic acid
paraquat
parathion
pesticides
phenols and derivatives
phenothiazine derivatives
phosphorus (yellow)

pilocarpine
poisonous plants
propoxyphene
quaternary ammonium compounds
ricin oil
salicylates
sodium monofluor acetate (1080)
solanine
toxalbumins
turpentine
vacor
veratrine
vitamins (vitamin A)
xylene
all other irritants and corrosives

Diseases

acidosis
appendicitis
brain tumor
enteritis
gastritis
infectious diseases, onset
intestinal obstruction
kidney disturbances
liver disturbances
pancreatic disturbances
pregnancy, early
ulcer, gastric or duodenal
uremia

EXCITATION, TWITCHING, CONVULSIONS

Poisons

absinthe
acetaminophen
aconitine
aldrin
aminophylline
ammonium salts
amphetamines
antipyrine
arsenic
aspidium
aspirin
atropine and similar compounds
barium
benzene

brucine
caffeine
camphor
cantharides
carbon disulfide
carbon monoxide
chlorates
chlordan(e)
chlorinated hydrocarbons
cicutoxin
cocaine
colchicine
coniine
cyanides
DDT

DFP (diisopropyl fluorophosphate)
Diamox
Dibenamine hydrochloride
dieldrin
endrin
ergot
fluorides
HETP (hexaethyltetraphosphate)
hexachlorophene
lead
lobeline
malathion
methaqualone
Metrazole
nicotine
nikethamide
Nupercaine
oxalates
parathion
phenols
picrotoxin
Priscoline
Privine
procaine
propoxyphene
pyrethrins
quaternary ammonium compounds

santonin
sodium monofluor acetate (1080)
strychnine
TEPP (tetraethyl pyrophosphate)
theophylline
toxaphene
tricyclic antidepressants
uracil derivatives (mixtine)
Xylocaine
other CNS analeptics or stimulants or convulsants
other local anesthetics

Diseases

birth injuries
brain tumors
CNS acute diseases or injuries (especially meningitis)
eclampsia
epilepsy
hydrophobia   .
sunstroke
temperature, high (especially children)
tetanus
tetany
uremia

DROWSY, SLEEPY, DEPRESSION, UNCONSCIOUS, COMA

Poisons

acetaldehyde
acetaminophen
alcohols
amyl nitrite
antihistamines
arnica
arsenic
arsine
aspirin
atropine
barbiturate derivatives
benzene
bromides
carbon dioxide
carbon disulfide
carbon monoxide
carbon tetrachloride

chloral hydrate
chloroform
codeine
corticosteroids
cyanide
Demerol
DFP
diazepam
Doriden
ether
heroin
HETP
hydrogen sulfide
insulin
kerosene and other petroleum distillates
lead
Librium

malathion
meprobamate
mercury (alkyl)
methadone
methaqualone
morphine and derivatives
nicotine
opium and opiate derivatives
organic solvents
paraldehyde
parathion
phenols
phenothiazines
Placidyl
propoxyphene
salicylates
santonin
scopolamine
sulfide
Sulfonal
TEPP
tricyclic antidepressants
Trional

vacor
Valium
vitamin A
xylene
other CNS depressants

Diseases

acidosis
Addison's disease
brain diseases
brain injury
cerebral embolism and thrombosis
cerebral hemorrhage
eclampsia
malaria
septicemia
shock due to hypo- or hyperglycemia, or
    due to chemicals or trauma
sunstroke
typhus
uremia
yellow atrophy of the liver, acute

DELIRIUM

Poisons

alcohols
aminophylline
amphetamines
antimalarials
arsenic
belladonna group (atropine, hyoscine)
benzene
camphor
cocaine
DDT
DET (diethyltryptamine)
DMT (dimethyltryptamine)
ergot
lead
LSD (lysergic acid diethylamide)
marihuana
methaqualone
PCP (phencyclidine)
solanine

terpenes
toluene
xylene

Diseases

delirium tremens
diabetes mellitus
diseases, terminal stages
epilepsy
fever, high
insanity
liver damage
nephritis
organic brain diseases such as meningitis
    and encephalitis
psychosis
Rocky Mountain spotted fever
uremia
yellow fever

GENERAL OR PARTIAL PARALYSIS

Poisons

aconite
alcohols
arsenic
barium
botulism
carbon dioxide
carbon monoxide
curare
cyanide
DDT
lead
mercury
nicotine
physostigmine

Diseases

brain and spinal cord (tumor, inflammation, hemorrhage)
meningitis
neuritis
tetanus
trauma
uremia

DILATATION OF PUPILS (MYDRIASIS)

Poisons

aconitine
alcohols
aminophylline
amphetamine
antihistamines
barium
belladonna group (scopolamine, atropine, hyoscyamine, stramonium)
Benadryl
benzene
camphor
carbon dioxide
carbon monoxide
chloroform
cocaine
cyanide
Demerol
dibutylene
ephedrine
epinephrine
Etamon
ether
gasoline
gelsemine
Isuprel
meperidine hydrochloride
Neo-Synephrine
nicotine
papaverine
petroleum distillates
phenothiazine
Privine
Pyribenzamine
solanine
thallium
tricyclic antidepressants
vacor
other parasympatholytics or sympathomimetics

Diseases

certain emotional stages, e.g. fear, acute pain, or sudden noise.
epilepsy
glaucoma
pheochromocytoma
rapid rotation of body along its long axis

CONSTRICTION OF PUPILS (MIOSIS)

Poisons

barbiturates
caffeine
chloral hydrate
Dibenamine hydrochloride
ergot
meprobamate
morphine and derivatives

muscarine
nicotine
opium and opiate derivatives
organic phosphate esters (malathion parathion, HETP, TEPP, DFP, OMPA pesticides)
physostigmine
picrotoxin
pilocarpine
Priscoline
propoxyphene
yohimbine

all other parasympathomimetic or sympatholytic drugs

Diseases

paralysis of sympathetic fibers (Horner's syndrome)
sunstroke
tabes dorsalis and certain other diseases of the central nervous system
typhus
uremia

SLOW RESPIRATION

Poisons

alcohols
carbon monoxide
chloral hydrate
cyanides
hypnotics

morphine
opium

Diseases

anoxia, profound
increased intracranial pressure and/or compression of brain for any cause

RAPID RESPIRATION

Poisons

adrenaline
amphetamine
belladonna group (atropine)
caffeine
camphor
carbon dioxide
cocaine
nikethamide
strychnine
xanthine

Diseases

acidosis
anemia
heat or cold applied to the skin
hysteria
muscular exercise
pneumonia
respiratory disease, acute

DYSPNEA

Poisons

carbon monoxide
cyanide
strychnine (during convulsions)
volatile organic liquids such as benzine

Diseases

allergies
anemias

cardiac diseases
diabetes mellitus
medulla lesions
psychosis
respiratory diseases
uremia
vagus lesions

CYANOSIS

Poisons

acetaldehyde
acetanilid
amyl nitrite
aniline and derivatives
barbiturates
chlorates
DFP
ergot
HETP
morphine
nitrites
nitrobenzene
opium
parathion
phenacetin
Plasmochin
sulfanilamides
sulfides
all poisons listed under Excitation, twitching, convulsions (if convulsions are prolonged)

Diseases

arterial anoxemia
bronchopneumonia
congenital heart defects (some)
convulsions (prolonged) due to any cause
methemoglobinemia
pulmonary difficulties with cardiac embarrassment
all diseases listed under Dyspnea

BLOOD CHANGES

APLASTIC ANEMIA

arsphenamine
benzene
γ-benzene hexachloride
carbutamide
chloramphenicol
chlorpropamide
colchicine
dinitrophenol
gold
mepazine
mephenytoin
meprobamate
nitrogen mustard
phenylbutazone
quinacrine hydrochloride
sulfamethoxypyridazine
tolbutamide
trimethadione
trinitrotoluene

THROMBOCYTOPENIA

acetazolamide
aprobarbital
arsphenamine
benzene
γ-benzene hexachloride
carbutamide
chloramphenicol
chlorpropamide
colchicine
gold
mephenytoin
meprobamate
phenylbutazone
pyrimethamine
quinacrine
quinidine
quinine
sulfamethoxypridazine
sulfisoxazole
tolbutamide
trimethadione
trinitrotoluene

AGRANULOCYTOSIS

acetanilid
aminopyrine
arsphenamine
benzene
γ-benzene hexachloride
carbutamide

chloramphenicol
chlorothiazide
chlorpropamide
colchicine
dipyrone
gold
imipramine hydrochloride
mepazine
mephenytoin
meprobamate
methimazole
perphenazine
phenindione
phenylbutazone
prochlorperazine
sulfadiazine
sulfamethoxypridazine
sulfanilamide
sulfisoxazole
thenalidine
thioridazine hydrochloride
Thiothyr
thiouracil
tolbutamide
triflupromazine hydrochloride
trimethadione
trinitrotoluene

HEMOLYTIC ANEMIA

acetanilide
aminopyrine
aminosalicylic acid
arsines
benzene
dimercaprol
furaltadone
fava bean
naphthalene
nitrofurantoin
phenacetin
phenols
procainamide
quinidine
salicylazosulfapyridine
saponins
snake venoms (some)
sodium sulfoxone
stibophen
sulfacetamide
sulfamethoxypyridazine

sulfanilamide
sulfapyridine
sulfisoxazole
trinitrotoluene
xylene

DECREASED COAGULABILITY

benzene
carbon monoxide
Coumadin
dicumarol (warfarin)
fluorides
heparin
phosphorus
salicylates

BASOPHILIC STIPPLING

arsenic
gold
lead

COLOR CHANGES

Cherry red blood

carbon monoxide (carboxyhemoglobin)
cyanide
monofluoroacetate

Dark red blood

nicotine

Chocolate blood (methemoglobin)

acetanilide
aniline and nitro derivatives
chlorates
methylene blue (high concentrations)
nitrites
nitrobenzene
phenacetin
Plasmochin
sulfa drugs
Sulfonal

AGGLUTININS

abrin
croton
poisonous mushrooms
ricin
snake venoms (some)

CARDIOVASCULAR CHANGES

BRADYCARDIA
aconite
barium
digitalis
eserine
muscarine
opiates
parasympathomimetics
parathion
pilocarpine
quinidine
quinine

TACHYCARDIA
alcohols
amphetamine
anesthetics in general
arsenic
aspirin
atropine
cocaine
ephedrine
epinephrine
nicotine
parasympatholytics
sympathomimetics

HYPERTENSION
amphetamine
barium
convulsant drugs
corticosteroids
ephedrine
epinephrine
ergot
lead
nicotine

HYPOTENSION
alcohols
aldrin
amidopyrine
aminophylline
arsenic
arsines
aspirin

barbiturates
carbon monoxide
chloral hydrate
chloroform
cyanide
dieldrin
Doriden
endrin
hexachlorophene
iron salts
Librium
meprobamate
muscarine
nitrates
nitrites
opiates
phenacetin
phenols
phenothiazines
quinine

CAPILLARY PERMEABILITY (HEMORRHAGE)
antimony
arsenic
aspirin
benzene
corrosives
dicumarol
Dilantin
gold
histamine
histaminelike substances
iodides
snake venom (some)
sulfa drugs
thiouracil

AURICULAR FIBRILLATION
aconitine
carbon monoxide
digitalis
fluoroacetate
Metrazole
nitroglycerin
quinine
squill, red

FLUSHING

aconitine
acrolein
alcohol
amphetamine
amyl nitrite
aniline
aspirin
atropine and belladonna group
camphor
codeine
curare
ephedrine
ethyl bromide
gasoline
gelsemine
mercury
nitroglycerin
paraldehyde
santonin
scopolamine
squill, red

DISTURBED VISION

PURPLE-YELLOW VISION

aspidium
digitalis
marihuana
santonin
parathion
solanine
TEPP
thallium

BLURRED VISION

belladonna group, especially atropine
carbon tetrachloride
ergot
DFP
ethyl alcohol
HETP
methyl alcohol

PARTIAL OR TOTAL BLINDNESS

aspidium
formic acid
methyl alcohol
methyl bromide
methyl chloride
solanine

OTHER CHANGES

ACIDOSIS

acetone
aspirin
ethylene glycol
ferrous sulfate
isopropyl alcohol
mercuric chloride
methyl alcohol
oil of wintergreen
oxalic acid
salicylates
sulfa drugs
ergot
radium
thallium
x-ray

BUZZING IN EARS (TINNITUS)

camphor
ergot
methyl alcohol
quinine
salicylates
streptomycin

ALOPECIA

alkali sulfide
arsenic
chemotherapeutic agents

COLITIS

arsenic
mercuric chloride

DRY MOUTH
anticholinergics
antihistamines
belladonna group, especially atropine
Benadryl
castor bean
Dramamine
ephedrine
morphine

INCREASED SALIVATION
acids
alkalies
arsenic
mercury
parasympathomimetics
parathion (cholinergics)
strychnine
thallium

INCREASED BODY TEMPERATURE
amphetamine group
arsenicals
atropine group
boric acid
camphor
cocaine
dinitrophenols
Doriden
thyroxin
toxaphene

DECREASED BODY TEMPERATURE
acetanilide
aconite
barbiturates

central nervous system depressants
chloral
chloroform
ether
morphine
nitrites
quinine
salicylates

INCREASED SWEATING
alcohols
ammonia
amphetamines
arecoline
arsenic
aspirin
bismuth
cholinergics
DFP
dieldrin
fluoride
HETP
insulin
LSD
mercuric chloride
morphine
muscarine
nitrites
parasympathomimetics
parathion
physostigmine
pilocarpine
poisonous mushrooms

HOT, DRY SKIN
belladonna group (atropine)
botulism toxin
stramonium

PERIPHERAL NEURITIS

Acute
antimony
arsenic
benzene
carbon monoxide
chenopodium oil
ciguatoxin (fish poisoning)

copper
cortisone
dinitrobenzene
dinitrocresol
dinitrophenol
Doriden
emetine

kerosene
lithium
methanol
methyl bromide
methyl chloride
opium
parathion and parathion group
quinine
TEPP
thallium

Chronic
aniline
arsenic
bismuth
carbon disulfide

chlorinated hydrocarbons
cocaine
cyanide
ergot
ethanol
gasoline
hydrogen sulfide
lead
manganese
mercury
methanol
sulfa drugs
Sulfonal
tetrachloroethane
trichloroethylene
tri-o-cresyl phosphate

RESTLESSNESS (EXCITEMENT)

Amanita muscaria or *phalloides*
arsenic (acute)
atropine
belladonna
benzene
caffeine
dinitrophenol

kerosene
methanol
mercury (chronic)
salicylates
stramonium
turpentine

RESTLESSNESS (INSOMNIA)

amphetamines
arsenic trioxide
benzene
caffeine
cocaine

lead (soluble salt)
mercury (chronic)
methyl bromide
nicotine (chronic)

NERVOUSNESS (IRRITABLE, "ERETHISM")

amphetamines
arsenic trioxide (chronic)
benzene
digitalis derivatives
Dilantin

gasoline
lead
mercury (chronic)
nicotine (chronic)
petroleum distillates

ANXIETY AND FEAR

arsenic trioxide
aspirin (salicylates)
caffeine
camphor

carbon monoxide
mercury (chronic)
nicotine (chronic)
PCP

paraldehyde (chronic)
parathion
pine oils
ricin

santonin
thiocyanate
turpentine

LIVER DAMAGE

acetaminophen
acetone
Amanita phalloides
ammonia
antimony
antipyrine
apiol
arsenic
Avertin
barium
benzene
borates
carbon disulfide
carbon tetrachloride
chloral hydrate
chlorates
chlorinated hydrocarbons
chloroform
chlorpromazine
chromates
cinchophen
DDT
Dilantin

dinitrocresol or phenol
ethyl chloride
fava bean
ferrous sulfate
isoniazid
Lethanes
mercurochrome
methyltestosterone
naphthalene
naphthol
nitrobenzene
phenols
phenothiazines
phosphorus
picric acid
Plasmoquine
pyridine
ricin
tannic acid
thiouracil
TNT (trinitrotoluene)
toluene
tri- and tetrachlorethylene

KIDNEY DAMAGE

acetic acid
acetone
alloxan
aloe
Amanita phalloides
amyl nitrite
aniline (chronic)
antimony
antipyrine
apiol
arsenic salts
arsine
aspidium
barium
benzene
boric acid (borates)

bromates
cantharidin
carbon tetrachloride
castor oil
chloral hydrate
chlorates
chloroform
chromates
cinchophen
colchicine
copper salts
cresol
p-dichlorobenzene
dinitrocresol or phenol
dioxane
ergot

ethylene glycol
fava bean
ferric chloride
fluorides
formaldehyde
gasoline
gold
iodine
Lysol
mercury salts
methapyrilene hydrochloride
methyl salicylate
morphine (chronic)
naphthalene
naphthol
nitrates
nitrobenzene
oxalic acid (oxalates)
phenolphthalein
phenols
phenothiazines

phosphorus (yellow)
picric acid
Plasmoquine
poison ivy
potassium permanganate
quinine
resorcinol
ricin
santonin
streptomycin
sulfanilamide derivatives (insoluble metabolites)
terpenes
thallium
thiocyanates
thujone
TNT
turpentine
uranium salts
vitamin D
zinc chloride

PULMONARY EDEMA

barbiturate derivatives and other hypnotics
chlorine gas or other gas irritants
kerosene and other petroleum distillates when aspirated into lungs
lung irritants
morphine and derivatives and other

narcotics
muscarinelike compounds
"narcotic lung" in narcotic overdose
parasympathomimetics
parathion and other similar organic phosphate esters
respiratory depressants

URINARY CHANGES

POSITIVE BENEDICT OR FEHLING'S TEST FOR SUGAR

amygdalin
ANTU (alphanaphthyl thiourea)
aspirin
carbon tetrachloride
chloral hydrate
chloroform
epinephrine
ether
glucosides
menthol
morphine
paraldehyde
phenacetin

phlorizin
salicylates
turpentine

ABNORMAL COLOR

Dark Color

blood
cascara
cresols
Flagyl
iron salts
levodopa
methemoglobinemia
naphthalene
naphthol

nitrobenzene
nitrofurantoin
pamaquine
phenacetin
phenols
porphyrins
pyrogallol
quinine
resorcinal
rhubarb
Robaxin
salol
senna
sulfanilamids
tannins

Wine or Red-Brown

aloin (in alkaline solution; is pink)
amidopyrine
antipyrine
benzene
caffeine
carbon tetrachloride
cinchophen
dinitrophenol
fava bean
lead (chronic)
mercury (chronic)
phenothiazines
phenolphthalein (in alkaline solution)
picric acid
Pyridium
santonin (in alkaline solution)
Sulfonal
TNT
warfarin

Green

bile
creosotes
methylene blue
phenols
phenyl salicylates
resorcinol
Robaxin

Green-Blue

amitriptyline
Doan's kidney pills

methylene blue
phenols
resorcinol
salol
Tetralin
thymol
tolonium

Yellow

carrots
phenacetin
picric acid
quinacrine hydrochloride
santonin

Yellow-Brown (Acid Urine)

acetanilide
aloe
aminopyrine
cascara
phenolphthalein
rhubarb
senna

Yellow-Pink (Alkaline Urine)

aloe
antipyrine
cascara
phenolphthalein
rhubarb
santonin
senna

Orange (Orange-Red)

aminopyrine
antipyrine
azogantrisin
beets
blackberries
cascara
Coumadin
deferoxamine
Dilantin
phensuximide
Pyridium
rhubarb
warfarin

OLIGURIA
acids
benzene
barbiturates
chlorates
cantharidin
carbon tetrachloride
chlorates

essential oils
ethylene glycol
mercury bichloride
oxalates
petroleum derivatives
phenols
sulfa drugs

ABNORMAL STAINING OR SKIN COLORING

STAINS (ESCHARS; PRECIPITATED PROTEINS)

Brown-Black
iodine
silver nitrate

Deep Brown
bromide

Yellow
atabrine
nitric acid
picric acid

White (Bleached)
phenols and derivatives

Ash Gray
mercuric chloride

COLORING OF SKIN

Cherry Red or Pink
carbon monoxide
cyanides
nitrites

Blue Gray
silver salts

Yellow
Atabrine
picric acid

Brown Bluish
acetanilids
chlorates

nitrobenzene
all those listed under Cyanosis

DISCOLORATION OF GUMS

Blue-Black Gum Line ("Burton's lines")
bismuth (usually chronic)
lead
mercury

SKIN RASH (DERMATITIS)
acetanilide
amidopyrine
antimony
antipyrine
arsenic
Atabrine
barbiturates
belladonna
borates
bromides
chloral hydrate
coal-tar derivatives
Dilantin
gold
iodides
methenamine
opium
phenacetin
phenolphthalein
propylthiouracil
quinine
sulfa drugs
Tridione
turpentine
many others, including drug allergies

ABNORMAL COLOR OF FECES*

Whitish or Gray

antacids
antibiotics
biliary obstruction
chocolate
cocoa
fats
jaundice
pancreatic disease

Black

anticoagulants (blood)
bismuth
blackberries
blood
charcoal
huckleberries
iron salts
lead salts
meat, red (in excess)
mercuric salts
salicylates

Green or Blue

biliverdin
borates

dithiazanine
mercurous chloride
spinach

Yellow

rhubarb
santonin
senna

Yellow-Green

anthroquinones
diarrhea
mercurous salts
senna

Red or Orange

anticoagulants
beets
Pyridium
salicylates
tetracyclines

Pink-Red

anticoagulants
blood
pyrvinium
salicylates

CHARACTERISTIC ODORS OF BREATH, VOMITUS OR BODY FLUIDS

Phenolic (Disinfectants)

creosotes
phenols

Ethereal (Sweet)

ether

Sweet (Penetrating)

acetone
chloroform

Bitter Almonds

cyanides

Violets

turpentine (in urine)

Stale Tobacco

nicotine

Pears

chloral hydrate

Alcohol (Fruity)

alcohols

Garlic

arsenic
malathion
parathion
phosphorus
tellurium

---

*Treuting

Shoe Polish
nitrobenzene

This list is not complete, but experience will enable you to recognize substances such as the following
acetone
benzene
camphor

carbon disulfide
carbon tetrachloride
chlorine compounds
formaldehyde
gasoline
hydrogen sulfide
mercaptans
methyl salicylate
naphtha
paraldehyde
pyridine
xylene

INFLAMMATION OF GASTROINTESTINAL TRACT

erosion
hemorrhage
perforation

ulceration
all listed under Nausea, vomiting, abdominal pain, or diarrhea

COLORED MATERIAL IN GASTRIC LAVAGE

INORGANIC SALTS

Purple or Pink
potassium permanganate

Pink
cobalt salts

Bright red
mercurochrome

Blue or Green
copper salts
dyes added to fluoride, strychnine, or
   bichloride or mercury
nickel salts (green)

Yellow
nitric acid
picric acid

Blue-Brown
iodine

Brown
hydrochloric acid

**Black and Granular
(Like Coffee Grounds)**
oxalic acid
sulfuric acid

Luminous Particles
phosphorus (yellow)

COLORED CAPSULES

Red
Seconal

Yellow
ephedrine
methapyrilene hydrochloride
Nembutal
Nods
Pronestyl

Blue
Amytal
Bentyl

Green
butabarbital
Ethobral
phenobarbital
secobarbital

Orange
Delvinal

White
Carbrital. (blue band)
Dilantin (red band)

See Physician's Desk Reference (PDR) for more complete descriptions.

GENERALIZED SYMPTOMS FROM DRUGS AFFECTING THE AUTONOMIC NERVOUS SYSTEM

PARASYMPATHOMIMETIC AGENTS (CHOLINERGIC)

acetylcholines
ambenonium chloride (Mytelase)
benzpyrinium bromide (Stigmonene)
bethanechol (Urecholine) chloride
carbachol (Carcholin; Doryl)
demecarium bromide (Humorsol)
echothiophate (Phospholine) iodide
edrophonium bromide (Tensilon)
furtrethonium (Furmethide)
isofluorphate (Floropryl; DFP)

methacholine (Mecholyl) chloride
muscarine
neostigmine (prostigmin)methyl sulfate
organic phosphate esters (parathion, methyl parathion, malathion, Diazinon, DFP, HETP, DDVP, EPN, OMPA, TEPP, others)
physostigmine (Escrine)
pilocarpine
pyridostigmine (Mestinon) bromide
quarternary ammonium compounds

GENERAL SYMPTOMS: Nausea, vomiting, pinpoint pupils, disturbed vision, abdominal cramps, increased sweating, tearing and lacrimation, bradycardia, gut motility, diarrhea, pulmonary edema, bronchiolar constriction, difficult breathing, muscular tremors, convulsions, coma, collapse, cardiac and respiratory failure.

(Toxin from the bufamarine toad may also produce above symptoms.)

PARASYMPATHOLYTIC AGENTS (ANTICHOLINERGIC)

adiphenine (Trasentine) hydrochloride
ambutonium bromide
aminopentamide (Centrine)
amolanone (Amethone)
amprotropine phosphate (Syntropan)
anisotropine methylbromide (Valpin)
atropine, scopolamine, stramonium belladonna group
benzomethamine chloride (Cotranul)
benztropine mesylate (Cogentin methanesulfonate)
biperidin hydrochloride (Akineton)
caramiphen hydrochloride (Panparnit, Toryn)
chlorphenoxamine hydrochloride (Phenoxene)
cyclopentolate hydrochloride (Cyclogyl)
cycrimine HCL (Pagitane)
dibutoline (Dibuline) sulfate

dicyclomine (Bentyl) hydrochloride
diethazine hydrochloride (Diparcol)
diethylaminoethyl diphenylacetate (adiphenine; Trasentine) hydrochloride
diphemanil methylsulfate (Prantal)
ethopropazine hydrochloride (Parsidol)
eucatropine (Euphthalmine)
glycopyrrolate (Robinul)
homatropine methylbromide (Homapin; Homatromide, Malcotran; Mesopin; Novatrin; Sethyl)
isopropamide (Darbid)
mepenzolate bromide (Cantil)
methantheline (Banthine) bromide
methixene hydrochloride (Trest)
methscopolamine (Pamine) bromide
methylatropine nitrate (Metropine)
nicotine (large amounts)
octatropine methylbromide (Valpin)
orphenadrine (Disipal)
oxyphencyclimine (Daricon)
oxyphenonium bromide (Antrenyl)

Pavatrine hydrochloride
pentapiperide (Quilene)
phenthienate (Monodral) bromide
pipenzolate bromide (Piptal)
piperidolate (Dactil)
poldine methyl sulfate (Nacton)
procyclidine hydrochloride (Kemadrin)
propantheline bromide (Pro-Banthine)

thiphenamil hydrochloride (Trocinate)
tricyclamol methosulfate (Elorine sulfate)
tridihexethyl chloride (Pathilon)
trihexphenidyl hydrochloride (Artane; Pipanol)
tropicamide (Mydriacyl)
valethamate bromide (Murel)

GENERAL SYMPTOMS: Dilatation of pupils, disturbed vision (cycloplegia for many hours), paralyzed accommodation, may induce, glaucoma, tachycardia, elevated temperature, dry mouth and throat, decreased secretions, decreased gut motility, difficult urination, excitement, agitation, hallucinations.

SYMPATHOMIMETIC AGENTS (ADRENERGIC)

amphetamine (Benzedrine)
cocaine
cyclopentamine (Clopane)
dextroamphetamine sulfate (Dexamyl; Obotan; Dadex; Dexedrine sulfate)
ephedrine
epinephrine (adrenalin; Supranephrin; Asthma-meter; Sus-Phrine)
hydroxyamphetamine (Paredrine)
isometheptene (Octin)
levarterenol (Levophed)
mephentermine (Wyamine)
metaraminal (Aramine)
methamphetamine (d-desoxyephedrine, Norodin)
methamphetamine hydrochloride (Amphedroxyn; Desoxedrine; Desoxyn; Desyphed; Drinalfa;Methedrine; Methoxyn)
methoxamine (Vasoxyl) hydrochloride
methoxyphenamine (Orthoxine)
2-methylaminoheptane (Oenethyl)
1-methylhexaneamine (Forthane)
1-methylhexylamine (Tuamine)
naphazoline (Privine hydrochloride)
nordefrin (Cobefrin) hydrochloride
phenmetrazine (Preludin)
phenylephrine (Isophrin; Neo-Synephrine; NTZ) hydrochloride
phenylpropanolamine (Propadrine) hydrochloride
phenylpropylmethylamine (Vondedrine)
propylhexedrine (Benzedrex)
racemic epinephrine (Vaponefrin)
tetrahydrozoline (Tyzine)
xylometazoline hydrochloride (Otrivin)

GENERAL SYMPTOMS: Insomnia, pallor, nervousness, nausea, vomiting, chills, fever, irritability, hallucinations, apprehensiveness, dilated pupils, blurred vision, difficult shallow breathing, cyanosis, elevated blood pressure (which may drop), spasms, tremors, convulsions, coma, collapse, respiratory failure.

SYMPATHOLYTIC AGENTS

azapetine phosphate (Ilidar)
bretylium tosylate (Darenthin)
dihydroergot alkaloids (Hydergine)
ergonovine
ergotamine
ergotoxine
guanethidine sulfate (Ismelin)
methyldopa (Aldomet)
phenoxybenzamine (Dibenzyline)

phentolamine (Regitine)
piperoxane (Benodaine)

tolazoline (benzazoline, priscoline, Vasimid)

GENERAL SYMPTOMS: Postural hypotension, tachycardia, hyperpnea.

ANTICHOLINERGIC DRUGS
Quaternary Ammonium
Amino Esters

Antrenyl
Banthine bromide
Malcotran
Marplan
Monodral bromide
Pamine bromide
Piptal
Pro-Banthine
Skopolate

Quaternary Ammonium
Compounds

Cotranul
Darstine
Elorine
Pathilon
Prantal
Tral
Tricoloid chloride

Tertiary Ammonium
Compounds

atropine
Centrine
Netrin
Pacatal
scopolamine

ANTICONVULSANTS

aminoglutethimide (Elipten)
diazepam (Valium)
diphenylhydantoin (Dilantin)
ethosuximide (Zarontin)
ethotoin (Peganone)
mephenytoin (Mesantoin)
mephobarbital (Mebaral)
metharbital (Gemonil)
methsuximide (Celontin)
paramethadione (Paradione)

phenacemide (Phenurone)
phenobarbital (Luminal)
phensuximide (Milontin)
primaclone (Msoline; Primidone)
trimethadione (Tridione)

HYPNOTICS
(NONBARBITURATES)

bromisovalum (Bromural; Isoval)
carbamide (Sedormid)
ectylurea (Nostyr)
emylcamate (Nuncital)
ethchlorvynol (Placidyl)
ethinamate (Valmid)
flurazepam dihydrochloride (Dalmane)
glutethimide (Doriden)
methapyrilene (Dormin; Histadyl; Nytol; Sleep-Eze; Sominex; Thenylene)
methaqualone (Quaalude)
methylparafynol (Dormison)
methyprylon (Noludar)
trichlorethanol (metabolite of chloral)

HYPNOTICS

barbiturates and derivatives
bromides
chloral hydrate
paraldehyde
Petrichloral (Perichlor)
toloxychorinol

ANALEPTICS

doxapram
Emivan (less toxic than amphetamine)
Meratran (less toxic than amphetamine)
Ritalin (less toxic than amphetamine)
Wyamine (less toxic than amphetamine)

CURARIFORM AGENTS

caramiphen hydrochloride (Panparnit)
diethazine hydrochloride (Diparcol)
gallamine triethiodide (Flaxedil)

hexamethonium (Hexameton) chloride
mephenesin (Tolserol)
meprobamate (Equanil)
T.E.A. (Etamon) chloride

TRANQUILIZERS
Phenothiazines
dimethylamino propyl compounds
  chlorpromazine hydrochloride (Thorazine
  promazine hydrochloride (Sparine)
  triflupromazine hydrochloride (Vesprin)
piperazine compounds
  acetophenazine dimaleate (Tindal)
  carphenazine (Proketazine)
  fluphenazine dihydrochloride (Permital, Prolixin)
  perphenazine (Trilafon)
  prochlorperazine dimaleate (Compazine
  thiopropazate dihydrochloride (Dartal)
  trifluoperazine dihydrochloride (Stelazine)
piperidine compounds
  mepazine hydrochloride (Pacatal)
  mesoridazine (Serentil)
  thioridazine (Mellaril)

Diphenylmethane Derivatives
benactyzine hydrochloride (Suavitil)
hydroxyzine (Atarax)

Others
acetyl serpasil (deserpidine)
azacyclonol (Frenquel)
  buclizine dihydrochloride (Softran)
captodiamine hydrochloride (Suvren)
clorazepate dipotassium salt (Tranxène)
chlordiazepoxide hydrochloride (Librium)
chlormezanone (Trancopal)
chlorprothixene (Taractan)
diazepam (Valium)
ectylurea (Levanil; Nostyn)
emylcamate (Striatran)
hydroxyphenamate (Listica)
hydroxyzine pamoate (Vistaril)
mephanoxalone (Lenetran; Trepidone)
meprobamate (Equanil; Miltown)
oxanamide (Quiactin)
oxazepam (Serax)
phenaglycodol (Ultran)
Rauwolfia serpentina (reserpine, Serpasil)
tybamate (Solacen)

ANTIDEPRESSANTS
Tricyclic Agents
amitriptyline hydrochloride (Elavil)
desipramine hydrochloride (Norpramin, Pertofrane)
doxepin hydrochloride (Sinequan)
imipramine hydrochloride (Tofranil)
nortriptyline (Aventyl)
protriptyline hydrocloride (Vivactil)

Tricyclic agents should not be given with, or soon after (2 weeks), any of the monoamine oxidase inhibitors because this combination may produce severe atropinelike reaction: high fever, tremors, convulsions, delirium, and even death.

Monoamine Oxidase Inhibitors
isocarboxazid (Marplan)
nialamide (Niamid)
phenelzine (Nardil)
tranylcypromine sulfate (Parnate)

Others
amphetamine (Raphetamine) phosphate
amphetamine (Benzedrine) sulfate
dextroamphetamine (Dexedrine) sulfate
methamphetamine hydrochloride (Desoxyn, Methedrine)
methylphenidate (Ritalin)

ANOREXIANTS

amphetamine (Raphetamine) phosphate
amphetamine (Benzedrine) sulfate
benzphetamine hydrochloride (Didrex)
chlorphentermine hydrochloride (Pre-Sate)
dextroamphetamine (Dexedrine) sulfate
diethylpropion hydrochloride (Tenate, Tepanil)
methamphetamine hydrochloride (Desoxyn, Methedrine)
phendimetrazine bitartrate (Plegine)
phenmetrazine (Preludin)
phentermine hydrochloride (Wilpo)

SKELETAL MUSCLE RELAXANTS

carisoprodol (Rela, Soma)
chlorzoxazone (Paraflex)
diazepam (Valium)
mephenesin (Tolserol)
metaxalone (Selkaxin)
methocarbamol (Robaxin)
styramate (Sinaxar)

HALLUCINOGENS

amphetamines and derivatives
antihistamines used for vertigo or antiemetics (some)
atropine derivatives
belladonna
cocaine
DET
DMT
Jimson weed
LSD (D-lysergic acid diethylamide)
marihuana
mescaline (mescal buttons or peyote)
morning glory seeds (some varieties)
parsley
PCP
psilocybin
STP
stramonium

GENERAL SYMPTOMS: Hallucinations (visual or auditory), distortion of time, space, and images; confusion, rambling speech, euphoria, irrational behavior, irritability, excitement, anxiety, panic.

ANTIDOTES AND TREATMENT

SOME POSSIBLE MECHANISMS OF INJURY OR DEATH

ACIDS OR ALKALI: Corrosion, stricture, or perforation of esophagus; cardiovascular collapse.

ARSENIC: Corrosion; cardiovascular collapse; inhibition of sulfhydril enzymes; liver and kidney damage.

ASPIRIN: Profound metabolic acidosis due to metabolite salicylic acid; hypoprothrombinemia; CNS depression; electrolyte imbalance.

BARBITURATES AND SIMILAR DEPRESSANTS: Profound CNS depression, especially respiratory; terminal pneumonia.

CARBON MONOXIDE: Carboxyhemoglobin produces a profound anoxia (anemic); brain and heart most vulnerable.

CARBON TETRACHLORIDE: CNS depression; profound liver and kidney damage.

CYANIDE: Anoxia (histotoxic); destroys cellular respiratory enzymes.

ETHANOL: Profound CNS depression (acute), especially respiratory.

ETHYLENE GLYCOL: CNS depression followed by a profound metabolic acidosis due to metabolite oxalic acid; kidney damage.

FERROUS SULFATE: *Immediate:* Corrosion. *Delayed:* (excessive) ferritin produces vasomotor depression (VMD); cardiovascular collapse; acidosis.

FLUORIDE SALT: Lowers blood calcium; destroys enzyme systems; ventricular fibrillation.

KEROSENE AND PETROLEUM DISTILLATES: Mild depressant; irritant, very damaging especially when aspirated into lungs (even

32

several drops); may produce a chemical pneumonitis.

LEAD: Deposits in bone marrow as phosphate and carbonate salt; depresses RBC formation; nerve, liver, and kidney damage.

MERCURY SALT: Corrosion; cardiovascular collapse. *Delayed, days later:* Kidney damage (nephrosis); acidosis; uremia.

MERCURY METAL VAPORS: Mild CNS and oral involvement.

MERCURY ORGANIC COMPOUNDS: Severe CNS damage.

METHANOL: CNS depression followed by a profound metabolic acidosis due to the metabolite formaldehyde and formic acid; retinal (edema) and nerve damage; electrolyte imbalance.

NICOTINE: Blocks ganglia (parasympathetic and sympathetics).

PARATHION: Profound respiratory depression (cholinergic action): massive pulmonary edema; constriction of bronchioles; respiratory center depression.

PHOSPHORUS (YELLOW) — (PASTA ELÉCTRICA): Severe corrosion; cardiovascular collapse. *Several days later:* Yellow atrophy of liver, severe liver damage; bone necrosis.

STRYCHNINE: Profound convulsions; anoxia (spasm and exhaustion of respiratory muscles).

GENERAL TREATMENT AND MANAGEMENT

Do not wait for *absolute identification* before giving supportive treatment *(maintain all vital signs).* Treat the patient and not the alleged poison.

MINIMIZE ABSORPTION

1. Lime water to precipitate fluorides or oxalates.
2. Citrus fruits to neutralize alkali.
3. $KMnO_4$ (1:10,000) to oxidize alkaloids and oxalates.
4. *Adsorbent charcoal* (activated)—and milk—to slow up absorption and then *gastric* lavage. *Gastric lavage* is contraindicated with acid, alkali, other strong corrosives, kerosene or other petroleum distillates, strychnine or other convulsants and when in coma; but it has been used when patient is depressed or unconscious, with careful use of inflated cuffed endotracheal tube to prevent aspiration into lungs. Gastric lavage even eight hours (or more) later may sometimes be helpful. Con-

vulsing patient *must* first be sedated. Save gastric lavage for identification of poison; look also for color, shape, and odor of poison; see pages 25 and 26.

5. Emetics—tablespoon of ipecac (syrup). Is contraindicated by cardiac diseases, aneurysm, convulsions, late pregnancy; acids, alkalis, or other corrosives; kerosene or other petroleum products, when depressed or in coma, or when immediate response is necessary (action may be delayed 20 minutes). Do not give with activated charcoal.

Emptying the stomach even six hours later may still be worth the effort. With a cooperative patient, a tongue blade tickling the back of the throat is also effective. When the patient is retching, keep his face down with his head lower than his hips in order to prevent aspiration into his lungs. Introducing some fluids, such as warm water or dilute milk, allows vomiting more easily.

6. Saline cathartics: Two tablespoons (30 gm) of Na_2SO_4 (Glauber salts) or $MgSO_4$ (Epsom salts) in a glass of warm water hastens elimination. $MgSO_4$ is contraindicated with kidney or heart disease.

7. Oil or fat demulcents are contraindicated when poison is oil soluble, as with acetone, aniline, benzene, cresol, CCl_4, chloroform, DDT, chlordane, toxaphene, aldrin, dieldrin and other chlorinated hydrocarbons, parathiontype insecticides, kerosene, Lysol, phenols, phosphorus, turpentine, xylene, etc.

Milk, cream, white of egg, gelatin solution, flour or cornstarch are better suited substitutes.

8. Epinephrinetype vasopressors are contraindicated when poisons such as CCl_4; chloroform; DDT and other chlorinated hydrocarbons; gasoline, kerosene, benzene and derivatives, and other petroleum distillates are suspected. They may sensitize the myocardium and this could then trigger a ventricular fibrillation.

SUPPORTIVE

1. Maintain a patent airway; clear with suction if necessary; maintain respiration, body heat, water and electrolyte balance;

prevent secondary infection, relieve pain, catheterize as needed; prevent and correct circulatory and respiratory difficulties; hemodialysis or regulating pH of urine may help to hasten elimination of some poisons, for example when maintaining—
   a. alkaline urine: Aspirin and barbiturates will be *more rapidly eliminated* as sodium salt.
   b. acid urine: Amphetamines will be *more rapidly eliminated* as acid salt.
2. For inhaled gases, remove patient to fresh air (*carry* horizontally); minimize oxygen demand by bed rest and no exertion; artificial respiration and/or oxygen therapy, as needed; cardiac and/or respiratory support as indicated.

SPECIFIC TREATMENT

Great caution must be exercised before administering a specific antidote. Some antidotes are capable of producing harmful effects themselves if the poison for which they are given is not actually present in the body. It would be well to correlate symptoms, history, analysis of vomitus or gastric lavage, and other findings and then proceed with prudence and close observation.

Once the nature of the poison is known, management can continue with more certainty. *Specific antidotes,* if available, may now be used safely. However, general symptomatic and supportive treatment is always equally important to insure survival and should not be under-estimated. Antidote package insert information should be followed.

There are only a few *specific* antidotes. The following list shows their possible application.

Lead Poisoning

The calcium salt of disodium ethylenediaminetetraacetic acid (EDTA, edathamil, Edatate, or Versene) is a specific (chelating) antidote for lead poisoning. This is significant, because lead poisoning occurs more frequently than is generally suspected, especially among the poor and among children. The alkaline treatment and acid elimination employed in the past were time-consuming, produced serious side reactions, and were of questionable effectiveness. The disodium calcium salt of Versene (EDTA) is a rapid, effective, chelating agent that allows for the safe elimination of lead. The dosage suggested in the package insert is followed. The blood and urine are studied to determine when the patient is completely deleaded. Several series of treatments may be indicated in cases of severe plumbism, with intermittent rest periods. It is not unusual for the amount of lead eliminated in the urine at its peak to be as high as 1 mg daily. Prompt improvement usually follows and, in children, encephalopathy subsides and usually does not recur. Clinical results indicate that Versene is the most effective agent so far proposed for treatment of plumbism. It may also be effective in poisoning due to cadmium, cobalt, nickel, iron, and copper.

Versene can be used as a diagnostic aid in cases in which the diagnosis of plumbism is equivocal (which is not too infrequent) especially in chronic cases. Partial (initial dose) treatment is given. If the urinary output of lead is markedly increased above normal (more than 0.100 mg of lead per day), lead is present at least at the time of testing in the soft tissue or the bones, and the signs and symptoms may be due to lead intoxication.

Heavy Metal Poisoning

British Anti-Lewisite (BAL, Dimercaprol) is an effective, specific (chelating) antidote for arsenic, mercury, gold, antimony, bismuth, nickel, and copper, but its use is contraindicated in cases of poisoning due to thallium, selenium, or cadmium. The dosage suggested in the package insert is followed. Occasional side reactions to BAL may occur: nausea, vomiting, headache; burning sensation of mouth, lips, throat, and eyes; lacrimation and salivation; constriction of throat and chest, muscular aches, and anxiety. These side reactions may be diminished with 50 mg of Benadryl or 25 mg of ephedrine given prior to treatment (follow package insert information).

Narcotics Poisoning

Naloxone hydrochloride (Narcan) is the *best* and *safest* specific antagonist for the cardiovascular and respiratory depression produced by morphine, heroin, codeine, Pantopon, Dionin, Demerol, methadone, and other pharmacologically related narcotic compounds. The dose suggested in the package insert is followed. It is relatively safe in that if it were *not* a morphinelike poisoning, the Naloxone would so indicate by a lack of response and would also *not* complicate the clinical picture by producing a further depression.

N-allylnormorphine (Nalline) or levallorphan tartrate (Lorfan) as antagonist has also been used with good results; the dose suggested in the package insert is followed. However, if Nalline or Lorfan is given in the absence of morphine or a related compound, a marked depression of the central nervous system affecting the cardiovascular and respiratory systems may develop, similar to but less intense than morphine poisoning.

In morphine poisoning, the effects of Naloxone or Nalline are dramatic and can be lifesaving. Respiration is restored toward normal within several minutes, and pupillary constriction and cyanosis also tend toward correction. Superficial and deep reflexes and blood pressure are improved.

Naloxone or Nalline is not effective against respiratory depression produced by other depressants such as barbiturates, ether, or cyclopropane.

The response to Naloxone or Nalline is so specific that it may be interpreted as a biologic test for the presence of morphine or a pharmacologically related compound in man (detection of drug addiction). There is aggressive competition for the same receptor sites.

Cholinergic-like Poisons

Atropine is a (lifesaving) specific antidote for the cholinergic-like poisons that inhibit or destroy the acetylcholinesterases. Atropine attaches to postganglionic receptors and thus blocks action of acetylcholine. These poisons have received much publicity as nerve gases for warfare or as powerful insecticides. They may be lethal in small doses (25 mg). Some of the early, commonly known of these organic phosphate ester insecticides are parathion, malathion, diisopropyl fluorophosphate (DFP), tetraethylpyrophosphate (TEPP), and hexaethyltetraphosphate

(HETP). However, other parasympathomimetic drugs such as muscarine, pilocarpine, physostigmine, Doryl, and Mecholyl also act generally in a similar manner, and their action can also be effectively counteracted with atropine—especially the respiratory distress. Carbamate anticholinesterase insecticides also respond to atropine.

The patient must be kept partially atropinized during the entire crisis. Repeat as needed to relieve symptoms. The acute emergency may last twenty-four to forty-eight hours. A favorable response to one dose does not guarantee against sudden and fatal relapse. Full atropinization is evidenced by a dry flushed skin, dilated pupils, and a tachycardia as high as 140 per minute. The atropine not only dilates the bronchioles and dries secretions of the respiratory tract, but also reduces heart block. Persons poisoned with these organic phosphates have an increased tolerance to atropine. However, *do not* attempt to give atropine while a patient is cyanotic. Relieve this condition first by clearing the airway and artificial respiration; then give atropine. Follow directions given in package insert for dosage.

PAM (2-pyridine aldoxime; Pralidoxime; Protopam) is used for parathionlike poisonings (organic phosphate ester insecticides). PAM helps to stimulate reactivation of cholinesterase but should be used only in conjunction with atropine therapy; cannot be used for carbamate poisonings. Follow package insert directions.

Cyanide Poisoning

Nitrites and thiosulfate, if given early enough, may act as a specific antidote for cyanide poisoning. Cyanide is rapidly fatal, producing a histotoxic anoxia by poisoning the oxidative enzymes at cell level. Immediate measures are necessary.

Gastric lavage should be done with 5% sodium thiosulfate, leaving about 10 gm in the stomach. Slow intravenous injection of 10 ml of 3% sodium nitrite solution and 10 to 20 ml of 10% thiosulfate will abate or prevent the cyanide from exerting its action on the oxidation enzymes by producing methemoglobin, which combines with cyanide to form cyanomethemoglobin and sodium thiocyanate, both of which are now relatively nontoxic conversion products of cyanide. A kit (Lilly) is available; follow package insert information.

To be effective, *treatment must be rapid.* Therefore, if sodium nitrite is not immediately available, the inhalation of several perles of amyl nitrite may be substituted temporarily.

Iron Poisoning

Desferal (deferoxamine methanesulfonate) will treat iron. It acts as a specific chelating agent.

Mercury Poisoning

N-acetylated DL-penicillamine acts as a chelating agent for mercury.

Metabolic Acidosis

Sodium bicarbonate $(NaHCO_3)$ —for metabolic acidosis (aspirin, salicylates, methanol, ethylene glycol, oxalates—neutralizes and also may hasten urinary elimination.

Drug-Induced Convulsions

Valium (diazepam) or intermediate-acting barbiturates are used for drug-induced convulsions as a sedation to help prevent convulsion.

Methemoglobinemia

Methylene blue (1%), for methemoglobinemia, reduces Fe^{+++} back to Fe^{++} (normal). Ascorbic acid also helps to reduce iron, but is a slower process.

Anticholinergic Crisis

Physostigmine salicylate is an antidote for acute anticholinergic crisis with atropine and atropine-like drugs, including tricyclic antidepressants, some of the antihistamine group, some of the phenothiazine group, and other drugs that produce atropine-like anticholinergic side effects. It is contraindicated with asthma and cardiac or vascular diseases. Follow package insert instructions.

Phosphorus (Yellow) Poisoning

Copper sulfate solution will help encapsulate yellow phosphorus as Cu_3P_2.

Iodine Poisoning

Starch or $Na_2S_2O_3$ interacts with elemental iodine causticity.

Methanol or Ethylene Glycol Poisoning

Ethanol slows down lethal conversion of methanol into formic acid and of ethylene glycol into oxalic acid.

GENERAL SUPPORTIVE MANAGEMENT SUGGESTIONS

General treatment for some of the major groups of common poisons follows.

Alkaloids (Morphine, Codeine, Atropine, Cocaine)

Induce vomiting with emetics (avoid when vital centers are depressed). Gastric lavage after giving activated charcoal, or dilute potassium permanganate (1:10,000). Watch for specific symptoms and treat supportively. Saline cathartics. Artificial respiration as indicated; oxygen therapy.

If specific alkaloid is known (or determined), proceed as directed for particular alkaloid.

Acids (Hydrochloric, Nitric, Sulfuric, Acetic)

Do not use stomach tube or emetic if severe corrosion is evident. Dilute with water or milk with caution. Neutralize with milk of magnesia, lime water, soap suds, Amphojel, Creamalin, or other mild antacid. *Do not use* sodium bicarbonate or other *carbon dioxide forming* compounds. Give milk, cream, or white of egg as demulcent. Keep patient warm and quiet. Give morphine for pain. Give sedatives, antibiotics, and treatment for shock as necessary. Give crushed ice to relieve thirst. If there are signs of asphyxia, tracheotomy may be indicated. Protect against respiratory obstruction, perforation, or stricture formations.

Guard against secondary infection. Cortisone therapy has been recommended in persistent shock.

If burns are external, wash with plenty of water and then apply a paste of sodium bicarbonate.

Caustic Alkalies (Sodium Hydroxide, Potassium Hydroxide, Lye)

Carefully dilute with water without delay; then neutralize with dilute vinegar or dilute (fresh or canned) lemon or lime juice. Milk, cream, white of egg, olive oil, and bismuth subnitrate are useful demulcents. Keep patient warm and quiet; give cracked ice to relieve thirst, morphine for pain, and sedatives as necessary. If there are signs of asphyxia, tracheotomy is indicated. Protect against esophageal obstruction, perforation, or stricture formations with corticosteroids.

Therapy is aimed to prevent infection, to minimize stricture, and to relieve pain once diagnosis is made. Esophageal strictures have sometimes developed even weeks later when corticosteroids were not given. Liquid broad-spectrum antibiotics and corticosteroid therapy are therefore suggested, and bismuth subnitrate powder may provide sufficient local analgesia to manage pain.

If burns are external, wash with ample water and then wash with dilute vinegar or lemon or lime juice.

Other similar strong alkalies producing the same general symptoms and requiring the same general treatment are thioglycolate (permanent hair wave), sodium carbonate, washing powders, sodium metasilicate, sodium perborate, sodium triphosphate, and sodium hexametaphosphate. Other caustics are Clorox, Drano, Saniflush, Ajax floor cleaner or bleach, E-Z bleach, paint removers, Clinitest tabs.

Since phosphate caustic preparations also deplete the body calcium, restore calcium with calcium gluconate given intravenously.

General

The suggestions for antidotes and treatment are to be followed with caution. Much will depend upon judgment as to what type and how much treatment is required.

Avoid aspiration when evacuating the stomach. In presence of strong irritants, emetics may be contraindicated. Use specific antidotes (with caution) whenever available in severe poisoning. Antibiotics may help patients exposed to noxious gasses, in prolonged coma, or with blood dyscrasias.

If particular poison is known, proceed as directed for specific poisons.

Supportive Measures (Support *all* Vital Signs)

Combat and prevent convulsions or hyperexcitement, preferably with diazepam, or short-acting barbiturates or ether as necessary. Maintain a patent airway, use suction to remove mucus, or tracheotomy as required. Maintain respiratory exchange, body heat, water and electrolyte balance, and blood pressure. Prevent secondary infection, relieve pain, catheterize as needed, prevent and correct circulatory and respiratory difficulties.

HEMODIALYSIS: It has been reported that forced diuresis can be helpful to hasten elimination of some drugs (*Bol Assoc Med de PR, 70:*332, 1978). The regulation of the pH of urine and hemodialysis may also hasten elimination in some cases:

> Alkaline urine: Barbiturates and salicylates (aspirin)
> Acid urine: Amphetamines
> Hemodialysis: May be effective to hasten elimination of some toxic agents.

Success has been reported for the following, but benefit versus risk must always be evaluated whenever hemodialysis is used.

Alcohol, methyl	chlorates
alcohol, isopropyl	chromates
amphetamines	ethylene glycol
Aureomycin	ferrous sulfate
barbiturates (long-acting)	oxalic acid
borates	salicylates
bromates and bromides	sulfa drugs
carbon tetrachloride	

Hypnotic, Sedative or Depressant Drugs

Carefully evaluate all reflexes (especially corneal and patellar). This is an excellent guide as to depth of depression. At all times, maintain adequate respiratory exchange. Keep air passages open; prevent aspiration. Give artificial respiration or oxygen, as indicated, using an endotracheal tube if airway is obstructed.

Remove as much of the drug as possible by gastric lavage, taking every precaution to avoid aspiration. Avoid emetics if patient is depressed. Saline cathartic (30 gm of sodium sulfate) into the gastrointestinal tract should further minimize absorption of drug.

Maintain adequate circulatory activity with measures just adequate to maintain near normal blood pressure, as needed.

Carefully evaluate all reflexes, respiratory pattern, skin color, and response to pain stimuli at frequent intervals to guide further therapy.

Guard against the dangers of aspiration and hypostatic pneumonitis (secondary infection).

Maintain nutritional fluids, electrolyte balance, body heat, and water balance. Catheterize as necessary.

Maintain a respiratory exchange with artificial respiration or oxygen therapy. The use of picrotoxin, Metrazole, amphetamine, or other strong analeptics is *ineffective and perhaps dangerous* for patients in deep depression and *unnecessary* for mild cases. Use mild analeptics *(if you must)* such as bemegride (Megimide), Emivan, or Ritalin just to maintain reflexes and to keep the E.E.G. active; however, these should *not* be used in an attempt to awaken the patient.

Use supportive measures as indicated.

"Intensive care" is vital, especially during the acute phase.

Coma may persist for days with the long-acting depressants or barbiturates (phenobarbital, barbital). Prognosis is good if anoxia and secondary infection can be prevented.

If the blood-drug level is high and life-threatening and the drug is a long-acting barbiturate, then hemodialysis may be used to advantage. Success has been reported for some other long-acting depressants.

The foregoing suggestions are for the markedly depressed. If, however, the depression or overdosage is mild, then treatment should also be "mild." If respiration is normal, color is good, and twitching and corneal reflexes present, it may suffice to let the patient sleep it off, carefully watching to prevent aspiration and for any possible later development of respiratory difficulties.

Gastric lavage may still be of some value even hours later, since depressants may delay emptying time. Supportive measures should be generally similar to those used for barbiturate intoxication and should include maintaining an adequate airway with mechanical support of respiration as needed. Maintain fluid and electrolyte balance, and blood pressure.

Good nursing care is essential, especially to avoid development of stasis pneumonia.

In general, it is better to provide mechanical and physiologic support of vital functions rather than to give stimulants or analeptics in an attempt to awaken the patient. Avoid vasopressor and antipyretic drugs. Diuretic drugs to correct oliguria should also be avoided. *Avoid* all *unnecessary* drugs.

ANALYSIS

URINE, VOMITUS, GASTRIC LAVAGE, and blood are especially suited for analysis for many of the common poisons; these should be collected and saved in clean containers. In addition, any residues in drinking glasses, or pills, tablets, capsules, other medicinals, containers of known or unknown chemicals, insecticides, food, drink, etc., found in the vicinity should also be saved for analysis.

Prior to doing the analysis, gather as much information as you can. This information helps you "spot" the poison you are dealing with. Labels on bottles; shape and color of capsules, etc.; information from witnesses; and typical signs, symptoms, and clues will by their very nature help rule out large groups of toxic agents and allow you to make rapid presumptive tests that, in conjunction with other findings, will strengthen your diagnosis immeasurably.

Time interval between exposure to poisons and time of examination and analysis is of great importance. It may be unfruitful to test for the presence of many common poisons in body fluids if more than 24 hours has elapsed. Many of these are detoxified, conjugated, and eliminated in less than 24 hours, especially if taken in small amounts. The most notable exceptions to this rule are the cumulative poisons such as the heavy metals, bromides, amphetamines, and long-acting barbiturates.

It is rarely wise to use all the available specimen for the first presumptive tests. It is far more judicious to save approximately half the sample (if possible) for later confirmation. Careful records should be kept of the specimens received, types of tests performed, and results obtained—especially in anticipation that this case may later become one of legal interest.

45

It is impractical to attempt to describe the many detailed specific tests or the various separation and purification techniques required to isolate all poisons. However, for emergency procedures, the most simple methods described under each poison in Section II, although not specific in some cases, will suffice for most practical purposes, especially when supported by history, signs, and symptoms.

Rapid screening tests should be performed first for those poisons more common to your area. This will save much time and will allow you to direct your attention toward a particular poison or group of poisons.

In some cases, as directed under methods, tests are described that can be performed *directly* on blood, urine, tablets, capsules, etc., with little or no previous preparation. However, often a simple, rapid isolation-purification is recommended that divides the vast numbers of possible poisons into several major groups depending upon their physical and chemical properties as described below. These may be performed serially or individually as the case may be.

ACID-STEAM DISTILLATION OF VOLATILE POISONS

Set up a *small steam distillation apparatus;* distill an aliquot acidified portion of the stomach contents, vomitus, etc. (acidified with tartaric acid to pH 5), and collect distillate, packed with an ice bath.

Use small portions of this distillate to test for the poisons in Table I.—page 79

Decomposed tissue or smoker's urine or tissue may yield tryptamine, phenylethylamine, and/or pyridine and exhibits spectra similar to amphetamine when alkaline distilled. (Levels usually are *very* high and out of reasonable range):

1. Detect by characteristic odor.
2. Refer to section on particular poison suspected.
3. Scan in ultraviolet (UV) spectrophotometer for characteristic maximum and minimum peaks. If solution is too dilute, then

concentrate by extraction with suitable solvents and scan again. (See Table VIII.—page 85) .

4. Concentrate by extraction with suitable solvents or use head space and scan with gas chromatography (GLC). (See Table XXI—pages 128 and 324) .

5. Special situations: (a) Cyanide should be collected in dilute sodium hydroxide. (b) Phosphorus should be collected in nitric acid or silver nitrate solution. (c) Carbon disulfide is not distilled over in the first 10 ml portion; it is the second portion that contains the greatest yield.

6. See Table II for rapid presumptive tests,—page 80.

MICRODIFFUSION TECHNICS

Conway-Feldstein-Klendshoj

APPARATUS:	Conway unit, Öbrink plastic type; Catalogue #40941, Bel-Art Products, Pequannock, New Jersey.
LIBERATING AGENT:	Spread 1–2 ml of liberating agent in outer chamber.
ABSORBENT OR REACTANT:	Two (2) ml in center chamber of absorbent or reactant. See under specific test for details; also Table III,—page 81.
SEALER:	In the *small* groove of the rim, put 1 ml of liberating agent, which will later act as a liquid seal.
SPECIMEN:	One (1) ml of blood, urine, gastric lavage, or homogenized tissue is spread in outer chamber, on top of liberating agent, and then lid quickly put in place. Gently twist to liquid trap-seal the lid; then gently swirl entire unit to mix specimen with liberating agent. Diffusion is started.
TIME:	One to two hours at room temperature (25°C).

1. Carbon monoxide: Palladium chloride (11 mg) is dissolved

in 25 ml 0.01N HCl; gentle heat may be required.

Sensitive to less than 10 percent carboxyhemoglobin saturation. Standards should be run simultaneously using 5, 10, 20, 40, and 60% "carbon monoxide-blood." A reliable estimation can be made easily. If more standards are prepared, comparison within less than 10 percent may be made.

Blood should be fresh; putrefaction may interfere. (Cohn suggests 5% $AgNO_3$ as liberant.)

2. Ethanol: See Section II under Ethanol for details and for confirmation of positive results. Negative results are absolute.

Any change (even slight) from yellow of blank may be positive. Compare color change with standards similarly prepared. Confirm for absence of methanol, formaldehyde, and isopropanol by referring to tests suggested under each in Section II.

3. Cyanides: Sodium hydroxide (10%) as absorbent; ferrous sulfate (20%) freshly prepared; hydrochloric acid; sulfuric acid (10%) as liberating agent and sealer.

One hour diffusion time at room temperature is sufficient for the 10% sodium hydroxide to absorb all liberated cyanide.

Now add 10 drops of fresh ferrous sulfate solution to center chamber. A precipitate forms; swirl to mix. Then dropwise (1 at a time) add hydrochloric acid to just dissolve this heavy precipitate. The appearance of a blue color (Prussian blue) is positive and specific for cyanide. This test is sensitive to less than 5 μg. Standards of cyanide are similarly treated, and a quantitative estimate may be made by comparison.

Fluorides (Frere and Rieders)

Plastic microdiffusion cell:
A H Thomas # 4472 S.

OUTER CHAMBER: 1 ml of blood + 1 ml of 80% H_2SO_4 with 0.25% Tergitol 4.

INNER CHAMBER: 0.25 ml of 10^{-3} M cerous nitrate in water. 0.25 ml 10^{-3} M alizarin complexone in 1M acetate buffer at pH 4.5.

SEAL LEDGE: 1.5 ml of 80% H_2SO_4 with 0.25% Tergitol 4.

PROCEDURE: Gently swirl so that blood and liberating acid will mix. Diffuse at room temperature for about three hours.

Dilute center reactant reagents to 3.0 ml with water.

Compare with standards similarly prepared: 0–5 μg (5 μg gives OD about 0.3); normal blood less than 50 μg% (Curry); normal tissue less than 80 μg%; normal urine less than 1000μg per day.

Urine is specimen of choice and should be stored and shipped only in polyethylene bottles.

Kerosene, Benzene, Toluene, Gasoline

Marquis' reagent → red color.

Conway microdiffusion (Hensel):
14 drops H_2SO_4, inner chamber
14 drops H_2SO_4, outer chamber
1 drop formaldehyde, inner chamber (Marquis reagent)
1 ml H_2SO_4 for sealing well.
2 ml of urine + 2 ml of ether + 2 gm $(NH_4)_2SO_4$ (anhydrous)

Shake and separate; then centrifuge and transfer the ether layer to another tube containing Na_2SO_4 (anhydrous) and quickly again shake, separate, and centrifuge. Transfer the ether very quickly to outer chamber of Conway cell.

Ether is soluble in H_2SO_4, and vapor tension is reduced so that only kerosene, benzene, toluene, and gasoline diffuse. Allow to diffuse for 1 hour at room temperature (30°C).

Red color is positive for all (Marquis' reagent in inner chamber).

A semiquantitative estimate can be made by comparison with standards.

Very sensitive reaction: 0.004 ml/ml blood for kerosene; 0.001 ml/ml blood for others.

VOLATILE POISONS BY NEAR INFRARED
SPECTROPHOTOMETRY (720–2800 nm)

Ice cold tissue (300 gm) and crushed ice (200 gm) are homogenized in a blender. This is transferred through a powder funnel into a distilling flask already containing a 1.5 inch Teflon-covered magnetic stirring bar and 450 gm of $(NH_4)_2SO_4$. Rinse blender and funnel with additional 100 gm of crushed (homogenized) ice. Set up vertical distillation with the flask set on a magnetically stirring hot plate. Swirl and mix before setting up heat. The collecting tip of the vertical condenser should be near the bottom of a 60 ml separatory funnel, which is immersed in crushed ice up to its neck.

Slowly increase heat. As the mixture is being stirred and heated, the $(NH_4)_2SO_4$ dissolves. Keep heat at the lowest possible level. When condensation starts forming in the neck of the flask, reduce heat so that the condensate rises into the trap head in no less time than 5 minutes. Brain tissue will produce a bad foaming. Intermittent rapid stirring may minimize this; other tissues or fluids do not foam so badly.

Collect 30 ml of distillate in about 20 to 30 minutes.

Minute (0.05–0.5 ml) portions are tested for the following:

1. Characteristic retention time, with GLC (see Table XXI—page 128).
2. Volatile *reducing* substances such as alcohols, aldehydes, acetone, sulfides (see ethyl alcohol).
3. Cyanide, phosphorus, halogenated hydrocarbons, organic nitrates (see Table II—page 80).

A 15 ml aliquot A of the distillate is extracted serially with the following:

1. Two (2) ml CCl_4. Fraction I is separated.
2. One-half (0.5) ml of saturated NaOH and 2 ml CCl_4 (for 5 min). Fraction II is separated.
3. Acidify residual distillate with 0.2 ml H_4SO_4, saturate with 10.5 gm $(NH_4)_2$, and extract with 3 ml CCl_4. Fraction III is separated.
4. Finally extract with 3 ml CCl_4 plus 1 ml of pyridine. Fraction

IV is separated.

5. The remainder, aliquot B of the original distillate, is now extracted with 2 ml of chloroform ($CHCl_3$). Fraction V.
6. Thirty (30) ml of distilled water is treated and extracted exactly as above (steps 1 through 5) to serve as reference blank.

Standards are used for comparison and identification. The fractions are examined in the near infrared (NIR) against corresponding reference:

FRACTION I: The NIR scan will show presence of ethers; methyl salicylate; essential oils, turpentine, etc.; hydrocarbons (kerosene, gasoline, etc.); halogenated hydrocarbons (except CCl_4 or chloral); ethchlorvynol (Placidyl).

FRACTION II: The NIR scan will show presence of chloral hydrate after the addition of NaOH, which will convert it to chloroform. *Now* you will get the $CHCl_3$ spectrum in the NIR.

FRACTION III: The NIR scan will show presence of isoamyl, isopropyl, and butyl alcohol, and large quantities of ethanol (over 0.4%).

FRACTION IV: The NIR scan will show presence of methyl, ethyl, or isopropyl alcohol.

FRACTION V: The NIR scan will show presence of carbon tetrachloride.

Reference: Rieders: *J Forensic Sci,* 6:401, 1961.

GENERAL SEPARATION

VOLATILES

1. An aliquot of stomach contents, vomitus, or urine is acidified with a saturated solution of tartaric acid and is then gently steam distilled. Collect an equal volume of distillate (1:1) into an Erlenmeyer flask packed with an ice bath.
2. Identify the volatile by its characteristic odor and UV curve: Take an aliquot of distillate and scan with a UV spectrophotometer (see Table VIII—page 85). Concentrate the distillate (if necessary) by extraction and repeat UV scan or use an aliquot to scan with gas chromatography (see Table XXI—page 128).

52 *Handbook of Emergency Toxicology*

ACIDS AND NEUTRALS

1. See Table IV. Five (5) ml of blood or urine is extracted with 25 ml of chloroform (or ether); allow to separate and re-extract the chloroform layer with 5 ml of 0.5N sodium hydroxide. Transfer the NaOH extract to a silica cuvette* and scan in UV spectrophotometer for the weakly acidic compounds (especially the barbiturates); reconfirm by GLC. Save the chloroform layer for neutral drugs that do not form a sodium compound.

2. The chloroform remaining from above (neutrals) is gently evaporated to dryness in a 37°C water bath with a constant flow of nitrogen. Pick up the residue with about 10 drops of chloroform or methanol. Spot an aliquot onto a TLC plate and determine the Rf of the *neutral* and weakly *basic* compounds; reconfirm by GLC. (See Tables XV and XVIII—pages 109 & 119).

3. The 0.5N NaOH extract after scanning in the UV (above, 1) is now made acidic with dropwise dilute sulfuric acid, and this is extracted with 30 ml of chloroform. Allow to separate and then gently evaporate the chloroform to dryness. Pick up the residue with about 10 drops of chloroform or methanol. Spot an aliquot onto a TLC plate and determine the Rf of the acidic compounds for reconfirmation of the UV scan; also reconfirm by GC (see Tables XV and XVIII—pages 109 & 119).

BASICS

1. Ten (10) ml of urine or blood or tissue homogenase is hydrolyzed with 1 ml of HCl on a boiling water bath for about five minutes. This is then made alkaline with NaOH (NH$_4$OH is better suited for some weak bases). This is extracted with 2 × 25 ml of chloroform (or ether**). Allow to separate and then extract the chloroform portion with 5 ml of 0.5N sulfuric acid.

*Note: When using 5 ml of blood and 25 ml of chloroform and reextracting with 5 ml of 0.5N NaOH or H$_2$SO$_4$ and then reading in a 1 cm light path, use the following factor to compensate for loss and correction.

$$\frac{100}{5} \times \frac{25}{20} \times \frac{5}{1} = mg/dl$$

**Ether must be used for Serax, Valium, Librium, some antihistamines, and phenothiazines; CHCl$_3$:isopropanol (3:1) is used for morphine (with buffer at pH 9). See under individual poison.

Transfer the sulfuric acid extract to a silica cuvette and scan in UV spectrophotometer for the basic compounds. (See Table X—page 90).

2. The 0.5N sulfuric acid extract after scanning in the UV (above, 1) is made definitely basic with NaOH and is extracted with 30 ml of chloroform. Allow to settle; separate; add 1 drop of HCl to the chloroform portion and then gently evaporate to dryness. Pick up the residue with about 10 drops of methanol. Spot an aliquot onto a TLC plate and determine the Rf of the basic compounds as a confirmation of the UV scan; also reconfirm by GLC. (See pages 111 and 119).

Basic drugs that may form a sulfate salt with 0.5N H_2SO_4 are listed in Tables X and XVI—pages 90 and 111.

For opiate derivatives, see morphine—page 405.

EXTRACTION, PURIFICATION, PRELIMINARY SCAN

See under each poison to select the most efficient solvent. Chloroform is more often better suited, but it emulsifies more frequently than ether. Ether, however, must be used for phenothiazines and benzodiazepines.

If extractions are made *vigorously,* emulsions are more certain to occur; centrifugation, adding drops of isopropanol, adding a foam breaker, adding more solvent, or swirling gently may help to break emulsion. Definite separation of layers and filtering the solvent through filter paper to remove droplets of water also will improve purity of the extract.

EXTRACT EXAMINATION

Gently evaporate the solvent and examine for presence of crystals. If crystals are too impure to study, then purify by re-extraction or microsublimation. Dissolve the impure crystals in ethanol and transfer to a sublimation tube. Gently evaporate the ethanol. The tube is then connected with a glass-joint upper tube, which is lined with a small strip of dialyzing membrane to make later removal of crystals easy. Connect the open end of the tube to a vacuum pump and place the sublimation tube into an aluminum block on a hot plate. (Aluminum block is so prepared to have two holes: one for a tube and one for a thermometer.) The crystals are then sublimed at reduced pressure at the lowest temperature possible. When sublimation is complete, remove the dialyzing paper carefully.

Another technic is to dissolve crystals in ether and pick up with a drawn-out microcapillary tube by capillary action. Allow ether to evaporate spontaneously and, as it does, it brings with it pure crystals that crust and seed around the capillary ends.

1. Examine the crystals for formation, shape, and color.
2. Determine the melting point (micro), mixed melting point, and derivatives.
3. Dissolve a few crystals in 0.5N NaOH, and also in 0.5N H_2SO_4, and scan with a UV spectrophotometer for characteristic maximum and minimum peaks (see Tables IX and X—page 86). These crystals may be recovered by re-extraction and may be available for further tests.
4. Several crystals may be dissolved in minimal solvent and then determined by TLC, GLC, and/or NIR spectrophotometry.
5. Determine the presence of halides (chlorine, bromine, iodine), sulfur, or nitrogen by performing a sodium fusion: Put a few crystals or residue in a small soft glass test tube; then add a *small* piece of metallic sodium and heat the bottom of the test tube vigorously until red-hot residue and sodium are entirely fused. Quickly dip hot bottom of test tube in a small beaker of water (approximately 5 ml). Test tube bottom will break. Filter this solution, which will contain NaX (chloride, bromide, or iodide) and/or NaCN (fused nitrogen) and/or Na_2S.

Sulfur

1. One (1) ml of filtrate plus 3 drops of dilute freshly prepared sodium nitroprusside solution (10%) produces an intense violet color, which eventually fades.
2. One (1) ml of filtrate plus 3 drops of dilute lead acetate produces a black precipitate of lead sulfide.

Sulfur is present in Pentothal, Sulfonal, sulfa drugs, Mellaril, and some others.

Nitrogen

Gently boil 3 ml of filtrate with 5 drops of 10% sodium hydroxide and 5 drops of dilute ferrous sulfate solution for about $\frac{1}{2}$ minute. Dropwise, add enough dilute hydrochloric acid (10%) to dissolve the brown precipitate; add 1 drop in excess. If nitrogen is present, it will produce a precipitate of Prussian blue.

Nitrogen is present in *all* the alkaloids, aminopyrine, phenacetin, barbiturates, and many other drugs.

Nitrogen is absent in salicylates, chloral hydrate, DDT, camphor, etc.

Halogens

1. When sulfur and nitrogen are both absent, acidify 2 ml of filtrate with dilute nitric acid and add 1 ml of dilute silver nitrate solution (10%) :
   Chlorine → Ag Cl (white precipitate)
   Bromine → Ag Br (brown precipitate)
   Iodine → Ag I (yellow precipitate)
2. If either sulfur or nitrogen is present, place remainder of filtrate in a small dish and add dilute sulfuric acid until faintly acid: filter if cloudy. To 2 ml of filtrate, add 1 ml of nitric acid plus 1 ml of silver nitrate solution (10%). A precipitate indicates halides.

   See Table V for other negative radicals—page 83.

HEAVY METALS

(A general scheme to identify and differentiate mercury, arsenic, antimony, and bismuth.) Mercury, arsenic, antimony, and bismuth will deposit onto a copper wire or sheet* (5 × 5 mm) (modified Reinsch's test). This test is rapid, specific, sensitive, reliable, and can be used directly on body fluids without any previous digestion, extraction, or other preliminary treatment. The following scheme will identify with specificity and will estimate each element in the presence of one another: Use 10 to 15 gm of body fluid or tissue homogenate, 3 ml concentrated hydrochloric acid, small copper spiral or strip; heat gently for 1 to 2

---

*Heavy Cu foil, 0.005 inches thick.

hours (Bismuth requires 2 hours.) Examine spiral for deposition; can be compared with standards. See Table VI—page 84.

DETAILED METHOD FOR DEPOSITION

Place a 20 gm sample of finely macerated tissue homogenate, water or stomach contents, urine, etc., in an Erlenmeyer flask; then add 4 ml of concentrated hydrochloric acid. A spiral is prepared by winding a length of 20-gauge copper wire tightly and closely over a piece of glass rod ten times. The copper spiral or a copper sheet* (5 × 5 mm), after being washed with alcohol and with ether, is introduced into the material contained in the flask. The contents of the flask are gently boiled for approximately 1 hour, and the original volume is maintained constant by a watch glass cover and addition of 10% hydrochloric acid from time to time. After at least 1 hour, the spiral is removed and washed with water. A large amount of mercury or bismuth may require a longer heating period. A silvery coating may indicate mercury. A dark discoloration may indicate antimony, arsenic, bismuth, selenium, sulfur, tellurium, or any combination of these substances. It is recommended that, even in the absence of a visible deposition, the identification procedures be carried out since sensitivities of suggested confirmation tests for these metals would detect smaller amounts than are visible on the copper spiral.

IDENTIFICATION AND ESTIMATION

Mercury

Mercury may be readily identified by a shiny silvery deposit and is confirmed by Gettler's test:

A small filter paper is placed on a watch glass and 2 drops of a suspension of cuprous iodide placed on the filter paper. The silver-coated spiral is placed upon the spot of cuprous iodide, covered with a watch glass, and allowed to stand for several hours.

A salmon pink color, due to the formation of cuprous mercuric iodide, develops if mercury is present in amounts even as small as 0.020 mg. A set of standard cuprous mercuric iodide stains, rang-

---

*Heavy foil 0.005 inches thick.

ing from 0.020 to 0.20 mg of mercury, may be made in a similar manner. By comparing the stain obtained from the sample with the standard stains, one can estimate the quantity of mercury in the sample. The test is specific for mercury. (Other metals that deposit on the copper spiral do not interfere.)

After determination of either the absence or presence of mercury, the procedure is continued with the original coated copper spiral. After the mercury test, the spiral is washed free of adhering cuprous iodide and transferred to a small test tube, or prepare a new deposit to test for bismuth.

Reagent: Cuprous iodide: Dissolve 5 gm of copper sulfate and 3 gm of ferrous sulfate in 10 ml of water; 7 gm of potassium iodide in 50 ml of water is added while stirring. The precipitate is filtered and washed with water. The precipitated cuprous iodide is then transferred to a brown bottle with the aid of a little water. It is kept in the form of a suspension.

Bismuth

Bismuth deposit on the copper spiral may be quantitatively dissolved with dilute nitric acid. The other deposited metals neither dissolve nor interfere with the subsequent test for bismuth, under the conditions of the procedure described. This test is sensitive to 0.010 mg of bismuth.

To the copper spiral, now in the small test tube, add 1 ml of 5% sodium sulfite solution and 1 ml of 15% nitric acid. This mixture is allowed to act on the spiral with frequent agitation. Approximately 5 minutes is sufficient if the deposit of bismuth is not too large. Arsenic and antimony do not dissolve under these conditions. The copper spiral is carefully removed from the test tube with the aid of a wooden applicator, washed with water, and retained for subsequent testing. To the solution remaining in the test tube, add 1 ml of distilled water and 1 ml of quinine-potassium-iodide reagent.

The suspension of quinine-bismuth iodide that results is orange-colored. This is compared with standard suspensions prepared as follows: Into each of six small test tubes, similar to the one used above, introduce 1 ml of 5% sodium sulfide solution and

1 ml of 15% nitric acid.   Then add respectively 0, 0.010, 0.020, 0.040, 0.070, and 0.100 mg of bismuth.   The contents of each test tube are then diluted to a volume of 3 ml with distilled water, and 1 ml of quinine-potassium iodide reagent is added.   The test tubes are then shaken and the turbidities compared.   The color of the blank is slightly yellow but clear; 0.010 mg of bismuth produces a slight turbidity and a faint orange color; 0.020 mg yields more turbidity and a more distinct orange color.   With higher concentrations the turbidity and color progressively increase.   The resulting turbidity is approximately 75 percent of the theoretical value as determined by recovery experiments.   Use of a correction factor of 4/3 gives a reliable estimation of bismuth content.   The method is specific for bismuth.   The addition of sodium sulfite inhibits any reaction of dissolved copper with the iodide.

Reagent: Quinine-potassium-iodide: Dissolve 1 gm of quinine sulfate in 100 ml of 0.5% nitric acid; add 2 gm of potassium iodide and allow to dissolve.   This reagent is stable if kept in a brown bottle.

Antimony

If the deposit on the copper spiral has a purplish sheen, the presence of antimony is suggested.   In any case the following procedure should be employed.

The copper spiral* is placed in a small test tube.   Add 0.5 ml of 10% potassium cyanide.   Shake contents of the tube gently for 5 minutes.   A deposit due partially or totally to the presence of arsenic, selenium, tellurium, or sulfur will be dissolved by this treatment while an antimony deposit will be unaffected.   The copper spiral is removed from the solution and washed with a little water.   The solution is preserved for the detection of arsenic, selenium, tellurium, and sulfur (see under next heading).   The copper spiral should be tested immediately, or prepare a new deposit for antimony since on standing (1 hour or more) the antimony becomes passive and its determination is difficult.

Under the conditions of the various procedures performed up to this point, only antimony will remain on the copper spiral.   A

---

*Spiral or strip 5 × 5 mm (0.005 inches thick) .

comparison with standard quantities of antimony deposited on copper spirals yields a fair estimation of the quantity of antimony present. It is well to proceed with the analysis of the antimony deposit on the copper spiral by means of the modified Gutzeit methods described for arsenic; these are sensitive to 0.010 mg of antimony. When testing for antimony, it is preferable to impregnate the disk of filter paper with a 5% solution of silver nitrate instead of the mercuric bromide solution, as suggested for arsenic, because antimony will not react with mercuric bromide if present in less than 0.200 mg.

If antimony is present, it is converted in the Gutzeit apparatus into stibine, which stains the silver nitrate paper a light gray to black color. The intensity of the stain is proportional to the quantity of stibine produced. In order to determine the quantity of antimony present in the sample, the stain on the paper disk is compared with a series of standard stains prepared in the same manner from known quantities of antimony, ranging from 0.01 to 0.10 mg. These standard stains are stable if stored in the dark.

Arsenic acts similarly to antimony in the Gutzeit test, but the former has been removed previously from the copper spiral by dissolving it with potassium cyanide solution. In order to be absolutely certain that the stain is due to antimony, it is exposed without delay to hydrochloric acid fumes. If due to antimony, the stain fades; if due to arsenic, the stain remains unchanged.

Arsenic, Selenium, Tellurium, and Sulfur

The potassium cyanide solution that was preserved is now tested for arsenic, and for selenium, tellurium, and sulfur if present in large amounts. Experiments have shown that large quantities of selenium, tellurium, and sulfur will darken a copper spiral in the Reinsch test. Under ideal conditions the darkening will take place with as little as 0.050 mg of these elements.

However, the conditions of the Reinsch test as previously described are not ideal for the quantitative deposition of selenium and tellurium. In the presence of 4 ml of concentrated hydrochloric acid, most of the volatile hydrides of selenium, tellurium, and sulfur are lost during the procedure. If 0.25 ml of concentrated hydrochloric acid is added, then these elements may be quantitatively deposited on the copper. However, if there is a large quantity of these elements (0.2 mg or more), the copper spiral would darken in spite of the excess of acid, and it is with this particular situation that we are now concerned. In the event that the spiral is tarnished and arsenic, bismuth, and antimony are absent, it would be of some importance to know whether the deposit is due to sulfur from decomposed biologic material or from administered sulfur-containing drugs such as sodium formaldehyde sulfoxylate, or whether it is due to selenium or tellurium.

If one is specifically interestd in the identification and estimation of selenium and tellurium, the deposition on the copper spiral should be carried out on 20 gm of the original material after adding only 0.25 ml of concentrated hydrochloric acid solution. To a 0.5 ml potassium cyanide solution, introduce the copper spiral; add 4 drops of ethyl alcohol and 5 drops of cadmium acetate reagent. Shake and let stand for 5 minutes. An orange precipitate indicates selenium and a black precipitate, tellurium; a yellow precipitate indicates sulfur. These three elements cannot be detected in the presence of one another but may be detected in the presence of mercury, antimony, bismuth, and arsenic.

These precipitates are distinctive and specific, and none of the other metals that deposit on the copper spiral interfere with the test. The cadmium acetate test, although sensitive to 0.050 mg in each case, does not give positive results with pure solutions of these elements. It appears that the deposition on the copper and solution of the deposit in the cyanide reagent comprise an integral part of the test.

In order to estimate the approximate quantity of selenium or tellurium present (if originally the smaller quantity of hydrochloric acid had been used in the Reinsch test), a series of standards is prepared ranging from 0.025 to 0.100 mg in 20 cc of water containing 0.25 ml of concentrated hydrochloric acid solution. These standard quantities of selenium or tellurium, as the case may be, are then deposited on a series of copper spirals as previously described. The deposit is dissolved in 0.5 ml of 10% potassium cyanide solution. To this solution, add 4 drops of ethyl alcohol and 5 drops of the cadmium acetate reagent; this solution is shaken and allowed to stand 5 minutes. By comparing the precipitated suspension obtained from the biologic sample with the suspensions obtained in the series of standards, a fair estimation of the quantity present is obtained.

Reagent: Cadmium acetate: Dissolve 2.5 gm of cadmium acetate in 20 ml of glacial acetic acid and dilute to 100 ml with distilled water.

Arsenic, although dissolved by the cyanide solution together with the selenium and tellurium, does not give any reaction with the cadmium acetate reagent. If the copper spiral was tarnished and if the cyanide solution of the deposit yielded a negative cadmium acetate test, there is a strong indication that arsenic was originally present.

For a quantitative estimation of arsenic, it is advisable to take another 20 gm portion of tissue or body fluid and allow all of the arsenic to deposit on a new copper spiral as already described. The coated copper spiral is then placed in the modified Gutzeit apparatus. The paper disk is impregnated with 5% mercuric bromide in 95% ethyl alcohol. The yellow stain produced by arsine is compared with standard arsenic stains prepared in a similar manner. Standards should range between 0.005 and 0.040 mg. Above 0.04 mg, the stain is so deep brown in color that an estimation is impossible. The presence of as little as 0.005 mg of arsenic may be detected, and differences of a few micrograms of arsenic are discernible. It was experimentally observed that in this method there is only a 50 percent recovery (which is a constant value), because one-half of the arsenic combines chemically with the copper while the other half deposits on the copper. It is this latter half that is converted into arsine. The value of the stain from the sample must, therefore be multiplied by a correction factor of 2.

More accurate analyses require previous digestion of organic material before specific tests can be performed.

ACID DIGESTION

For metals such as arsenic, lead, bismuth, antimony, copper, zinc, barium, cadmium, and thallium, transfer 50 ml of urine or 10 ml of blood, etc., to a 100 ml Kjeldahl flask. Add several glass beads; then add 100 ml of nitric acid, c.p. and 4 ml of sulfuric acid, c.p. Heat the contents gently at first to prevent foaming. When the foam is broken, increase the heat and continue heating until the volume is approximately 50 ml. Remove flame and add 50 ml more of nitric acid; *carefully* and slowly, add 3 ml of concentrated perchloric acid (72%).* Heat again until the solution clears and white sulfur trioxide fumes are copiously evolving. This usually occurs when volume is below 3 ml. (Sometimes, several more small portions of concentrated nitric acid may be necessary, in addition, at this point.) Continue heating for an additional several minutes. The solution is now completely digested and should be clear and *free* from nitric acid. Volume is approximately 2 ml. Allow to cool. Dilute with distilled water to exactly 20 ml. Final solution contains approximately 10% sulfuric acid. Tests for metals may be made on aliquots of this solution. Proceed as directed under each specific metal.

ATOMIC ABSORPTION

Detection limits have been suggested by Perkin-Elmer in μg/ml for the elements shown in Table VII page 84. Details for lead and mercury are described under each.

ULTRAVIOLET (UV) SPECTROPHOTOMETRIC ANALYSIS

Many organic drugs, chemicals, or poisons show characteristic absorption curves with maximum and minimum peaks in the UV (Ultraviolet) region of the spectrum. These spectra can be plotted with a spectrophotometer with a UV source of light.

This is a very useful technic to screen out or scan for large

---

*Perchloric acid is highly explosive under certain conditions; this method is not for the inexperienced.

groups of possible poisons (drugs or chemicals) in a small sample of blood, gastric contents, tissue homogenate extracts, etc.; many compounds are sensitive to trace amounts (micrograms).

The *identity* of a particular compound is made by comparison with standard absorption curves. The absorption spectrum is plotted—optical density against wavelength (nm). Normal blood would show a straight line, whereas many organic compounds plot a characteristic curve that is compared with standard established curves for known compounds. A collection of as many known compounds as possible is desirable. The larger the collection, the more certain is the identification. These are compared as to maximum and minimum densities (number and intensity of peaks), and the degree and character of slope between peaks. Peaks can be duplicated within 2 nm, but impurities and pH can make a big difference.

NEUTRAL OR WEAKLY ACIDIC ORGANIC COMPOUNDS

Twenty-five (25) ml of redistilled chloroform (or purified ether) is transferred to a Squibb-type separatory funnel; then 5 ml of blood is added and *gently* shaken for several minutes. The chloroform will not only precipitate the protein but will also quantitatively extract most organic acidic compounds (and also neutral organic compounds). The chloroform layer is allowed to settle and is then carefully separated and filtered through several layers of filter paper to remove excess water droplets. Collect exactly 20 ml, extract this with 5 ml of 0.5N sodium hydroxide. The sodium hydroxide is allowed to stand and is then carefully separated. Excess droplets of chloroform are removed by centrifugation. This extract should be colorless. (Slight yellow is occasionally encountered if blood is hemolyzed.) Three (3) ml of NaOH extract is transferred to a silica cuvette and is scanned in the UV region of the spectrophotometer using a 0.5N sodium hydroxide reference blank saturated with chloroform. Normal blood displays a relatively straight line, whereas many organic aryl drugs may show characteristic peaks. Compare with known standards.

Quantitative determinations can be made by reading the

optical density at its maximum and comparing this with a standard curve prepared in a similar manner.

Reagent: 0.5N sodium hydroxide: 3 ml of saturated (70%) NaOH diluted to 110 ml to make 0.45–0.5N.

BASIC ORGANIC COMPOUNDS

Five (5) ml of blood, urine, or tissue homogenate are added to 25 ml of chloroform or ether in a separatory funnel. This is made alkaline with sodium hydroxide and is gently extracted for several minutes. Allow layers to separate and then filter the chloroform through filter paper to remove droplets of water. Twenty (20) ml of chloroform is extracted with 5 ml of 0.5N sulfuric acid. Allow layers to separate and the chloroform droplets are spun down by centrifugation. The sulfuric acid is transferred to a 3 ml cuvette and scanned in the UV spectrophotometer. Examine and compare with standard curves, as above for the acidic compounds.

Normal blood would plot an approximate straight line. If blood is old or hemolyzed, it may show a maximum optical density at 260 nm and a minimum at 240. Putrefied tissue may show a maximum at 258 nm and a minimum at 230 (looks like amphetamine, but in far greater concentrations than could be possible for amphetamine) (see Amphetamine).

However, some unknowns show characteristic curves that can be compared and matched with standard organic compounds with great reliability. These are compared as to maximum and minimum density (number and intensity of peak); the degree and character of slope between peaks prove very helpful in identification and differentiation (see characteristic curves in Fig. 1; also see Tables VIII–XIII—pages 85 to 107).

Reagent: 0.5N sulfuric acid: 1.5 ml H_2SO_4 (conc.) diluted to 100 ml.

Quantitative determinations of the acid-neutral (Table IX) and basic (Table X) compounds can be made by reading the optical density at its maximum and comparing this with a standard curve prepared in a similar manner.

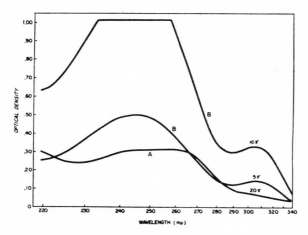

FIGURE 1a. Chlordiazepoxide hydrochloric (Librium): 7-chloro-2-(methyl-amino)-5-phenyl-3H-1,4-benzodiazepine-4-oxide hydrochloride. *A*. In 0.5N NaOH (µg/ml). *B*. In 0.5N H_2SO_4 (µg/ml).

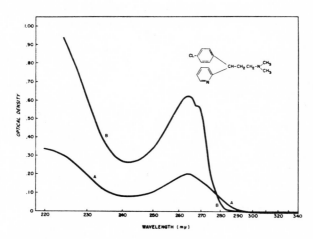

FIGURE 1b. Chlorpheniramine maleate (Chlor-Trimeton, Teldrin). *A*. Acid (H_2SO_4) 10nm. *B*. NaOH, 50 µg/ml.

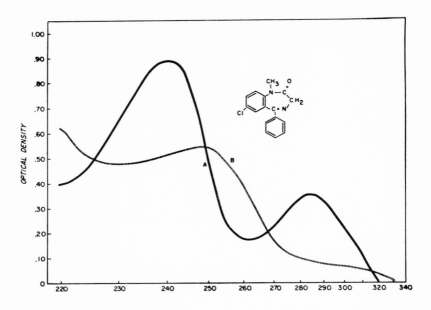

FIGURE 1c.   Diazepam   (Valium): 7-chloro-1,3-dihydro-1-methyl-5-phenyl-2*H*-1,4-benzodiazepin-2-one.   *A*. 0.5N H_2SO_4.   *B*. 0.5N NaOH.   (10μg/ml.)

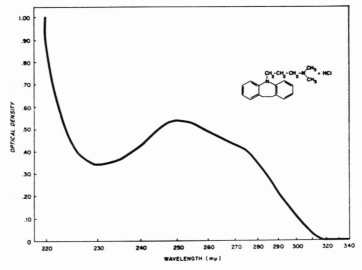

FIGURE 1d.   Imipramine hydrochloride (Tofranil).   20μg/ml of 0.5N H_2SO_4.

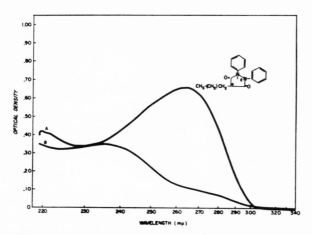

FIGURE 1e. Phenylbutazone (Butazolidin) : 4-butyl-1, 2-diphenyl-3, 5-pyrazoli-dinedione. *A*. Solvent:0.5N NaOH *B*. Compound was insoluble in 0.5N H_2SO_4. (10μg/ml.)

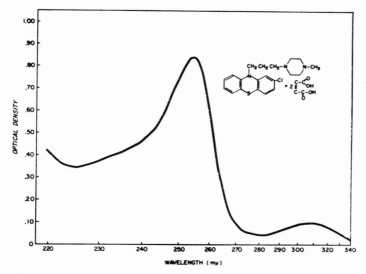

FIGURE 1f. Prochlorperazine • dimaleate (Compazine). 10μg/ml of 0.5N H_2SO_4.

To compute on a basis of milligrams per 100 ml when using a 5 ml original specimen, and to correct for aliquot; multiply microgram reading by 125 for mg/dl.

References—UV Analysis

Andrea, C.N. and Snow, S.W.: *Interbureau By-Lines.* DEA, 1967.

Bradford, Lowell W.: Personal communications.

Clarke, E.G.C.: *Isolation & Identification of Drugs.* London, Phar Press, 1969.

Johnson, C.A. and Thornton-Jones, A.D. (Eds.): *Drug Identification.* London, Pharmaceutical Press, 1966.

Siek, Theodore J.: Merrifield, Virginia, Bureau of Forensic Sciences.

Sunshine, I. (Ed.): *Handbook of Analytical Toxicology.* Cleveland, Chemical Rubber Co, 1969.

Sunshine, I. and Gerber, S.: *Spectrophotometric Analysis of Drugs.* Springfield, Thomas, 1963.

U.S. Environmental Protective Agency (EPA): *Manual of Chemical Methods,* 1975; and Vol. I & II, 1977. Washington, D.C. EPA.

White, R.G.: *Handbook of Ultraviolet Methods.* New York, Plenum, 1965.

CHROMATOGRAPHY

PAPER CHROMATOGRAPHY

Wet a 55 to 60 cm length of Whatman #2 filter paper with a buffer and allow to dry.   (A different pH for each strip.)

Spot an alcohol solution of the basic drug near one end of the paper along with a control compound (codeine) .

Immerse the spotted end in the buffered butyl alcohol of corresponding pH and allow to develop for about 15 hours.

Remove and mark the solvent front.

Locate the drug spot with a beam of UV light or by spraying with iodoplatinate reagent.

Using the front of the drug spot, calculate the Rf of the drug by using the following formula:

$$Rf = \frac{\text{distance traveled by drug}}{\text{distance traveled by solvent}}$$

For identification, compare with known standards. See Table XIV—page 108.

To recover the drug, cut out the spot; place in a separatory funnel and cover with 5 ml of sodium sulfate solution.   When the paper is decolorized, add a suitable solvent and shake.

Evaporate the solvent to dryness. Other tests may now be made to confirm the identity of the drug, including a UV spectra scan.

Spot may be examined by (a) behavior in UV light (quinine and Pentothal fluoresce); (b) use of chemical reagents designed to produce *color* or changes in behavior under UV; (c) eluted spot dissolved in either 0.5N sodium hydroxide or sulfuric acid and analyzed by UV spectrophotometry.

Reagents (Goldbaum and Kazyak)

- *MacIlvaine's buffers:* pH, 3.0; 790 ml of 0.1M citric acid diluted to 1.0 liter with 0.2M sodium dibasic phosphate. pH, 5.0: 480 ml of 0.1M citric acid diluted to 1.0 liter with 0.2m sodium dibasic phosphate.
- *Sorenson's buffers:* pH, 6.5; 680 ml of M/15 potassium monobasic phosphate diluted to 1.0 liter with M/15 sodium dibasic phosphate. pH, 7.5; 164 ml of M/15 potassium monobasic phosphate diluted to 1.0 liter with M/15 sodium dibasic phosphate.
- *Iodoplatinic acid reagent:* Mix 45 ml of 10% potassium iodide, 5 ml of 5% platinum chloride, and 100 ml of distilled water.
- *Sodium sulfite reagent:* A 4% sodium sulfite solution in half-saturated sodium borate solution.
- *Developing Solution:* *n*-butyl alcohol saturated with buffers.

References—Paper Chromatography

Algeri, E.J. and Walker, J.T.: *Am J Clin Path,* 22:37, 1952. (Barbiturates)

Block, R.J., Durrum, E.L., and Zweig, G.: *Manual of Paper Chromatography and Electrophoresis,* 2nd ed. New York, Acad Pr, 1958.

Curry, A.S.: The application of paper chromatography to forensic chemistry. *J Crim Law Police Sci,* 44:787, 1954.

Curry, A.S. and Powell, H.: *Nature,* 173:1143, 1954. (Alkaloids.)

Davidow, B. *et al.: Am J Clin Path,* 46:58, 1966.

Dybing, F.: *Acta Pharm Toxicol,* 11:72, 1955. (Barbiturates.)

Goldbaum, L.R. and Kazyak, L.: *Anal Chem,* 28:1289, 1956. (Alkaloids.)

Leiserson, L. and Walker, T.B.: *Anal Chem,* 27:1129, 1955. (Nicotine.)

McBay, A.J.: Chromatographic methods in forensic problems. *Forensic Sci,* 3:364, 1958.

McBay, A.J. and Algeri, E.J.: *Amer J Clin Path,* 24:1139, 1954. (Barbiturates.)

Metcalf, R.L. and March, R.B.: *Science, 117:*527, 1953. (Parathion.)
Randerath, K.: *Thin Layer Chromatography.* New York, Academic, 1966.
Sabatino, F.J.: *JAOAC, 37:*1002, 1954. (Barbiturates.)
Wright, J.T.: *J Clin Path,* 7:56, 1954. (Barbiturates.)

THIN LAYER CHROMATOGRAPHY (TLC)

TLC is now considered one of the more useful and effective technics for the isolation and identification of many toxic agents. It is equally effective in the presence of multiple agents (which is sometimes the case). It can also identify metabolites in relation to parent compound; this is a further assistance in identification. TLC combines the speed of gas chromatography and the reliability of paper chromatography. It possesses a great sensitivity, even to small traces, and allows the sharpness of separation when dealing with metabolites or combined agents. This technic is simple, rapid, reliable, inexpensive to perform. Spots may be removed later (scraped off), re-extracted with methanol and then rerun (reconfirmed) using another developing system, or by GLC. TLC *should* be reconfirmed.

When precision is exercised, comparison with calibrated standards may permit a reliable estimate of concentration, when color intensity and area are considered.

The Rf reported are *averages* and *will vary* from plate to plate. Internal standards are run in parallel with samples; this will help standardize tests.

General Procedure

Glass plates (20 × 20 cm) may be purchased or may be easily prepared. A good standard plate for general use is a 250μ thickness of silica gel G. Sometimes, aluminum oxide (Al_2O_3) or other absorbents may be used for special purposes. Thickness, composition, and pH can be varied to suit special situations.

Vertical lines are drawn 1.5 cm apart to allow individual "runways" for each sample. Purified tissue extracts dissolved in 0.5 ml of methanol are serially spotted with a micro pipette and dried in a *small* circle in the lower center of a runway, 1.5 cm from the bottom. Other samples, including reference standards, are similarly spotted in other runways. A horizontal line (stop point) is drawn exactly 10 cm or 15 cm above these starting points.

A TLC tank is filled with suitable developing solvents to a depth of about 1 cm from the bottom. The selection of solvent mixtures depend upon polarity and solubility of solute. Polar solvents travel a greater distance than nonpolar. The ideal solvent is one that moves the samples about one-half the distance of the solvent front (10 cm) and resolves it into a discrete small area (no tails). If the sample is a mixture of drugs or if it is a drug that produces metabolites, the solvent should allow for separate small areas to be detected. If the drug does not move much from starting point, or if the sample migrates too close to the solvent front, another developing solvent should be tried (see Tables XV and XVI—pages 109 to 117).

The plate properly spotted is then dipped 1 cm into the solvent; the lid is *firmly* closed and the atmosphere is allowed to saturate with vapor. When the solvent front just touches the 10 cm horizontal mark (this usually takes about thirty minutes), quickly remove the plate and allow it to *air dry*.

Examine the plate under a UV light at 350 and 254 nm for characteristic fluorescence or absorbance. Some drugs are visible by this means. Calculate the Rf. Rf is the ratio of the $\frac{\text{(solute front)}}{\text{(solvent front)}} \times 100$.

The plate is then sprayed with appropriate reagents to bring out characteristic color spots. It is now much easier to see and measure the Rf. The reagents sprays used will vary with groups being tested.

Approximate quantitation may be made by comparison with standards (similarly prepared on the same plate) for intensity of color and area size.

The spot can sometimes be scraped off, extracted with methanol, purified (gentle heat, filter, wash residue with 2 × 2 ml methanol; and 25μl acetic acid (20%), gently evaporate to dryness. Pick up with 0.5 ml of methanol, and then retest by UV spectrophotometry, gas chromatography, crystal structure, color tests, or by another TLC solvent system.

Varying the nonpolar solvents and their ratios may be used

to further differentiate the Rf values between the various compounds.

The following precautions should be taken:

a. Solvents should be of the purest quality and should be freshly prepared at regular intervals.

b. Plates should be prepared properly and should be activated by heating prior to use.

c. Do not overload plates with specimens.

d. Jar should be *firmly* sealed so that its atmosphere can be saturated with solvent vapors.

e. Confine the spotting to very small spots in a line of dots about 1.5 cm from the bottom of the plate. A micropipette is useful to make these serial drops; allow to dry before next addition.

f. Area is equally as important as color intensity in the estimation of approximate quantity.

g. The Rfs suggested in the literature (Tables XV and XVI) are to be used only as a guide. Each analyst should prepare and establish his own Rf according to his own conditions and technic. Rf will vary for each, and will vary from plate to plate.

h. Each plate should contain "probable" knowns (standard concentrations) to be run with the unknown, for comparison.

i. Rf is given by whole number (ratio × 100).

j. The (TLC; Rf) spot represents a fairly pure separation and concentration of drug. This spot can be carefully scrapped and collected into a beaker. The same solvent (developing solvent) used originally (or methanol) may be used to dissolve the drug to separate it from the silica gel. No one solvent may be ideal for all situations and not all scrapings will produce a recovery, but it is worth a try especially when specimen quantity is meager. Evaporate solvent. Reconstitute in manner best suited for proposed confirmation: GLC or TLC with another solvent system or even UV if the $E^{1\%}_{1cm}$ sensitivity is adequate.

k. The spot, if in the upper one-third of plate, may be made to migrate again by turning the plate 180° and using another solvent system or turn only 45 degrees (two dimensional TLC).

1. The spot, if "grouped" with several other spots in the lower one-third of plate, may be made (perhaps) to separate from the group—if the plate is removed, dried, and another solvent system now is used. This new migration (with new solvent system) may unbunch the group.

Developing Solvents for Drugs — see pages 109 & 111

* $CHCl_3$:acetone (9:1) (Sunshine).
  Spray: $HgSO_4$ and diphenylcarbazone.
* Ethyl acetate:methanol:NH_4OH (85:10:5) (Davidow; and DOT H5-801-016 Feb. 1974).
* Cyclohexane: $CHCl_3$:acetic acid (40:50:10) (Gänshirt in Stahl).
  Spray: 0.2% fluorescein in ethanol, and look under UV.
* Methyl ethyl ketone (Gänshirt in Stahl).
* $CHCl_3$: ether (85:15) (Machata).
* $CHCl_3$: ethanol (9:1) (Machata).
* $CHCL_3$: ethanol (8:2) (Machata).
* Ethyl acetate:methyl alcohol:ammonium hydroxide (90:7.3) (Modified Davidow for acids) (Quantum Assays).
  Spray: Mercuric sulfate, diphenylcarbazone.
* Benzene:ethyl acetate:diethylamine (70:20:10) (Schnackerz-Munter-Waldi in Stahl).
* Chloroform:acetone:diethylamine (50:40:10) (Schnackerz-Munter-Waldi in Stahl).
* Chloroform:diethylamine (90:10) (Schnackerz-Muter-Waldi in Stahl).
* Cyclohexane:chloroform:diethylamine (50:40:10) (Schnackerz-Munter-Waldi in Stahl).
* Ethyl alcohol:dioxane:benzene:NH_4OH (5:40:50:5) (Steele).
  Spray: Potassium iodoplatinate (10 ml $PtCl_3$ to 250 ml of 4% KI diluted to 500 with water).
* $CHCl_3$:dioxane:ethyl acetate:NH_4OH (25:60:10.5) (Steele).
  Spray: Potassium iodoplatinate.
* Ethyl acetate:benzene:NH_4OH (60:35:5) (Steele).

Spray: Potassium iodoplatinate.
* a. Etheyl acetate:methanol:NH$_4$OH (85:10:5) (Davidow, et al.
  Spray: H$_2$SO$_4$ (5% v/v) (expose to UV).
  b. (Davidow, Li Petri, Quame, Searle, Fastlich, and Savitsky).
  Spray: Potassium iodoplatinate, dried and then Drangendorff's reagent.
  c. (Dole, Kim, Glitis).
  Spray: Potassium iodoplatinate, 4% nihydrin in acetone.
  d. D.O.T. HS-801 016.
  e. Sunshine CRC 1973.
  f. Change ratio to (85:10:1) (better).
* Methanol:acetone:triethanolamine (100:100:3) (Randerath).
  Spray: UV light, then Dragendorff's reagent.
* Pyridine:petroleum ether:CHCl$_3$ (1:1:5:0.1).
* Benzene:acetone.NH$_4$OH (50:10:5) (Paulus).
* Methanol (Machata).
* CHCl$_3$:EtOH (10%) (Machata).
* *n*-Hexane:acetone:NH$_4$OH (80:20:1) (Osorio).
* Methanol:NH$_4$OH (100:1.5) (Sunshine, Bastas, Kananen, Montforte).
  Spray: 5% H$_2$SO$_4$; then potassium iodoplatinate. (Serax, meprobamate, Librium, Valium do not stain very well).
* Ethyl acetate:methyl alcohol:ammonium hydroxide:water (85:13.5:0.5:1).
  Modified Davidow for Basics. (Quantum Assays)
  Spray: Ninhydrin, Iodoplatinate.

Reagents (Sprays for TLC) for Drugs

* Ninhydrin: 0.4% in acetone (or 0.2% in *n*-butanol). Store in brown bottle in refrigerator (for 1° and 2° amines).
  Expose plate to 254 and 366 nm for 3–5 minutes; then gently heat → pink-red.
* Sulfuric acid: 5% in ethanol (for phenothiazines).
* Forrest and Forrest spray for tricyclic antidepressants. See tricyclic antidepressants.
* Potassium iodoplatinate: 1 gm platinic chloride in 100 ml water, mix with 300 ml of water containing 10 gm potassium iodide;

dilute to total of 400 ml with water; age for 24 hours. Store in a dark bottle and in a refrigerator. Stores better without acid, but acidify plate before spraying if required.

* Mercuric sulfate: Suspend with mixing 5 gm of mercuric oxide (HgO) in 100 ml of water. Add, while stirring, 20 ml of H_2SO_4. Cool the suspension, then dilute it to 250 ml with water (for acidic and neutral).
* Diphenylcarbazone (DPC): Dissolve 5 mg DPC in 50 ml of chloroform. Store in a dark bottle and in a cool place (for acidic and neutral).
* Dragendorff's reagent: 1.3 gm bismuth subnitrate in 60 ml of water containing 15 ml of glacial acetic acid; this is then mixed with 12 gm KI in 30 ml water. To final mixture, add 100 ml H_2O and 25 ml glacial acetic acid (for alkaloids).
* Potassium permanganate: 1% in water (to show unsaturation in barbiturate groups).
* FPN: 5 ml 5% $FeCl_3$ + 45 ml 20% $HClO_4$ + 50 ml 50% HNO_3 for phenothiazines.
* p-Dimethylaminobenzaldhyde: Saturated in concentrated HCl (for amines and methylene groups).

References—TLC

Clarke, E.G.C.: *Isolation and Identification of Drugs.* London, Pharm Press, 1969.

Quantum Assays Corp., *Procedural Bulletins.*

Sunshine, I. (Ed.): *Handbook of Analytical Toxicology,* Cleveland, Chemical Rubber Co, 1969.

Sunshine, I. (Ed.): *Methodology for Analytical Toxicology.* Cleveland, Chemical Rubber Co, 1974.

Stahl, E. (Ed.): *Thin Layer Chromatography: A Laboratory Handbook.* New York, Acad Pr, 1965.

Strobbe, M.: *Environmental Science Laboratory Manual.* St. Louis, Mosby, 1972.

U.S. Dept. of Transportation: DOT, HS-801-016. Washington, D.C., 1974.

U.S. Environmental Protective Agency (EPA), *Manual of Chemical Methods.* Washington, D.C., 1977.

TLC TECHNIC FOR PESTICIDES

Organic Phosphate Esters: Stomach contents or residue, etc., is extracted with n-hexane or petroleum ether. Separate, filter, and then carefully evaporate to dryness. Pick up residue with a minimum of chloroform or methanol; then spot onto a 250μ silica gel G plate, confining the spot with a capillary pipette in the usual manner. Select solvent system and allow to run for about 30 minutes, or until solvent front reaches 10–15 cm; then quickly remove from tank.

Plate is allowed to air dry, then is placed into another tank saturated with bromine vapors for 1 or 2 minutes. An open bromine bottle at the bottom of the tank will suffice, but extreme care is urged with bromine, which is very toxic to skin or by breathing.

Plate is removed and aerated free from bromine vapors, under a fume hood, and then sprayed with fluorescein solution or rhodamine B solution. The presence of blue-white spots on a bright pink background will demonstrate organic phosphate insecticides. These spots will fluoresce a brilliant purple when placed under a UV light. Compare Rf with standards.

Chlorinated Hydrocarbons: If the above procedure is negative for the organic phosphate insecticides, then proceed by spraying with 5% silver nitrate. Allow to air dry, and then expose plate to UV light at 254 nm for about 15 minutes or until brown or gray spots are observed.

See Table XVII.—page 118

Developing Solvents for Pesticides
* Hexane:acetone (4:1) (Machata from Baumski, Baumler, and Rippstein)
* Hexane:acetone (5:1)
*Hexane:acetone (9:1)
* Chloroform:acetic acid (9:1)
* Cyclohexane:chloroform (4:1) (Machata, Stahl, Gänshirt and Waldi)
* Hexane 100%
    Others
* Acetone:benzene (10:90)
* Cyclohexane:acetone:chloroform (70:25:50)
* n-Hexane:acetone (99:1) for chlorinated hydrocarbons
* Benzene:ethyl acetate (90:10)

Sprays for Pesticides
* Bromine fumes for organic phosphate esters (take great care; extremely toxic; use in hood) .
* Rhodamine B (0.5% in ethanol); then sodium carbonate (10%); examine under UV light.
* Fluorescein (0.2% in ethanol); examine under UV light.
* Silver nitrate (5%) .

References—TLC for Pesticides
Clarke, E.G.C.: *Identification of Drugs.* London, Pharm Press, 1969.
Randerath, K.: *Thin-Layer Chromatography.* New York, Acad Pr, 1966.
Stahl, E. (Ed.): *Thin-Layer Chromatography: A Laboratory Handbook.* New York, Acad Pr, 1969.
Strobbe, M.A.: *Environmental Science Laboratory Manual.* St. Louis, Mosby, 1972.
Sunshine, I. (Ed.): *Handbook of Analytical Toxicology.* Cleveland, Chemical Rubber Co, 1969.
Sunshine, I. (Ed.): *Methodology for Analytical Toxicology.* Cleveland, Chemical Rubber Co., 1975.
U.S. Environmental Protection Agency: *Manual of Methods for Pesticides,* Vol. I and II. Washington, D.C., EPA, 1975.

GAS LIQUID CHROMATOGRAPHY (GLC)
GLC is sensitive, accurate, rapid, and simple for the separation, identification, and quantitation of many volatile compounds.

There are many thousands of references in the literature and this is continuously growing at a rapid rate.

The following GLC data and suggestions for screening of drugs is suggested as a guide to be used in conjunction with the facilities available.

Method A*
Instrument: Perkin-Elmer Model 3920 with flame ionization detector. Column 3% OV-17, on 100–120 mesh Gas Chrom Q (Applied Science), on a 6 foot, 4 mm i.e. glass column.

The retention times are given for two temperatures: 250°C and 220°C. At 250°C the retention times are relative to cocaine. All

*Reproduced with permission of U.S. Dept. of Justice, Drug Enforcement Administration; Charles B. Teer, Forensic Chemist (Tabulated 1976) .

drugs having a relative retention time at 250°C of less than 1.00 were reinjected at 220°C, relative to diphenhydramine. The retention time is measured from the point of injection. The data is presented in three tables (see pages 119 to 128) :

1. Retention times at 250°C relative to cocaine (Table XVIII).
2. Retention time at 220°C relative to diphenhydramine (Table XIX).
3. Drug index (alphabetical) (Table XX).

Method B*

Instrument: Dual column F & M model 402, FID nitrogen carrier gas; inlet pressure 40 pound/square inch, 6 feet × 4 mm i.d. glass coiled column, 5% Hallcomid M-18 and 0.5% Carbowax 600 on 40/60 mesh Teflon 6 HC.

Column temperature approximately 50°C adjusted so that ethanol standard has a retention time of 1.9 ± 0.1 minute. Injection port: 150°C; Detector: 75°C; carrier gas rate: approximately 40 cc/minute. The injection port is fitted with a removable precolumn glass linear to facilitate cleaning.

Data is listed in Table XXI. The data has been also reported by Dubowski (Methodology for Analytical Toxicology) as appropriate for head space analysis. Data in Table XXII is taken from the literature and also may be used as a guide.

References—GLC

Clarke, E.G.C.: Isolation and Identification of Drugs. London, Pharm Pr, 1969.

Finkle, B.S., Cherry, E.J., and Taylor, D.M.: Forensic toxicology. *J Chrom Sci, 9:*393, 1971.

Sunshine, I. (Ed.): *Handbook of Analytical Toxicology*. Cleveland, Chemical Rubber Co., 1969.

---

*From Finkle, B.S., Cherry, E.J., and Taylor, D.M.: Forensic toxicology. *J Chrom Sci, 9:*393, 1971.

APPENDIX—TABLES

TABLE I
VOLATILES

I. Barely acidified with tartaric acid (sat), then steam distillated; catch distillate in ice bath to minimize loss.

acetone (Seba Nil)

aldehydes

arsenic (As_2O_3)

benzene*

benzyl alcohol (Foille)

camphor (Panalgesic; Rhuligel) *

carbon disulfide (best yield is in second portion)

carbon tetrachloride (pyrene; Carbona)

chloral hydrate (Aquachloral; Felsules; Kessodrate;Noctec)

chloroform (catch in CCl_4 and read in NIR)

cresols*

croton oils

cyanide (potassium, sodium or ammonium) ; must be collected and trapped in dilute NaOH)

p-dichlorobenzene*

ethchlorvynol (Placidyl)

ethyl alcohol (alcoholic beverages and as an industrial or tincture solvent)

ether (catch in CCl_4 and read in NIR

formaldehyde (Formalin)

fusel oils

gasoline*

isopropanol (Cetylside; Komed HC; Tinver; Xerac)

kerosene*

methyl alcohol (wood alcohol, or solvent)

methyl parafynol (Dormison)

methyl salicylate (oil of wintergreen) *

naphthalene*

α-naphthol*

β-naphthol*

nitrobenzene*

paraldehyde

paranitrophenol (parathion precursor) *

petroleum distillates (benzine, charcoal igniting fuel, gasoline, kerosene, mineral seal oil, mineral spirits, naphtha, spindle oil, stoddard solvent, toluene)*

79

TABLE I — (Cont'd)

phenols (Chloraseptic; Oraderm) *
phosphorus (yellow)
thymols (Bensulfoid) *
turpentine (oleoresin from pinus) *

II. Alkaline with NaOH, and then steam distill; carefully concentrate.
amphetamines*
aniline*
chloral hydrate → chloroform
nicotine*
benadryl
chlortrimeton

---

*Read in UV spectrophotometer; give characteristic absorption curves.

TABLE II

GROUP REACTIONS FOR POISONS ISOLATED IN THE ACID-STEAM DISTILLATE
(For technic and reactions, see under poison indicated.)

---

1. Add bromine water:
   aniline
   phenol
   cresol

2. Add Millon's reagent, plus heat:
   aniline
   phenol
   cresol

3. Add silver nitrate solution:
   cyanides
   phosphorus

4. Prussian blue reaction:
   cyanides

5. Aniline+NaOH+heat:
   chloroform
   chloral hydrate
   carbon tetrachloride

6. Pyridine+NaOH+heat:
   chloroform
   chloral hydrate
   carbon tetrachloride

7. Direct Nicloux:
   ethyl, methyl, isopropyl
      alcohol
   formaldehyde
   acetaldehyde

8. Direct Schiff's reagent:
   acetaldehyde
   formaldehyde

9. Schiff's reagent (after
   oxidation) :
   ethyl alcohol
   methyl alcohol
   acetaldehyde
   formaldehyde

10. Direct chromotropic acid:
    formaldehyde

11. Chromotropic acid (after oxidation) :
    methyl alcohol
    formaldehyde

12. Chloroform+NaOH+heat:
    pyridine

TABLE II — (Cont'd)

13. Deniges' reagent (H_2SO_4) direct:
    acetone

14. Deniges (after oxidation) + heat:
    isopropyl alcohol
    acetone

15. $PbAc_2$ + KOH + formaldehyde:
    carbon disulfide

16. Iodine crystals:
    turpentine

17. Pellet of NaOH→ yellow
    (after heating) :
    parathion

Sensitivities of the foregoing tests are sufficient to detect these various poisons when present in toxic amounts.

Directions for performing these tests will be found under the individual poisons in Section II.

TABLE III
MICRODIFFUSION TECHNIC

Poison	Liberating Agent	Absorbent and/or	Reactant
1. carbon monoxide	H_2SO_4 10%		$PdCl_2$ turns gray to black; proportional to carbon monoxide concentration.
2. ethanol (methanol & isopropanol)	Na_2CO_3 (sat.)		Anstie's reagent: yellow to green; proportional to concentration.
3. cyanide	H_2SO_4 10%	NaOH (10%)	$FeSO_4$ (20%); HCl: Prussian blue.
4. CCl_4 & $CHCl_3$	None	Toluene (reagent grade)	NaOH + purified pyridine +Δ: → pink-red.
5. phenols	H_2SO_4 10%	NaOH (10%)	Folin phenol reagent: → blue.
6. sulfides	H_2SO_4 10%	NaOH (10%)	a) Pb (Ac)$_2$ (10%: → B'K ppt. b) Cd (Ac)$_2$ (10%): → yellow ppt.
7. paraldehyde	H_2SO_4 10%	$NaHSO_3$ (10%)	p-hydroxydiphenyl → blue color in H_2SO_4 (keep cool).
8. methanol	Na_2CO_3 (sat.)	H_2SO_4	Chromotropic acid → blue.
9. isopropanol	Na_2CO_3 (sat.)	H_2SO_4	Salicylaldehyde (fresh, 0.1% in absolute alcohol) + 2 ml KOH (sat.) + Δ in water bath (2 min) + cool → red color.

TABLE IV
ACID AND NEUTRAL DRUGS
(extraction)

acetaminophen (Tylenol; Tempra;
Paracetamol)
acetanilid
acetazolamide (Diamox)
acetophenetidin (Phenacetin)
acetylsalicylic acid (aspirin)*
allopurinol (Zyloprim)
aloin
p-aminobenzoic acid (PABA)*
aminophylline
aminopyrine (Pyramidon)
p-aminosalicylic acid (PASA)
amobarbital (Amytal)
antipyrine
appretrol
ascorbic acid (vitamin C)*
banthine
barbiturate derivatives
bemegride
bendroflumethiazide
benzonatate (Tessalon)
benzthiazide (Aquatag; Exna)
bishydroxycoumarin (Dicoumarol)
bromisovalum
bromural
butabarbital (Butisol)
butalbital
caffeine
camphor
cantharidin (Spanish flies)
carbromal
carisoprodol (Rela; Soma)
carmol (Ingram)
chloral hydrate
chlorambucil (Leukeran)
chlordiazepoxide (Librium)
clorobutanol
chlorothiazide (Diuril)
chlorpropamide (Diabinase)
chlorthalidone Hyproton)
chlorzaxone (Paraflex)
chrysazin
cinchonine
cinchophen
citric acid*

colchicine
coumarin (Coumadin as Na salt)
p-cresol
cyclothiazide (Anhydron)
2,4 D; 2,4,5 T
(Flurazepam) Dalmane
diallylbarbituric acid
diazepam (Valium)
digitoxin
dimenhydrinate (Dramamine)
4,6-dinitrocresol
diphenylhydantoin (Dilantin;
phenytoin)
disulfiram (Antabuse)
doxepin (Sinequan)
ectyl urea (Levanil)
emetine (ipecac)
estrone (Coumadin; dicumarol;
warfarin)
ethclorvynol (Placidyl)
ethinamate (Valmid)
5-ethyl-5-phenyhydantoin (Nirvanol)
furosemide (Lasix)
glutethimide (Doriden)
isoproterenol (Isuprel)
heptabarbital
hexethal
hexobarbital (Evipal)
hydrochlorothiazide (Esidrex;
Hydrodiuril)
hydroflumethiazide (Saluron)
p-hydroxybenzaldehyde
p-hydroxybenzoic acid*
hydroxycoumarin derivatives
hydroxyphenolic acids
mebutamate (Capla)
meconin
mefenamic acid (Ponstel)
mephenesin (Tolserol; Nebralin)
mephobarbital (Mebaral)
meprobamate (Equanil; Miltown)
mercaptans
mercaptopurines (Purinethol)
methantheline bromide (Banthine)
metharbital (Gemonil)

TABLE IV — (Cont'd)

methaqualone (Quaalude; Sopor)
methitural (Neveral)
methocarbamol (Robaxin)
Methychlorthiazide (Enduron)
methyl-*p*-bensalicylate
methyl parcophymol (Dormision;
  Meparfynol; methyl parafynol)
methylprylone (Noludar)
methyl salicylate (oil of wintergreen)
milontin (Phensuximide)
nikethamide (Coramine)
oxazepam (Serax)
oxalic acid*
pentachlorophenol
pentobarbital (Nembutal)
phenacemide (Phenurone)
phenacetin (Phenaphen; Fiorinal;
  Soma comp.)
phenaglycodol
phenols and derivatives (carbolic acid)
phenylbutazone (Butazolidin)
phenyl salicylate (Salol)
picric acid*
picrotoxin (CHCl₃) (fish-berries)
polythiazide (Renese)
primidon (Mysoline)
saccharin*
salicylamide
salicylic acid*
santonin
schlererythin*
secobarbital (Seconal)

sedormid
strophanthin
succinylsulfathiazole
sulfadiazine
sulfadimethoxine
sulfaguanidine
sulfamerazine
sulfamethaxazole
sulfanilamide
sulfapyrazine
sulfapyridine
sulfathiazole
sulfisoxazole
sulfonamide
2,4,5 T (herbicide)
talbutal (Lotusate) (barbiturate)
tetrachlormethiazide
theobromine (Theocalcin)
theophylline (Tedral; Quibron)
thiamylal (Surital) (barbiturate)
thioguanine
thiopental sodium (Pentothal)
thymol
tolbutamide (Orinase)
trichlormethiazide (Methahydrin)
trichloroethanol
tricyclamol (Tricoloid)
trimethadione (Tridione)
tybamate (Solacen; Tybatran)
ureides
urethane
vasodilan (Isoxsuprine)

*Acidic (strong); for other acidic or neutral drugs see Table IX for UV spectrophotometric screening. See page 86.

TABLE V
DETECTION OF NEGATIVE RADICALS

Using silver nitrate (AgNO₃), nitric acid (HNO₃), and barium chloride (BaCl₂).
  ↓Precipitation formed
  ↑No precipitation formed (or disappeared)
1. AgNO₃ ↓ + HNO₃ ↓ chloride, bromide, iodide, thiocyanate,
  BaCl₂ ↑   hypochlorous acids.

TABLE V — (Cont'd)

2. AgNO₃ ↓ + HNO₃ ↑ BaCl₂ ↑	nitrous acid, cyanide, phosphate —
3. AgNO₃ ↓ + HNO₃ ↑ BaCl₂ ↓ + HNO₃ ↑	sulfite, phosphorus, carbonic, oxalic, iodic, boric, selenic, telluric acids.

4. AgNO₃ ↑ + HNO₃ ↑
   (colored)
   BaCl₂ ↓ + HNO₃ ↑
	arsenic, arsenous.
	chromic acids; thiosulfate.
	—

5. AgNO₃ ↑ BaCl₂ ↑	nitric, chloric, perchloric acids. —
6. AgNO₃ ↑ BaCl₂ ↓ + HNO₃↓	sulfate, fluoride. —

TABLE VI

HEAVY METALS

A. CONFIRMATORY TEST

silvery deposit	shiny black	dull black	purple
	+		
+	nitric acid (15%)	+	+
	+		
Cu₂I₂	Na₂SO₃ (5%)	Gutzeit's test	Gutzeit's test
↓	+	↓	↓
	quinine iodide	yellow	black
	↓		(fades with hydro-
salmon pink	orange		chloric acid
	precipitate	↓	fumes)
↓	↓		↓
Mercury	Bismuth	Arsenic	Antimony

B. SENSITIVITY

APPEARANCE	SENSITIVITY	CONFIRMATION TEST SENSITIVITY
mercury — silvery deposit	0.050 mg/20 ml	0.025 mg/20 ml
arsenic — dull black*	0.005 mg/20 ml	0.002 mg/20 ml
bismuth — shiny black	0.020 mg/20 ml	0.010 mg/20 ml
antimony — dark purple sheen	0.020 mg/20 ml	0.010 mg/20 ml

*Arsenic deposit dissolves in 1 ml KCN 10%; others do not.

TABLE VII

ATOMIC ABSORPTION DETECTION LIMITS

aluminum	0.03	lithium	0.0006
antimony	0.1	magnesium	0.0001
arsenic	0.1	manganese	0.002

TABLE VII — (Cont'd)

barium	0.02	mercury	0.5
beryllium	0.001	molybdenum	0.03
bismuth	0.04	nickel	0.01
boron	2.5	phosphorus	100.
cadmium	0.001	potassium	0.005
calcium	0.001	selenium	0.1
chromium	0.003	silicon	0.08
cobalt	0.01	silver	0.002
copper	0.002	strontium	0.01
gallium	0.1	tellurium	0.09
gold	0.02	thallium	0.03
iron	0.01	tin	0.02
lead	0.02	zinc	0.002

TABLE VIII
STEAM DISTILLATE
(H_2O)

	Maxima (nm)	$E_{1cm}^{1\%}$	Minima (nm)	$E_{1cm}^{1\%}$
aniline	280		260	75
	230	920		
benzene	228		229	
	233		234	
	238		240	
	242		245	
	248		250	
	254	6	257	
	260			
camphor	282	3	244	
cresol	273	143	260	107
kerosene	270		244	
	Varies with constituent mixtures as also does gasoline			
methyl salicylate	303			
	238	820	262	30
naphthalene	265		238	
	275		269	
	283		281	
	308			
α-naphtol	295	350	250	90
β-naphthol	330		295	
	285		280	170
	274	250	248	

TABLE VIII — (Cont'd)

	Maxima (nm)	$E_{1cm}^{1\%}$	Minima (nm)	$E_{1cm}^{1\%}$
nitrobenzene	270	780	228	240
p-dichlorobenzene	264		244	
	271		266	
	279		276	
phenol	270	147	238	
thymol	274	131	245	11
normal (tissue)	(270-280)			

Many of the above compounds have a distinct characteristic odor; many more aromatic compounds can fit into this scheme, i.e. gasoline, pine oil, methol, other phenols, etc.

If compounds are too dilute, these can be concentrated by extraction with a small volume of n-hexane (first purify n-hexane by passing it through silica gel). Read in n-hexane.

TABLE IX
ACID OR NEUTRAL COMPOUNDS

As Salt	0.5N NaOH				0.5N H₂SO₄			
	Max. Den.	$E_{1cm}^{1\%}$	Min. Den.	$E_{1cm}^{1\%}$	Max. Den.	$E_{1cm}^{1\%}$	Min. Den.	$E_{1cm}^{1\%}$
strophanthin	222	200						
aminopyrine (pyramidon)	225 260	400	250	120	257	440	233	310
tolbutamide	226 Shoulder: 255 to 275	400						
cinchonine	226 287 315	170	244 310	17	316 335	180	259	5
chlorthalidone (Hygroton)	228	600						
phenol	234 286	1100 370	260	110	270	180	238	20
theobromine	236 274	230	234 252	160	272	230	244	63
cresol	238 292	1500	228 268	1400	227	660	256	370
acetanilide	239	900			238	800		
picrotoxin	240	180			250	22		

TABLE IX — (Cont'd)

As Salt	0.5N NaOH				0.5N H$_2$SO$_4$			
	Max. Den.	$E\,^{1\%}_{1cm}$	Min. Den.	$E\,^{1\%}_{1cm}$	Max. Den.	$E\,^{1\%}_{1cm}$	Min. Den.	$E\,^{1\%}_{1cm}$
hexobarbital (Evipal)	242	250						
salicylamide	242 238	350	234 270		236 299	250	262	
phenacetin (acetophenetidin)	243	900			243	900		
chlorozoxazon (Paraflex)	243 287	580	229 263	80	279	320	246	
chlordiazepoxide (Librium)	243 260	1000 1080			245 306	1100 310		
metharbital (Gemonil)	244	320	231					
mephobarbital (Mebaral)	244	300	229					
1-naphthyl-*N*-methyl-carbamate (Sevin)	246	60	230	36				
methohexital (Brevital)	247		228					
methantheline (Banthine)	251 281	134	235 273					
pentobarbital (Nembutal)	253	310	234					
amobarbital (Amytal)	254	320	232					
hexethal	254	280	232					
butisol	254 221	234						
heptabarbital	254	229						
phenobarbital (Luminal)	254	355	236					
acetaminophen (Tylenol; paracetamol)	256	770	none		243	660 Shoulder at 275–285 nm		
butallylonal (Pernoston)	256		235					
chlorambucil (Leukeran)	256 300	380	286					
secobarbital (Seconal)	256	280	234					

TABLE IX — (Cont'd)

As Salt	0.5N NaOH				0.5N H$_2$SO$_4$			
	Max. Den.	$E_{1cm}^{1\%}$	Min. Den.	$E_{1cm}^{1\%}$	Max. Den.	$E_{1cm}^{1\%}$	Min. Den.	$E_{1cm}^{1\%}$
allopurinol	256	410	240					
(Zyloprim)	225		270					
	276							
tricyclamol	257	140	254					
(Tricoloid)	251							
	263							
paraquat	257	854			257	854		
cinchophen	258	1900	238	1100	244	1100	226	
	320		290		267		258	900
					343		294	
milontin	258	740	241					
	252							
	264							
disulfiram	262	19	236	8	262	11	248	9
(Antabuse)								
p-aminobenzoic acid	263	1340	230	280	225		252	1000
(PABA)*								
p-aminosalicylic acid	265	856	244	235	235	480	217	
(PAS)*	299		285		300		235	
methaqualone	263		288		273		257	
(Quaalude)	304		250		293			
	Shoulder at:		317					
phenylbutazone	265	600						
saccharin	268	98	245					
furosemide	270		293		273		296	
(Lasix)	228		248		234		251	
	330							
4,6-dinitrocresol	273	727	252					
	220		310					
caffeine	272	450	245		273	450	245	
theophylline	275	640	244	220	270	550	242	170
aminophylline	274	560	244	210	270	550	243	160
thymol	275	140	252	45				
dimenhydrinate	278	300	244	276	300		245	
(Dramamine)								
ethchlorvynol	280		257					
(Placidyl)								
2,4-D	283	97	258	22	282	20	249	30
dichlorphenoxyacetic acid	292		288		290		287	
2,4,5-T	Same as 2,4-D							

TABLE IX — (Cont'd)

As Salt	0.5N NaOH				0.5N H$_2$SO$_4$			
	Max. Den.	$E_{1cm}^{1\%}$	Min. Den.	$E_{1cm}^{1\%}$	Max. Den.	$E_{1cm}^{1\%}$	Min. Den.	$E_{1cm}^{1\%}$
N-(2,3-xylyl-anthranic acid (Ponstel)	283	347	253 316	180	White precipitate			
dexamethasone (Decadron)	286		262					
protriptyline (Vivactil HCl)	287		250		287		248	
benzonatate (Tessalon)	290	284	243	17	270	97	255	71
chlorothiazide* (Diuril)	291 227 310	330	256	277 226				
acetazolamide (Diamox)	292 241	523	254 228	86	265	420	228	
methyl-p-bensalicylate	293 300	1370	240 274	100	255 237 302	1050	225	200
phenyl salicylate* (Salol)	294 340	740	270 320	490	240 307	2200	272	260
methyprylon (Noludar)	294	5	248		294	5	248	
benthiazide (Naclex)	295 224		260 307					
salicylic acid*	300	275	265	65	235	680	265	45
thiopental sodium (Pentothal)	303	1150	245	8	285 238	900	252	
thiamylal (Surital)	304	886	246					
methitural (Neveral)	305	820	241	90				
ergotamine tartrate (Gynergen)	306	86	270	1				
warfarin Na (Coumadin)	308 Shoulder 290-294	420	258	110	304 280		290	
mercaptopurine (Purinethol)	309 232	670	270					
bishydroxycoumarin (Dicumarol)	313	690	260					
thioguanine	319 229	610	282					
penta-chlorophenol	325							
appetrol	327		265		297		263	
picric acid*	356	650	285	123				

*Strong acids

TABLE X
BASIC COMPOUNDS

As Salt	0.5N H_2SO_4				0.5N NaOH			
	Max. Den.	$E\,^{1\%}_{1cm}$	Min. Den.	$E\,^{1\%}_{1cm}$	Max. Den.	$E\,^{1\%}_{1cm}$	Min. Den.	$E\,^{1\%}_{1cm}$
yohimbine	220	1076	242					
(corynine)	272	320						
ethyl amino-	226	840	254		283	1750	238	
benzoate	270	100	274					
(Benzocaine)	276							
thyroxine	226	18	256		226	3	290	
(tetra-								
iodothyronine)								
cyclizine	227	400	245	10	227	260	246	
(Marezine)	257				253		256	
	262				259			
	269							
tetracaine	227	500	277		305	900	246	
(Pontocaine)	309	960						
procaine	227	450	254		283	600	239	
(Novocaine)	279							
berberine	228	820	246	380	228	610	246	380
	262	800			264			
phenocaine	228	530			260	460	250	440
Prothiaden	228	750						
	265	250						
	300	62						
chlorcyclizine	231	500	254		230	425	246	
(Perazil)	257		260					
	262	250	267					
	269							
cocaine	232	520	260					
	274	40						
diothane	232	260						
(Diperodon)								
eucaine	232	370	262	23	224	300		
	274							
hydroxyzine	232	320			230	325		
(Vistaril; Atarax)								
aconitine	234	200	262	16	224	140		
	275							
thonzylamine	235	800	261		241	775	270	
(Anahist)	273		287		273		289	
	213				279			
					312			

TABLE X — (Cont'd)

As Salt	0.5N H$_2$SO$_4$				0.5N NaOH			
	Max. den.	$E_{1cm}^{1\%}$	Min. den.	$E_{1cm}^{1\%}$	Max. den.	$E_{1cm}^{1\%}$	Min. den.	$E_{1cm}^{1\%}$
chloroquine (Aralen)	235 257 330 344	580	230 245 285 337	570	257 330	520	245 280	
phenylbutazone (Butazolidin)	235	350			263	675	231	350
cinchonine (Chinchonidine)	235 316	1200	268	40	227 290	1200	250	80
phenyramidol (Analexin)	236 308	675	260		240 297	620	267	
acetanilide	237	500			237	600		
pyrilamine (Neoantergan)	237 314	550	260		248 311	540	232 288	
salicylamide (Sabrin)	237 300	580	262		242 328	540	234 270	
chlorothen citrate (Tagathen)	237 312	360	272		243 308	400	282	
aminopyridine (Thenylpyramine)	237 312	690	264		240 308	700	280	
methaphenilene (Diatrin)	238	420			248	490		
amitriptyline hydrochloride (Elavil)	238	550	228		238	440		
methapyrilene (Histadyl)	238 315	640	265	50	240 310	600	278	
tripenolennamine (Pyribenzamine)	238 314	560	262		250 314	635	274	48
thenfadil (Thenyldiamine)	238 312	940	262		246 310	940	274	
ergotamine (Gynergen)	240 310	430	238 292					
corticosteroids	241				247			
diazepan (Valium)	241 283 331	1000 400	262	190	250	540	228	480
antazoline (Antistine)	242 290	510	223 275		248 295	600	223 275	
prothipendyl	242	800	270	50	249	810	274	

TABLE X — (Cont'd)

As Salt	0.5N H_2SO_4				0.5N NaOH			
	Max. den.	$E\frac{1\%}{1cm}$	Min. den.	$E\frac{1\%}{1cm}$	Max. den.	$E\frac{1\%}{1cm}$	Min. den.	$E\frac{1\%}{1cm}$
acetaminophen (Tempra; Tylenol; Paracetamol)	242	610	(Shoulder 275–285)		256	760		
	(249 in methanol)							
isothipendyl	244	860	274		249 315	850	275	
acetophenetidin (Phenacetin)	244	800			244	800		
colchicine	246	1200	289	170	245	1000	287	
	does not easily form salts							
Read in CHCl₃ (extraction from tissue)	240 261		250					
Directly in CHCl₃	245							
chlordiazepoxide (Librium;	246 306	1020	290		260 243	1050 1000		
physostigmine	246 302	420	270		244 300	460	260	
dibucaine (Nupercaine)	246 320	550	232 267	260	238 325	450	235 295	
chlorzoxazone (Paraflex)	246 290	580	229 264					
haloperidol	249	230	233					
promethazine (Phenergan)	249 298	980	230 274		253 305	1100	276	89
pyrathiazine (Pyrrolazote)	249 298	810	274		253 298	690	273	
hydrastine	250 306							
methotrimeprazine (Levoprom)	250							
quinidine	Same as quinine							
quinine	250 318	853	231 270 325	340	230 285	980	260 305	88
isoquinoline (Papaverine)	250 284 310	1800 250	269 290					
ethaverine	Similar to Papaverine							
methoxypromazine (Tentone)	250 302	500	230		252 304	850	277	

TABLE X — (Cont'd)

As Salt	0.5N H₂SO₄				0.5N NaOH			
	Max. den.	E 1% 1cm	Min. den.	E 1% 1cm	Max. den.	E 1% 1cm	Min. den.	E 1% 1cm
imipramine (Tofranil)	250	270	231	170	253	250	231	
allopurinol (Zyloprim)	250	360	232		256 276	290	240 270	160
papaverine	251 285 310							
promazine (Sparine)	251 300	1280	277		252 304	1250	277	
trimeprazine tartrate (Temaril)	251 299	800	274					
gelsemine	252	220	226	84	255	210	232	100
desipramine HCl (Norpramin; Pertofrane)	252	280	231		251	340		
diethylpropion (Tenuate Tepanil)	252	500			248	800		
mepazine (Pacatal)	253 301	930	275					
perphenazine (Trilafon)	253 303	850	278		255 308	850	225 280	
prochlorperazine (Compazine)	254 305	820	280 224	80	255 304	710	283	
thiopropazate (Dartal)	254 304	630	278		255 306	650	278	
pipamazine (Mornidine)	254 304	800	278					
strychnine	254 (286 shoulder)	390	228	376	256	380	233	180
chlorpromazine (Thorazine)	254 305	950	224 277		257	425	238	
fluphenazine (Permitil)	255 305	660	279		256 305	700	278	
phenmetrazine (propantheline; Preludin)	255 249 260 265	10	228 252 258 264		250 255	10	247 252	

TABLE X — (Cont'd)

As Salt	0.5N H_2SO_4				0.5N NaOH			
	Max. den.	$E\frac{1\%}{1cm}$	Min. den.	$E\frac{1\%}{1cm}$	Max. den.	$E\frac{1\%}{1cm}$	Min. den.	$E\frac{1\%}{1cm}$
trifluoperazine (Stelazine)	255 304	680	278		257 304	680	278	
triflupromazine (Vesprin)	255 304	820	222 278		(no curve)			
benactyzine (Suavitil)	256	110	248					
piperilate (Sycotrol)	256	34	242					
amphetamine (Benzedrine)	257 252 263	14	226 254 261	20	258 253 267	30	232 254 266	25
trihexyphenidyl (Artane)	257 251 261	7	230	4				
atropine	257 251 263	8	245 254 262	6	258 264 266	11	255 263 269	9
diphenhydramine (Benadryl)	257 252	15	244	1	258	15	244	1
propoxyphene (Darvon)	257 251 263	12	233 254 262	3	no curve			
meperidine (Demerol)	257 251 263	9	248 254 261	6	257 251 263	7	249 254 263	7
methamphetamine (Desoxyn)	257 252 263	14	226 254 261	7	257 252 263	12	238 254 263	
ephedrine ("ma huang")	257 251 263	10	228 254 261	7	256 251 262	10	240 254 261	7
azacyclonol (Frenquel)	257 253	18	247		257 253	17	247	
paraquat	257	850			257	850		
procyclidine (Kemadrin)	257 251 261	6	236	3				
chlorambucil (Leukeran)	257 252	14	233 254	6				

TABLE X — (Cont'd)

As Salt	0.5N H_2SO_4				0.5N NaOH			
	Max. den.	$E\,{1\% \atop 1cm}$	Min. den.	$E\,{1\% \atop 1cm}$	Max. den.	$E\,{1\% \atop 1cm}$	Min. den.	$E\,{1\% \atop 1cm}$
meratran	257 252	16	246					
phenelzine (Nardil)	257 251 263	10	227		257 266	11	234	
α-prodine (Nisentil)	257 251 262	7 9	235 254 260	 2	258 263 288	15 10 14	254 262 270	 8
prodeine (Primidone)	257 263	14 10	254 261					
aminopyrine (Pyramidon)	257	480	230	300	225 261	400	250	120
methylphenidate (Ritalin)	257 251 263	10	243 253 261	10 8	257 251 263	8	246	
glycopyrrolate (Robinul)	257 251 261	6	254 261	6				
hyoscine (Scopolamine)	257 252 263	9	248 254 261	 7	257 252 263	10	244 254 262	 7
trimethobenzamide (Tigan)	257	350	239		257	400	238	
tricoloid	257 251 261	5	233	3	257 251 262	14	254	
mephentermine (Wyamine)	257 252 263	9	227		257 252 263	13	232	
ethoheptazine (Zactane)	257 251 263	5	247		257 251 263	6	247	
piperidolate (Dactil)	258 252 264	11	243 250 268		258 252 262	12	243 250 268	
doxapram	258 253 262	2	245 255 262	1	253	117	242	
hyoscyamine	258	9	246	6				

TABLE X — (Cont'd)

As Salt	0.5N H_2SO_4					0.5N NaOH			
	Max. den.	$E\frac{1\%}{1cm}$	Min. den.	$E\frac{1\%}{1cm}$	Max. den.	$E\frac{1\%}{1cm}$	Min. den.	$E\frac{1\%}{1cm}$	
anileridine	258	12	245	8	288			
(Leritine)	251		253					
	263		261					
α-(methylphenethyl)	258	11	227		258	13	237	
hydrazine-HCl	252				254			
	263				267			
phenylpropanolamine	258	10	227	1	256	12	240	8
(dl-norephedrine;	251				251			
Propadrine)	263				262			
propyl-paraben	258	900			300	650	242	30
benztropin	259	15						
(Cogentin)								
methadone	259	19	250		290	65	288	64
(Amidone)	251		257		294		292	
	265		262	18				
	292		274					
cetylperidinium	259	5	232					
(Cepacol)								
nicotine	259	343	228	51	261	260	236	140
phenindamine	259	240	241		262	250	244	
(Thephorin)								
chiniofon	259	550	237		262	810	235	
(Yatren)	325		307		337		297	
melphalan	260	4	230					
(Alkeran)								
desipramine	260	247	234					
neostigmine	260	32	238	14	260	41	238	31
(Prostigmine)					280		278	
					292		286	
betahistine HCl	261	200			261	50		
pargyline	261	130	265	90				
(Eutonyl)	250		253					
	256		259					
	267							
niacin	261	424	233	71	263	268	240	125
(nicotinic acid)					269	207	267	200
nicotinic acid	261	396	238					
hydrazide								
veratrine	261							
	291							

TABLE X — (Cont'd)

As Salt	0.5N H_2SO_4				0.5N NaOH			
	Max. den.	E 1% 1cm	Min. den.	E 1% 1cm	Max. den.	E 1% 1cm	Min. den.	E 1% 1cm
anileridine	262	31	256	27	262	33	259	31
lidocaine	269		259		271			
(xylocaine)	271							
mepivacaine	262	22	256		262	18	254	
(Carbocaine)	272		270		270		270	
doxylamine succinate (Decapryn)	262	210	234	45	260	100	236	
thioridazine	262	1000	240	387	276	850		
(Mellaril)	305		285					
adenine	263	970	230	190	269	930	238	230
chlorpheniramine (Chlortrimeton)	263	200	242	100	261	125	242	55
carbinoxamine (Clistin)	263	260	243		260	170	246	
orphenadrine (Disipal)	263	15	244		263	15	244	
bisacodyl (Dulcolax)	263		245					
captodiamine	263	410	240	150	229	750	251	350
(Suvren; Covatin)					272			
nikethamide (Coramine)	264	700	242	380	263	220	246	190
rotoxamine	263	275	240	75	225	230	243	65
(Twiston)					261	120		
pheniramine (Trimeton)	264	300	238	100	262	160	245	
tranylcypromine	264	55	262		267		263	
(Parnate)	257		238	30	260		254	
	271		268		273		271	
brucine	265	328	235	165	265	320	240	90
	300		285		305		285	
phenybutazone (Butazolidin	265	680	230	320	235	460	224	
chlormethazanone	265	22	261					
	258		249					
acetazolamide	265	200	227	75	241	520	228	85
(Diamox)					292		254	

TABLE X — (Cont'd)

As Salt	0.5N H_2SO_4				0.5N NaOH			
	Max. den.	E 1% 1cm	Min. den.	E 1% 1cm	Max. den.	E 1% 1cm	Min. den.	E 1% 1cm
isoproniazid phosphate (Marsilid)	265	250	235	200				
nialamide (Niamide)	265	200	236	110	310	200	256	
chlorphentermine (Pre-Sate)	266	240						
	274	170						
	259	205						
picolinic acid hydrazide	266	238	244					
deserpidine (Harmonyl)	266	150	238					
	214							
deanol acetamido- benzoate (Deaner)	267	800	226		260	800		
isoniazid (INH) (Nydrazid; Rimifon)	267	374	235	215	296	292	252	187
methyclothiazide (Enduron)	268	250	244	70				
	310		295					
mescaline (peyote "buttons")	268	39	255					
mephenesin (Tolserol)	268	18	240		Same			
	275		272	9				
amolanone (Amethone)	270	55	255					
	276							
butacaine (Butyn)	270	33	255	27	280	410	240	90
dicapthon (Dicaptan)	270	350	240					
ISNA (isonicotinic acid)	270	355	238					
methoxalone (Skelain)	270	42	245					
	276		274	40				
Taractan	270		255					
	325		305					
apocodeine	271							
metaxalone (oxazoirdinone)	271	40	244		Same curve			
	278		275	32				
procainamide (Pronestyl)	271		257		275			
	224							

TABLE X — (Cont'd)

As Salt	0.5N H_2SO_4				0.5N NaOH			
	Max. den.	E 1% 1cm	Min. den.	E 1% 1cm	Max. den.	E 1% 1cm	Min. den.	E 1% 1cm
apomorphine	272	780			263	460	242	350
pyrimethamine (Daraprim)	272	136	260	110				
phenylephrine (Neosynephrine)	272	85	241	3	238 291	140	262	35
methocarbamol (Robaxin)	272	100	245		279	19	247	
tranylcypromine	272 264 258		270 262		273 266		270	
clemizole (Allercur)	274	300	235		250 274 281	200	235 262 278	
Bemidone	275	38	248	8	236	150	232	140
hydroxyamphetamine (Paredrine)	275 222	100 500		243 212	274 238		270	
metronidazole	276	440			320			
amydricaine (Alypin)	277 236		266		275 232		262	
zoxazolamine (Flexin)	277 283	400	282 248		240 283	750	228 260	
ketamine	277 268		275 239		277 267 260		275 265	
pentazocine (Talwin)	277	71	245		298	110	278	
Tyramine	277 221		248		293 237		268 228	
adrenalin (epinephrine)	278	222	249		282	150	262	
norepinephrine (Arterenol)	278	140	251	22	304 245	360	276 243	330
Botaperrine	278 244	409	367					
dimenhydrinate (Dramamine)	278	300	244		276	300	245	
diethyltryptamine	278 287 218		239		280		260 241	

TABLE X — (Cont'd)

As Salt	0.5N H_2SO_4				0.5N NaOH			
	Max. den.	E 1% 1cm	Min. den.	E 1% 1cm	Max. den.	E 1% 1cm	Min. den.	E 1% 1cm
digitalis (preferable in ethanol)	278 323	35	268 304	33	286	40	268	37
levallorphan tartrate (Lorfan)	278	73	244		239 298	360	268	
phentolamine	278			250	292			263
alphamethyldopa (Aldomet)	279	120	251					
ibogaine	279		250		295			255
isoproterenol (Isuprel)	279	110	249		285	450	215	
benzthiazide (Naclex)	279	80	248		295 310	250	261 306	
chlorzoxane (chlorzoxazone; Paraflex)	279	320	246		243 287	600	229 263	
tubocurarine (Tubarine)	279	130	256	43	292	200	263	110
quinacrine (Atabrine)	280 220	337	243		270 230		250	
chloramphenicol (Chloromycetin)	280	500	235	150	280	500	235	150
Cobefrin	280	170	250	17	246 295	450	232 274	360
curare	280	65	255	39				
dihydromorphinone (Dilaudid)	280	41	265	25	290	82	275	64
oxycodone (Eucodal)	280	39	262	22	280	38	262	25
heroin	280	86	255	54	278	47	250	16
lorazepam (Antivan)	281	150	272					
oxazepam (Serax)	282 237	168	261		(*In ethanol*) (230 (315	1000 100	))	
cyproheptadine	283		265		283 222		265	
acenocoumarol (Sintrom)	283 304	700	242 295	600	300	600	253	

TABLE X — (Cont'd)

As Salt	0.5N H_2SO_4				0.5N NaOH			
	Max. den.	E 1% 1cm	Min. den.	E 1% 1cm	Max. den.	E 1% 1cm	Min. den.	E 1% 1cm
codeine	285	58	262	22	284	52	262	20
ethylmorphine (Dionin)	285	59	260	27	285	49	265	22
methylene dioxy amphetamine	285		257		285		257	
methylene dioxy-amphetamine	285		257		285		257	
ergonovine maleate (Ergotrate)	285	660	280					
Morphine	285	55	260	17	250 300	246	247 280	240
propanolol	288 305 318	220 131						
protriptyline	290 237		257	257	288		259	
triprolidine	290 230		270		288 232		270	
Vasoxyl	290	110	253		289	190	251 260	
methyprylon (Noludar)	291	5	251		291		251	
doxepin	292	130	272					
methadone	292 258	19	274 262					
derris root (Rotenone)	292 235	550	256					
griseofulvin (Fulvicin)	294 221		271 228					
pyridone (Dornwal)	300		252		296		260	
LSD	312		270					
	Preferably in Tartrate							
narcotine	312							
chloroquine	330							

TABLE XI
UV Curves in Ethanol

Compounds	Max. den.	$E_{1cm}^{1\%}$	Min. den.
tyrothricin	220		
	281		
	288		
gramicidin	221		
	281		
	289		
Aramite	223		243
	275		
	282		
Chloroparacide	223		249
	263		
hydroquinone	225	450	
sodium levothyroxine (Synthroid)	225	616	218
β-p-hydroxyphenylpropionic acid	226	470	
	278	110	
methylbenzethonium chloride (Disparene)	227	37	264
	270		272
tubocurarine chloride	227		
	278		
	283		
dichlorophene	228	540	
	287		
methoxychlor	228		238
	245		265
	272		280
	282		
tolbutamide	228		500
amylocaine	230	550	
vanillin	231		
	309		
	280		
cocaine	233	200	217
	274		260
	281		279
crytopine	234	280	
	286	160	
quinidine	235	900	
quinine	235	900	
salicylamide	236	224	
	302	263	548

TABLE XI — continued

Compounds	Max. den.	$E_{1cm}^{1\%}$	Min. den.
Rotenone	237	500	238
	295	310	257
Sedormid	237		227
methyl salicylate	238	588	
	306	282	
p,p-DDT	238		228
	260		257
	268		264
	277		275
(phenylbutazone) Butazolidin	239	519	223
papaverine	239	1000	
	279	215	
	314	110	
	327	150	
corticosteroid (Prednisone)	240		
ergonovine maleate	240		
	311		
ethisterone	240	610	
hydrocortisone	240	435	
methyltestosterone	240	490	
stilbesterol	240	600	
acetanilide	241	1000	
veratrum	241	20	
prednisolone	241	450	
testosterone	242		
antazoline phosphate (Antistine)	243	580	
p-phenylene diamine	243	900	
pyrilamine maleate	247	310	
ascorbic acid	248		
acetaminophen	249	900 (methanol)	
phenacetin	250	1000	
benzophenone	252		
strychnine	255	380	234
	280	130	
	290	101	
benzene	255	28	

TABLE XI — continued

Compounds	Max. den.	$E_{1cm}^{1\%}$	Min. den.
nicotine	256		
	262		
glutethimide	257		
	261		
	251		
propoxyphene HCl	257		
	251		
	263		
amphetamine	258		
	253		
	264		
methyl-*p*-hydroxybenzoate	258	1000	
sulfisoxazole	260		221
anabasine	261		234
chlorpheniramine	261		240
sulfanilamide	261	1100	
tolbutamide	262		
tolazoline	263		
brucine	264	300	
orthocaine	265	520	
	308	250	
DNC	266		22
lidocaine	266		
methaqualone	266	300	
	305		
aminosalicylic acid	265	760	
	300	570	
reserpine	267	200	
TMA	267		
DMC	268		252
mescaline	269	25	231
benzhydrol	269		
o,p-DDT	269		253
	276		
narceine	270	210	
o-o-DDT	270		250
	278		275
Paraoxon	270		236
EPN	270		250
	274		272

TABLE XI — continued

Compounds	Max. den.	$E_{1cm}^{1\%}$	Min. den.
chloramphenicol	272		237
chlorotoluene	272		
nitrotoluene	272		
o-nitrophenol	272	400	
p-dichlorobenzene	272	824	243
Baygon	272		248
sulfacetamide	272	878	
Phenocaine	272	520	
	235	380	
	257	500	
benzoyl chloride	273		268
	279		277
methylparathion	273	420	234
parathion	274	328	234
phenol	274	175	
Placidyl	274		263
caffeine	275	160	
5,3-dichlorosalicylanilide	275	490	249
			313
5-chlorosalicylanilide	276	452	249
DMT	276		278
	282		287
	290		
dichlorobenzene	280		
DET	280	340	
Sevin	280	300	240
	271		272
heroin	281	60	
hexylresorcinol	281	120	
Cannabis sativa	283	280	
laudanine	283	200	
mefenamic acid	284	350	
racemorphan	283	90	
dihidrocodeine	284		260
ethylmorphine	285		
thebaine	285	230	
Guthion	286	260	261
	301		299
	315		311

TABLE XI — continued

Compounds	Max. den.	$E_{1cm}^{1\%}$	Min. den.
morphine	287	50	
(α-naphthylthiourea)	288	500	
ANTU			
protopine	290	275	
acetyl sulfisoxasole (Gantrisin)	290		248
narcotine	291	90	
	309	100	
Benzocaine	293		
methadone	295		
methylprylon	295		
hexachlorophene	298	150	
methyl-parafynol	300	3	250
procaine	300	900	
ergotamine	316	180	
ergotoxine	316	160	
Dipterex	323		326
	334		300
	280		261

TABLE XII
UV CURVES IN CHLOROFORM

Compounds	Max. den.	$E_{1cm}^{1\%}$	Min. den.
colchicine	241	465	
TACE	241	465	310
(chlorotrianisene)	310		

TABLE XIII
UV CURVES OF INSECTICIDES
n-hexane, n-heptane, ethanol

Compound	Max Den	$E_{1cm}^{1\%}$	Min Den
Sevin			
n-hexane	280	310	242
ethanol	280	300	241
DDT			
n-hexane	238	510	226
n-heptane	238	509	226
ethanol	237	523	226
parathion			
n-hexane	267	252	231
n-heptane	267	553	231

TABLE XIII — continued

Compound	Max Den	$E \, {}^{1\%}_{1cm}$	Min Den
ethanol	274	328	235
methyl parathion			
n-hexane	266	377	231
n-heptane	266	367	230
ethanol	272	420	234
Diazinon			
n-hexane	246	125	233
Guthion			
n-hexane	281	301	260
n-heptane	281	215	260
ethanol	285	260	261
malathion	265		243
n-hexane	268		251
	272		267
	285 (shoulder)		270
Nemagon	265		257 (shoulder)
n-hexane	268		267
	272		270
Di-Systox	268		267
n-hexane	272		270
methoxychlor	275 (shoulder)		265
in ethanol	244 (shoulder)		280
	282		
Baygon in ethanol	271		245
Certithion	249		247
n-hexane	274		252
DDVP	265		262
n-hexane	271		275
	278		
Dipterex	279		261
in ethanol	334		300
heptachlor	283		267
n-heptane	292		289
ronnel	281		253
in ethanol	290		287
Triox	241		243
n-hexane	247		249
	252		254
	258		261
terpene	253 (shoulder)		252
n-hexane	260		262
	264		265
	267		269
	272		

Aldrin, dieldrin, endrin, heptachlorhepoxide, lindane, toxaphene, chlordane do not exhibit characteristic curves.

TABLE XIV
PAPER CHROMATOGRAPHY Rf AT VARYING pH

Basic Drugs	pH 3	pH 5	pH 6.5	pH 7.5
codeine	.19	.20	.34	.78
Dilaudid	.12	.12	.16	.61
morphine	.15	.13	.26	.73
brucine	.15	.15	.21	.57
chloroquine	.15	.16	.26	.89
Dionin	.29	.29	.55	.86
Metapon	.24	.22	.37	.82
heroin	.31	.33	.56	.86
Nalline	.32	.39	.73	.88
atropine	.29	.37	.34	.62
adenine	.19	.39	.39	.41
emetine	.21	.27	.45	.89
strychnine	.25	.23	.31	.74
quinacrine	.31	.35	.48	.95
procaine	.30	.36	.53	.90
pilocarpine	.15	.22	.67	.84
scopolamine	.22	.26	.58	.86
nicotine	.19	.32	.69	.92
cocaine	.40	.52	.69	.96
doxylamine	.26	.56	.61	.90
Trimeton	.35	.59	.55	.89
methapyrilene	.35	.60	.65	.92
pyribenzamine	.37	.68	.70	.96
Chlor-Trimeton	.41	.68	.62	.91
quinine	.47	.74	.72	.92
quinidine	.46	.79	.75	.95
cinchonine	.50	.72	.68	.91
Demerol	.50	.60	.72	.90
tetracaine	.53	.50	.68	.91
thonzylamine	.50	.56	.62	.92
yohimbine	.55	.52	.74	.90
Dromoran	.60	.56	.54	.82
diphenhydramine	.65	.63	.67	.91
methadone	.71	.74	.68	.93
Ambodryl	.67	.75	.76	.95
Antihistine	.66	.71	.60	.78
chlorcyclizine	.71	.77	.87	.96
Cyclaine	.79	.83	.84	.94
Nupercaine	.83	.80	.83	.95
Coramine	.85	.92	.90	.91
Tranquilizing Drugs				
codeine (control)	.19	.17	.34	.80
Atarax	.70	.79	.92	.96
Clistin	.22	.45	.86	.88

TABLE XIV — continued

	pH 3	pH 5	pH 6.5	pH 7.5
Compazine	.29	.58	.88	.92
Dartal	.64	.79	.94	.95
Deaner	—	—	—	—
Frenquel	.68	.54	.41	.46
Harmonyl	—	—	—	—
Miltown	—	—	—	—
Moderil	—	—	—	—
Pacatal	.70	.72	.86	.94
Polaramine	.24	.48	.88	.87
Quiactin	—	—	—	—
Raudixin	—	—	—	—
Serpasil	—	—	—	—
Softran	—	—	—	—
Sparine	.72	.64	.80	.93
Stelazine	.31	.71	.92	.96
Suavitil	—	—	—	—
Suvren	.68	.71	.95	.95
Sycotrol	—	—	—	—
Thorazine	.80	.77	.90	.93
Tofranil	.68	.64	.75	.94
Trilafon	.35	.60	.76	.90
Ultran	—	—	—	—
Vesprin	.74	.74	.90	.96
Vistaril	.74	.74	—	.96

TABLE XV

Rf

NEUTRAL OR ACID COMPOUNDS

Developing No.	1	2	3	4	5	6	7	8
aminopyrine (Pyramidon)	85				62	81	90	
amobarbital (Amytal)	55	59			43	76	81	54
antipyrine (Tympagesic)			15		19			
Aprobarbital (Alurate)	50				43	70	80	
aspirin	40	18	42	11	20	22	30	27
cinchophen (Atophan)				24	03			
butalbital (Sandoptal)	55	58			40	71	85	85

TABLE XV — continued

Developing No.	1	2	3	4	5	6	7	8
butabarbital (Butisol)	50	55						
carbromal (Adalin)						42	75	87
chlordiazepoxide‡ (Librium)	55							66 61*
chlorpromazine‡ (Thorazine)								84 79*
diallylbarbital (Dial)					33	66	80	
diazepam (Valium)	69							84 77*
diphenylhydantoin (Dilantin)	30	54			23	64	75	50
glutethimide (Doriden)	85	95			60	84	92	86
ethchlorvynol (Placidyl)	95							
ethenzamidum				40	58			
heptabarbital (Medomin)	40				38	67	78	
hexobarbital (Sombucaps)	70				56	76	87	
diphenoxylate (Lomotil)								46
meprobarbital					60	81	90	
meprobamate (Equanil; Miltown)	21	74						85
methaqualone (Quaalude; Sopor; Parest)	90							53* 59†
methylprylon (Noludar)	35				24	68	81	85
paracetanol (Tylenol; Acetaminophen)			00	60				89
pentazocine‡ (Talwin)	40							75* 51*
pentobarbital (Nembutal)	55	65			47	80	89	56

TABLE XV — (Con'td)

Developing No.	1	2	3	4	5	6	7	8
phenacetin (Acetophenetidin)			24	57	26	62	73	
phenobarbital (Luminal)	40	28			28	70	82	33
phenylbutazone‡ (Butazolidin)			57	65				97 61* 14*
mefanamic acid (Ponstel)	47							·30
promethazine‡ (Phenergan)			24	03				
salicylamide (Salrin)			27	69				80
salicylic acid	25	18			30	40	58	
secobarbital (Seconal)	65	63						56
thioridazine‡ (Mellaril)								64 54* 45*
trifluoperazine‡ (Stelazine)								75
Valamin					38	70	82	

*Metabolite
†Hydrolyzed
‡Basic

TABLE XVI
Rf
BASIC COMPOUNDS

Developing No.	9	10	11	12	13	14	15	16	17	18	19	20	21	22	23	24
aconitine (aconite root)	44	65	90	32												
alphaprodine (Nisentil)					83	79	25									
priminodine (Alvodine)					97	98	93									
amitriptyline (Elavil)							98				56			56	64 21* 14*	

TABLE XVI — continued

Developing No.	9	10	11	12	13	14	15	16	17	18	19	20	21	22	23	24
amphetamine (Benzedrine)								80						38	45	
anileridine (Leritine)					95	95	77									
antipyrine															65	
antazoline phosphate (Antistine)												27	20			
atropine	12	38	40	16				45	17					04	24	
benactyzine (Suavitil)														14	75	
benthiazide								95								
benzocaine															73	
brucine	19	43	63	18				80								
butyryl perazine										10						
caffeine (neutral)								80	69			64	61	06	73	
captodiamine (Subren)											51	59	79			
carbinoxamine (Clistin)								78							37	14
chlorcyclizine (Perazil; DiParalene)								90								
chlordiazepoxide (Librium)								90	85			76	79		78	66
chloroquine (Aralene)								57								
chlorperphenazine									12							
chlorpheniramine (Chlortrimeton)								90							42	20
chlorpromazine (Thorazine)							67	90	48	38	05				62	61
chlorprothixene (Taractan)										69	45	57	72			
cinchonine	27	38	44	17											55	
clemizole (Allercur)												80	81	91		
cocaine	58	73	90	65	86	84	68	97	61			60	70	57	74	76

6*

TABLE XVI — continued

Developing No.	9	10	11	12	13	14	15	16	17	18	19	20	21	22	23	24
codeine	26	38	53	16	28	42	05	54	43		18	20	07		42	34
colchicine	04	47	41	04												
cyclazocine								82								
Dalmane															80	80
Dargactil											24	37	39			
dextro-amphetamine (Dexedrine)															40	40
diazepam (Valium)								94							73	79
hydrocodone bitartrate (Dicodid)					36	35	05									
dicyclomine								98								
diethazine (Diparcol)									81							
dihydrocodeine	28	38	54	18												
dihydro-ergotamine (DHE-45)	03	21	12	00												
dihydromorphine (Dilaudid)	11	51	65	21	18	19	02	24								
diphenhydramine (Benadryl)								95			42	22	31	50	33	
diphenylpyraline (Diafen)											35	42	49			
dorsacaine (Benoxinate-HCl)											64	58	73			
dimethyl tryptamine								84								
emetine	45	67	90	40												
ergometrine	02	14	06	00												
ethoheptazine (Zactane)															32	
ergotamine (Gynergen)	03	24	16	00												
ethopropazine (Parsidol)									94							
ethyl morphine (Dionin)					40	46	05	63				31	34			

TABLE XVI — continued

Developing No.	9	10	11	12	13	14	15	16	17	18	19	20	21	22	23	24
haloperidol (Haldol)															70	
halocaine											49	46	55			
halopyramine												19	21			
Heptodon											29	35	55			
heroin (diacetylmorphine)					74	67	16	90			34			09	54	57
homatropine	23	37	45	15												
hydroxyzine (Atarax)											52	56	71	11		
imipramine (Tofranil)								82			47	37	44		55	
ketamine															72	
levo-dromoran (levorphanol tartrate)					57	54	20									
levo-mepromazine											44	45	54			
lidocaine (Xylocaine)									71	68	86				73	
lobeline		68	90	48				98								
mepazine (Pacatal)								95		22	45				60	
meperidine (Pethidine; Demerol)					63	70	27	84	56			50	60	37	68	60
meprobamate (Miltown)														03	53	
mescaline					21	23	04	60								
methadone (Dolophine)					79	81	58	99	48					64	53	70 64*
methapyrilene (Histadyl)								90						23	65	
methamphetamine (Methedrine; Desoxyn)								58			13	11	14		37	
methaqualone (Quaalude)								92			89	79	79		75	42* 73*
mephentermine (Wyamine)														28	28	

TABLE XVI — continued

Developing No.	9	10	11	12	13	14	15	16	17	18	19	20	21	22	23	24
methyl dilaudid (metapon HCl)					28	30	03								60	
methylphenidate (Ritalin)								82			54	55	65	40	60	
methyprylon (Noludar)								90								
monoacetyl morphine					50	55	11									
morphine	03	10	08	00	18	20	02	35	40		15	06	00	43	23	
narcotine (Noscapine)	57	72	90	51	80	83		99			65	83		46		
nalorphine (Nalline)								60								
nicotine								90	57						68	57 19*
norpramine												38	53	66		
nortriptyline (Aventyl)															38	
nurcaine										59	46	57				
octamylamine											23	32	37			
oxymorphone (Humorphan)					56	56	15									
papaverine	17	67	90	42	73	77	53	95				78	82		80	
pentazocine (Talwin)								88							75	69 63* 56*
pentocaine								84								
perazine											07	17				
Peronine					53	51	09									
perphenazine (Trilafon)								84	09	00	48	29	33		62	70
phenazocine (Prinadol)					96	96	80									
phenelzine (Nardil)														34	50	
pheniramine (Trimeton)								90				11	12		43	
phenmetrazine (Preludin)											57	43	51	23	50	

TABLE XVI — continued

Developing No.	9	10	11	12	13	14	15	16	17	18	19	20	21	22	23	24
phenylpropano-lamine (Propadrine)								60						51	55	35
physostigmine (Eserine)	44	65	90	32											68	
phenylbutazone (Butazolidin)														08		
phenycyclidine															60	
pilocarpine	13	41	52	09												
pipamazine (Mornidine)															70	
tolazoline HCl (Priscoline)												16	10			
prochlorperazine (Compazine)								60	82		26				62	
procaine (Novocaine)					67	69	41	84	61			53	37		61	
promazine (Sparine)								90	38	17	37					
promethazine (Phenergan)								95	56	27	52	38	49			
d-propoxyphene (Darvon)								98						83	74	76 61*
propylhexedrine (Benzedrex)											13	11	14		23	
prothipendyl											18	20	25			
pyrilamine								90				30	47	57	60	
quinacrine (Atabrine)								92							50	
quinidine	25	33	40	15				62							60	
quinine	17	19	26	07	41	42	04	68	56			41	25	04	60	45 38* 18*
Reactivan												25	19			
scopolamine	34	56	60	19				84						06	27	
oxazepam (Serax)										12					65	96
reserpine (Serpasil)	46	72	80	25					86							

TABLE XVI — continued

Developing No.	9	10	11	12	13	14	15	16	17	18	19	20	21	22	23	24
clopenthixol (Sordinol)												36	39			
sparteine (Tocosamine)		70	90	68												
strychnine	38	42	63	18				60	19			13	24		30	
diethylpropion (Tepanil)											38	53	66			
tetracaine (Pontocaine)					68	70	33								67	
thebaine	50	65	90	51	65	73	23									
thenalidine (Sandostene)											40	51	65			
theobromine (Theocalcin)											50					
thioridazine (Mellaril)								82	30	45	24	38	44		55	63 54* 46*
trifluoperazine (Stelazine)								83							70	52 41* 36*
triflupromazine (Vesprin)								92	54	62			65			63 54* 46*
tripelennamine (Pyribenzamine)								96							93	
tutocaine (Aphrodine)												57	48		79	
yohimbine (Aphrodine)	37	63	62	18												

*Metabolite

TABLE XVII
TLC — Pesticides
Solvent System Rf

	1	2	3	4	5	6
aldrin	0		0		0	95
azinphos-methyl	14					
Baygon	40-78		24-80		12-30	75
BHC					0	50
Bromophos						65
chlordane	0					0
Chlorthion		34		0		
Co-ral	33					
coumaphos				78		
Cygon 267	12					
DDE	10					0
DDT	91		0		0	60
DDVP	54					5
demeton O		50		65		
demeton S		13		23		
Diazinon	50	49	32	67	30	15
dieldrin	0		0		53	17
dimethoate		3				
Dipterex	20		0		0	3
Di-siston	10					
endosulfan	40					85
endrin	0		45		30-60	24
ethion	93			85		62
Guthion	44	18	18	65	10	10
heptachlor	0	60	0		0	85
heptachlorhepoxide	97				68	18
Lindane	10	60	95		78	24
malathion	29	33	47	77	22	12
Meta-Systox	32					
methoxychlor	70		80		45	5
methyl parathion	47		42	84	24	55
methyl trithion	82					72
MIRPX						55
Mirey	0					
naled	50					
parthion	65	45	69	86	53	55
phorate	95	65		89		
Phosdrin	30					0
ronnel	10					72
Sevin	30		20		7	2
Strobane	0					0
TDE	95					65
terpene	0					0
Thymet						65
toxaphene	10					25
Trithion						75
2-4D	14		10		25	0

TABLE XVIII*

RETENTION TIMES AT 250°C RELATIVE TO COCAINE

Chlormethazanone	0.17	p-Acetylmethamphetamine	0.25
3,3-Dimethylglutarimide	0.17	Apresoline	0.26
Mephentermine	0.17	Aprobarbital	0.26
Oxanamide	0.17	Cantharidin	0.26
Tetramethylsuccinimide	0.17	Itobarbital	0.26
Tranylcypromine	0.17	5-Methoxyindole	0.26
Aletamine	0.18	Butabarbital	0.27
Chlorphentermine	0.18	Dyclonine	0.27
Dicyclohexylamine	0.18	Ethambutol	0.27
3-Methylglutarimide	0.18	p-Aminobenzoic Acid	0.28
Bemegride	0.19	Amobarbital	0.28
Cypenamine	0.19	Dicyclomine	0.28
Ethinamate	0.19	N,N-Dimethyl (MDA)	0.28
Metharbital	0.19	N,N-Dimethylmescaline	0.28
Methoxyphenamine	0.19	Methsuximide	0.28
Nicotine	0.19	Anisotropine MeBr	0.29
Norpseudoephedrine	0.19	Meperidine	0.29
Diethylpropion	0.20	Glyceryl Guaiacolate	0.29
Flubanilate	0.20	Mescaline	0.29
Diisopropylurazole	0.20	Methocarbamol	0.29
Hordenine	0.20	N-Methylmescaline	0.29
Dichlormethazone	0.21	Pentobarbital	0.29
Acetylcarbromal	0.21	Tiletamine	0.29
Ethylephedrine	0.21	Acetophenetidin	0.30
Hydroxyamphetamine	0.21	Methylphenidate	0.30
M.D.A.	0.21	Metronidazole	0.30
Modaline	0.21	Pentylenetetrazole	0.30
Phenmetrazine	0.21	Chlorphenesin Carbamate	0.31
Tyramine	0.21	Etryptamine	0.31
Methylparaben	0.21	Eucaine	0.31
Clofibrate	0.22	Phenylephrine	0.31
Phenacemide	0.22	Methohexital	0.31
Phendimetrazine	0.22	Phensuximide	0.31
Barbital	0.22	Secobarbital	0.31
Dimethoxyamphetamine	0.23	Sparteine	0.32
Nicotinamide	0.23	Vinbarbital	0.32
Propylparaben	0.23	Fenimide	0.33
Phenaglycodol	0.23	Pheniramine	0.33
Prolintane	0.23	Acetaminophen	0.34
Salicylamide	0.23	Benzphetamine	0.34
Encyprate	0.24	Lobeline	0.34
Mephenesin	0.24	Butamben	0.35
Methyprylon	0.24	Dimethyltryptamine	0.35
STP	0.24	Neostigmine Bromide	0.36
Zylofuramine	0.24	Piperoxan	0.36
Benzocaine	0.25	Prilocaine	0.36
Diallylbarbituric acid	0.25	Tryptamine	0.36
Oxyphencyclimine	0.25	Chlorzoxazone	0.37
Probarital	0.25	Cotarnine Cl	0.37

*From C.B. Teer: Gas chromatographic data for screening drugs. *Microgram*, IX(2): (1976).

TABLE XVIII — continued

Diphenhydramine	0.37	diperodon	0.63
Ethoheptazine	0.37	Acetylenheptine	0.64
Lobeline	0.37	Dolitron	0.64
Pellotine	0.37	Phenyramidol	0.64
Lidocaine	0.38	5-methoxytryptamine	0.64
Phencyclidine	0.38	Alverine	0.65
Cyclandelate	0.39	Brompheniramine	0.66
N-methyl-1-methyl-		Diphenylpyraline	0.66
tryptamine	0.39	Cycrimine	0.66
Mesantoin	0.40	Mepivicaine	0.66
Carisoprodol	0.40	Phenelzine	0.66
Hexobarbital	0.40	Heptarbital	0.67
Anhalonidine	0.41	Methadone	0.67
Desipramine	0.41	WIN-2299	0.67
Lophophorine	0.41	Bromdylamine	0.67
Orphenadrine	0.41	Chlophedianol	0.69
Thiamylal	0.41	Cyproximide	0.69
Doxylamine	0.42	Triflutrimeprazine	0.69
Ethamoxytriphetol	0.42	Parabutethamine	0.70
Glutethimide	0.43	Bromdiphenhydramine	0.72
Ketamine	0.43	Dextromethorphan	0.72
Anhalonine	0.45	Theophylline	0.72
Diethyltryptamine	0.45	Butriptyline	0.77
Tetrahydrozoline	0.45	Psilocybin	0.77
Ethotoin	0.45	Propranolol	0.78
Phenyltoloxamine	0.45	Triflupromazine	0.79
Tetrahydrozoline	0.45	Naphazoline	0.80
Mephobarbital	0.45	Amitriptyline	0.81
Caffeine	0.46	Adiphenine	0.82
Azapetine	0.47	Domiphen	0.82
Trimecaine	0.48	Perphenazine	0.82
Ethomoxane	0.49	Pipradrol	0.83
Atropine MeBr	0.51	Carbetapentane	0.86
Chlorpheniramine	0.51	Chlorcyclizine	0.87
Methastyridone	0.51	Phenindamine	0.86
Tripellenamine	0.51	Thozalinone	0.87
Aminopyrine	0.52	Pilocarpine	0.88
Antipyrine	0.53	Trimipramine	0.88
Methapyrilene	0.53	Thiabendazole	0.90
Thenyldiamine	0.53	Imipramine	0.90
Theobromine	0.53	Tetracaine	0.90
Cyclobarbital	0.54	Atropine	0.93
Cyclizine	0.55	Nortriptyline	0.93
Metabutethamine	0.58	Phenoxybenzamine	0.93
Phenobarbital	0.58	Thonzylamine	0.94
Isocarboxazine	0.59	Doxepin	0.95
Propylthiouracil	0.59	Pramoxine	0.95
Chlorphenoxamine	0.59	Hyoscyamine	0.98
Procaine	0.62	Pyrilamine	0.98
Carbinoxamine	0.62	Benactyzine	1.00
Isomethadone	0.62	Cocaine	1.00

TABLE XVIII — continued

Oxymetazoline	1.00	Elymoclavine	1.87
Methaqualone	1.02	Mazindol	1.88
Pentazocine	1.02	Carbamazepine	1.90
Desipramine	1.05	Ethylmorphine	1.90
Dimethindene	1.07	Dihydroergotamine	1.93
Protriptyline	1.07	Ergotamine (base)	1.94
6-Methoxyharmalan	1.09	Methixene	1.96
Metaxalone	1.10	Neopine	1.97
Promethazine	1.14	Chlorpromazine	2.02
Medazepam	1.16	Chlorprothixene	2.05
Isothipendyl	1.17	Diphenylhydantoin	2.08
Physostigmine	1.17	Morphine	2.16
Iprindole	1.19	Neocinchophen	2.16
Iproniazide	1.19	Diazepam	2.19
Mephenoxalone	1.19	Acetylidihydrocodeine	2.22
Benztropine	1.20	Methotrimeprazine	2.22
Homochlorcyclizine	1.22	Tetrabenazine	2.26
Proparacaine	1.22	Prenylamine	2.34
5-Benzyloxyindole	1.29	Melatonin	2.38
Harmine	1.29	Dihydrocodeinone	2.42
Methazolamide	1.29	Thiopental	2.46
Hexestrol	1.30	Hydromorphone	2.53
Azacyclonol	1.31	Mepazine	2.54
Promazine	1.34	Acetylcodeine	2.55
Imidoline	1.38	Pyrathiazine	2.57
Trioxazine	1.39	Dihydroergocristine	2.60
Secergan	1.40	O6-Acetylmorphine	2.67
Dioxadrol	1.41	Ergocristine	2.68
Dexoxadrol	1.42	O3-Acetylmorphine	2.68
Legoxan	1.42	Methoxypromazine	2.69
Prothipendyl	1.43	Loxapine	2.83
Diethazine	1.44	Trifluorperazine	2.84
Pyrrobutamine	1.49	Demoxapam	3.12
Cyproheptadine	1.50	Chlordiazepoxide	3.12
Cintriamide	1.52	Oxymorphone	3.12
Acetylprocaine	1.58	Thebaine	3.12
Oxazepam	1.57	Methopholine	3.16
Diphenidol	1.60	Methyltestosterone	3.25
Cyheptamide	1.60	Thiazesim	3.29
Phenazopyridine	1.62	Cinchonidine	3.46
Tropicamide	1.63	Cinchonine	3.46
Antazoline	1.64	Dibucaine	3.50
Diamthazole	1.66	Metiapine	3.58
Phenylbutazone	1.68	Alphaprodine	3.71
Butacaine	1.69	Amoxapine	3.76
Tetrahydrocannabinol	1.69	Prazepam	3.76
Dihydrocodeine	1.76	Heroin	3.89
Primidone	1.77	Captodiame	4.05
Codeine	1.81	Acepromazine	4.19
Citenamide	1.85	Laudanosine	4.24

TABLE XVIII — continued

Naloxone	4.49	Prochlorperazine (base)	7.77
Flurazepam	4.71	Doxapram	7.81
Laudanine	4.76	Papaverine	8.75
Progesterone	5.07	Meclizine	8.91
Oxomemazine	5.31	Dioxyline (base)	9.07
Propiopromazine	5.46	Ethaverine	9.64
Oxyphenbutazone	5.81	Cryptopine	13.5
Chlortrianisene	5.83	Protopine	11.2
Hydroxyzine	6.22	Hydrastine	15.2
Quinine	6.32	Buclizine	17.1
Piminodine Base	7.00	Strychnine (sulfate)	18.7
Anileridine	7.55	Noscapine	21.7

TABLE XIX*

RETENTION TIMES AT 220°C RELATIVE TO DIPHENHYDRAMINE

Amphetamine	0.26	Metharbital	0.37
Acetylcarbromal	0.25, 0.28	Tyramine	0.37
Pargyline	0.26	Diethylpropion	0.38
Chlormethazanone	0.27	Ethylephedrine	0.38
Tranylcypromine	0.27	Hydroxyamphetamine	0.38
Aletamine	0.28	Phendimetrazine	0.38
Benzoic Acid	0.28	Modaline	0.39
Mephentermine	0.28	Phenmetrazine	0.39
Oxanamide	0.28	Diisopropylurazole	0.40
Tetramethylsuccinimide	0.28	Clofibrate	0.40
3,3-Dimethylglutarimide	0.30	Methylparaben	0.41
3-Methylglutarimide	0.30	M.D.A.	0.42
Chlorphentermine	0.31	Phenacemide	0.42
Dicyclohexylamine	0.31	Barbital	0.44
Salicylic Acid	0.31	Nicotinamide	0.45
Methoxyphenamine	0.32	Prolintane	0.45
Nicotine	0.32	DMA	0.48
Ephedrine	0.32	N-Methyl MDA	0.48
Norpseudoephedrine	0.33	Encyprate	0.50
Cypenamine	0.34	Phenaglycodol	0.50
Phenelzine	0.34	Probarbital	0.50
Dichlormethazone	0.34	S.T.P.	0.50
Ephedrine (base)	0.34	p-Acetylmethamphetamine	0.51
Phenylpropanolamine	0.34	Mephenesin	0.51
Bemegride	0.36	Methyprylon	0.51
Ethinamate	0.36	Salicylamide	0.51
Flubanilate	0.37	Oxyphencyclimine	0.52
Hordenine	0.37	Zylofuramine	0.54

*From C.B. Teer: Gas Chromatographic data for screening of drugs. *Microgram, IX(2):* 1976.

TABLE XIX — continued

Propylparaben	0.54	Prilocaine	0.98
Cantharidin	0.55	Ethoheptazine	0.99
5-Methoxyindole	0.55	Pellotine	0.99
Benzocaine	0.56	Tryptamine	0.99
Diallybarbituric acid	0.56	Diphenhydramine	1.00
Apresoline	0.57	N-Methyl-1-Methyl-	
Aprobarbital	0.58	trytamine	1.00
p-Aminobenzoic acid	0.62	Piperoxan	1.00
Itobarbital	0.62	Cyclandelate	1.06
Butabarbital	0.63	Lidocaine	1.07
Dicyclomine	0.63	Phencyclidine	1.07
Methsuximide	0.64	Anhalonidine	1.11
N,N-Dimethyl MDA	0.67	Thiamylal	1.14
Amobarbital	0.67	Lophophorine	1.14
Dyclonine	0.68	Femmide	1.16
Anisatropine Methyl		Mesantoin	1.15
bromide	0.69	Thiamylal (Surital)	1.15
N,N,-Dimethylmescaline	0.69	Carisoprodol	1.17
Meperidine	0.69	Ketamine	1.17
Tiletamine	0.69	Hexobarbital	1.19
Methocarbamol	0.70	Glutethimide	1.20
Glyceryl Guaiacolate	0.71	Etryptamine	1.21
Pentylenetetrazole	0.71	Orphenadrine	1.21
Mescaline	0.74	Doxylamine	1.23
Pentobarbital	0.74	Diethyltryptamine	1.26
N-Methylmescaline	0.75	Anhalonine	1.27
Methylphenidate	0.75	Phenyltoloxamine	1.28
Metronidazole	0.75	Ethotoin	1.31
Phensuximide	0.76	Tetrahydrozoline	1.32
Sparteine	0.76	Mephobarbital	1.37
Acetophenetidin	0.78	Azapetine	1.37
Eucaine	0.79	Caffeine	1.39
Chlorphenesin carbamate	0.80	Acetylenheptine	1.40
Methohexital	0.80	Trimecaine	1.42
Phenylephrine	0.81	Ethomoxane	1.52
Ethambutol	0.82	Tripellenamine	1.52
Vinbarbital	0.82	Aminopyrine	1.56
Secobarbital	0.83	Methastyridone	1.56
Benzphetamine	0.88	Chlorpheniramine	1.57
Acetaminophen	0.89	Methapyrilene	1.62
Dimethyltryptamine	0.92	Antipyrine	1.62
Lobeline	0.92	Cyclizine	1.67
Pheniramine	0.92	Thenyldiamine	1.67
Butamben	0.94	Theobromine	1.69
Cotarnine Chloride	0.95	Cyclobarbital	1.73
Chlorzoxazone	0.96	Metabutethamine	1.86
Neostigmine Bromide	0.98	Ethamoxytriphetol	1.87

TABLE XIX — continued

Chlorphenoxamine	1.88	Naphazoline	2.66
Phenobarbital	1.93	Propranolol	2.74
Procaine	2.03	Triflupromazine	2.74
Carbinoxamine	2.04	Pipradrol	2.78
Dolitron	2.04	Thiabendazole	2.81
Alverine	2.05	Amitriptyline	2.83
Perphenazine	2.06	Phenindamine	3.08, 2.87
Phenyramidol	2.07	Trimipramine	2.90
Cycrimine	2.12	Adiphenine	2.97
5-Methoxytryptamine	2.14	Thozalinone	2.98
Mepivicaine	2.15	Pilocarpine	3.04
Diphenylpyraline	2.19	Domiphen	3.05
Brompheniramine	2.20	Chlorcyclizine	3.09
Bromdylamine	2.24	Carbetapentane	3.11
Isomethadone	2.24	Imipramine	3.22
Methadone	2.25	Phenoxybenzamine	3.22
Cyproximide	2.29	Atropine	3.30
Triflutrimeprazine	2.31	Nortriptyline	3.36
Heptarbital	2.32	Tetracaine	3.36
Dextromethorphan	2.40	Doxepin	3.38
Chlophedianol	2.42	Thonzylamine	3.42
Psilocybin	2.43	Pramoxine	3.54
Parabutethamine	2.43	Cocaine	3.67
Bromdiphenhydramine	2.48	Oxymetazoline	3.70
Theophylline	2.64	Pyrilamine	3.71
Butriptyline	2.65	Desipramine	3.88

TABLE XX*

INDEX

Compound	250°C	220°C	Compound	250°C	220°C
Acepromazine	4.19	—	Alverine	0.65	2.05
Acetaminophen	0.34	0.89	p-Aminobenzoic Acid	0.28	0.62
Acetophenetidin	0.30	0.78	Aminopyrine	0.52	1.56
Acetylcarbromal	0.21	0.25	Amitriptyline	0.81	2.83
		0.28	Amobarbital	0.28	0.67
p-Acetylmethamphetamine	0.26	0.51	Amoxapine	3.76	—
Acetylcodeine	2.55	—	Amphetamine	sf	0.26
Acetyldihydrocodeine	2.22	—	Anhalonidine	0.41	1.11
Acetylenheptine	0.64	1.40	Anhalonine	0.45	1.27
Acetylprocaine	1.58	—	Anisotropine		
Adiphenine	0.82	2.97	Methylbromide	0.29	None
			Anileridine	7.55	—
Aletamine	0.18	0.28	Antazoline	1.63	—
Alphaprodine	3.71	—	Antipyrine	0.53	1.62

*From C.B. Teer: Gas Chromatographic data for screening of drugs. *Microgram, ix(2)*: 1976.

TABLE XX — continued

Compound	250°C	220°C	Compound	250°C	220°C
Apresoline	0.26	0.57	Cintriamide	15.25	—
Aprobarbital	0.26	0.58	Citenamide	1.85	—
Atropine	0.93	3.30	Clofibrate	0.22	0.40
Atropine Methylbromide	0.51	None	Codeine	1.81	—
Azacyclonol	1.31	—	Cocaine	1.00	—
Azapetine	0.47	1.37	Cotarnine Chloride	0.37	0.95
Barbitol	0.22	0.44	Cryptopine	13.5	—
Bemegride	0.19	0.36	Cyclandelate	0.39	1.06
Benactyzine	1.00	—	Cyclizine	0.55	1.67
Benzocaine	0.25	0.56	Cyclobarbital	0.54	1.73
Benzoic Acid	sf	0.28	Cyheptamide	1.60	—
Benzphetamine	0.34	0.88	Cypenamine	0.19	0.34
Benzquinamide	10.6	—	Cyproheptadine	1.50	—
5-Benzyloxyindole	1.29	—	Cycrimine	0.66	2.12
Bromdylamine	0.68	2.24	Cyproximide	0.69	2.29
Bromidiphenhydramine	0.72	2.48	Demoxapam	3.11	—
Brompheniramine	0.66	2.20	Desipramine	0.41	3.88
Buclizine	17.1	—	Dexamethazone	9.03	—
Butabarbital	0.27	0.63	Dexoxadrol	1.43	—
Butacaine	1.69	—	Dextromethorphan	0.72	2.40
Butamben	0.35	0.94	Diallyylbarbituric Acid	0.25	0.56
Butriptyline	0.77	2.65	Diamthazole	1.66	—
Caffeine	0.46	1.39	Diazepam	2.19	—
Cannabinol	2.12	—	Dibucaine	3.50	—
Cantharidin	0.26	0.55	Dichlormethazone	0.21	0.34
Captodiame	4.05	—	Dicyclohexylamine	0.18	0.31
Carbamazepine	1.90	—	Dicyclomine	0.28	0.63
Carbetapentane	0.86	3.11	Diethazine	1.44	—
Carbinoxamine	0.62	2.04	Diethylpropion	0.20	0.38
Carisoprodol	0.40	1.17	Diethyltryptamine	0.45	1.26
Cholphedianol	0.69	2.42	Dihydrocodeine	1.76	—
Chlorcyclizine	0.87	3.09	Dihydrocodeinone	2.42	—
Chlordiazepoxide	3.12	—	Dihydroergocristine	2.60	—
Chlormethazanone	0.17	0.27	Dihydroergotamaine	1.93	—
Chlorotrianisene	5.83	—	Diisopropylurazole	0.20	0.40
Chlorphenesin			Dimethindene	1.07	—
Carbamate	0.31	0.80	3,5-Dimethoxyamphetamine	0.23	0.48
Chlorpheniramine	0.51	1.57	mine	0.23	0.48
Chlorphenoxamine	0.59	1.88	3, 3-Dimethylglutarimide	0.17	0.30
Chlorphentermine	0.18	0.31	*N*, N-Dimethylmescaline	0.28	0.69
Chlorpromazine	2.02	—	*N*, *N*-Dimethyl M.D.A.	0.28	0.67
Chlorprothixene	2.05	—	Dimethyltryptamine	0.35	0.92
Chlorzoxazone	0.37	0.96	Dioxadrol	1.41	—
Cinchonidine	3.46	—	Dioxyline (base)	9.07	—
Cinchonine	3.46	—	Diphenidol	1.60	—
			Dipedrodon	0.63	None

TABLE XX — continued

Compound	250°C	220°C	Compound	250°C	220°C
Diphenhydramine	0.37	1.00	Iprindole	1.19	—
Diphenylhydantoin	2.08	—	Iproniazid	1.14	—
Diphenylpyraline	0.66	2.19	Isocarboxazide	0.59	None
Dolitron	0.64	2.04	Isomethadone	0.62	2.24
Domiphen	0.82	3.05	Isothipendyl	1.17	—
Doxapram	7.81	—	Itobarbital	0.26	0.62
Doxepin	0.95	3.38	Ketamine	0.43	1.17
Doxylamine	0.42	1.23	Levoxan	1.41	—
Dyclonine	0.27	0.68	Laudanine	4.76	—
Elymoclavine	1.87	—	Laudanosine	4.24	—
Encyprate	0.24	0.50	Lidocaine	0.38	1.07
Ephedrine (base)	sf	0.34	Lobeline	0.37	0.92
Ergocristine	2.68	—	Lophophorine	0.41	1.14
Ergotamine (base)	1.94	—	Loxapine	2.83	—
Ethambutol	0.27	0.82	Mazindol	1.88	—
Ethamoxytriphetol	0.42	1.87	Meclizine	8.91	—
Ethaverine	9.64	—	Medazepam	1.16	—
Ethinamate	0.19	0.36	Melatonin	2.38	—
Ethoheptazine	0.37	0.99	Mepazine	2.54	—
Ethomoxane	0.49	1.52	Meperidine	0.29	0.69
Ethotoin	0.45	1.31	Mephenesin	0.24	0.51
Ethozolin	0.24	None	Mephenoxalone	1.19	—
Ethylephedrine	0.21	0.38	Mephentermine	0.17	0.28
Ethylmorphine	1.90	—	Mephobarbital	0.45	1.37
Etryptamine	0.31	1.21	Mepivicaine	0.66	2.15
Eucaine	0.31	0.79	Mesantoin	0.40	1.15
Fenimide	0.33	1.16	Mescaline	0.29	0.74
Flubanilate	0.20	0.37	Metabutethamine	0.58	1.86
Flurazepam	4.71	—	Metaxalone	1.10	
Glutethimide	0.43	1.20	Methadone	0.67	2.25
Glyceryl Guaiacolate	0.29	0.71	Methamphetamine	sf	
Harmine	1.29	—	Methapyrilene	0.53	1.62
Heptarbital	0.67	2.32	Methaqualone	1.02	
Heroin	3.89	—	Metharbital	0.19	0.37
Hexestrol	1.30	—	Methastryidone	0.51	1.56
Hexobarbital	0.40	1.19	Methazolamide	1.29	
Homochlorcyclizine	15.2	—	Methixene	1.90	
Hordenine	0.20	0.37	Methocarbamol	0.29	0.70
Hydrastine	51.2	—	Methohexital	0.31	0.80
Hydromorphone	2.53	—	Methopholine	3.16	
Hydroxyamphetamine	0.21	0.38	Metopon	2.51	
Hydroxyzine	6.22	—	Methotrimeprazine	2.22	
Hyoscyamine	2.88	—	6-Methoxyharmalan	1.09	
Imidoline	1.38	—	5-Methoxyindole	0.26	0.55
Imipramine	0.90	3.22	Methoxyphenamine	0.19	0.32

TABLE XX — continued

Compound	250°C	220°C	Compound	250°C	220°C
Methoxypromazine	2.69		Pellotine	0.37	0.99
5-Methoxytryptamine	0.64	2.14	Pentazocine	1.02	
Methsuximide	0.28	0.64	Pentobarbital	0.29	0.74
MDA	0.21	0.42	Pentylenetetrazole	0.30	0.71
3-Methylglutarimide	0.18	0.30	Perphenazine	0.82	2.06
Methylparaben	0.21	0.41	Phenacemide	0.22	0.42
N-Methylmescaline	0.29	0.41	Phenaglycodol	0.23	0.50
N-Methyl-1-Methyl			Phenazopyridine	1.62	
tryptamine	0.39	1.00	Phencyclidine	0.38	1.07
N-Methyl MDA		0.48	Phendimetrazine	0.22	0.38
Methylphenidate	0.30	0.75	Phenindamine	0.86	2.87
Methyprylon	0.24	0.51			0.38
Methyltestosterone	3.25		Phenelzine	0.66	0.34
Metiapine	3.28		Pheniramine	0.33	0.92
Metronidazole	0.30	0.75	Phenmetrazine	0.21	0.39
Modaline	0.21	0.39	Phenobarbital	0.58	1.93
Molindone	2.59	0.55	Phenoxybenzamine	0.93	3.22
O₃-Monacetyl-			Phensuximide	0.31	0.76
morphine	2.67		Phenylbutazone	1.68	
O₆-Monoacetyl-				2.29	
morphine	2.68		Phenylephrine	0.31	0.81
Morphine	2.16		Phenylpropanolamine	sf	0.34
Naloxone	4.49		Phenyltoloxamine	0.45	1.28
Naphazoline	0.80	2.66	Phenyramidol	0.64	2.07
Neocinchophen	2.16		Physostigmine	1.17	
Neopine	1.67		Pilocarpine	0.88	3.04
Neostigmine Bromide	0.36	0.98	Piminodine (base)	7.00	
Nicotinamide	0.23	0.45	Piperoxan	0.36	1.00
Nicotine	0.19	0.32	Pipradrol	0.83	2.78
Norpseudoephedrine	0.19	3.33	Pramoxine	0.95	3.54
Nortrijstyline	0.93	3.36	Prazepam	3.76	
Noscapine	21.7		Prenylamine	2.34	
Orphenadrine	0.41	1.21	Prilocaine	0.36	0.98
Oxanamide	0.17	0.28	Primidone	1.77	
Oxazepam	1.57		Probarbital	0.25	0.50
Oxomemazone	5.31		Procaine	0.62	2.08
Oxycodone	2.97		Prochlorperazine (base)	7.77	
Oxymetazoline	1.00	3.70	Progesterone	5.07	
Oxymorphone	3.12		Prolintane	0.23	0.45
Oxyphencyclimine	0.25	0.52	Promazine	1.34	
Oxomemazone	5.31		Promethazine	1.14	
	7.51		Proparacaine	1.22	
Papaverine	8.75		Propiopramazine	5.46	
Pargyline	sf	0.27	Propanolol	0.78	2.74
Parabutethamine	0.70	2.43	Propylparaben	0.23	0.54

TABLE XX — continued

Compound	250°C	220°C	Compound	250°C	220°C
Protopine	11.2		Thenyldiamine	0.53	1.67
Prothipendyl	1.43		Theobromine	0.53	1.69
Protriptyline	1.07		Theophylline	0.72	2.64
Psilocybin	0.77	2.43	Thiabendazole	0.90	2.81
Pyrathiazine	2.57		Thiamylal	0.41	1.14
Pyrilamine	0.98	3.71	Thiazesim	3.29	
Pyrrobutamine	1.49		Thiopental	2.46	
Quinine	6.32		Thonzylamine	0.94	3.42
Salicylic Acid	sf	0.31	Thozalinone	0.87	2.98
Salicylamide	0.23	0.51	Tranylcpromine	0.17	0.27
Scopolamine	1.48		Trifluoperazine	2.84	
Secergan	1.40		Trifluopromazine	0.79	2.74
Secobarbital	0.31	0.83	Triflutrimeprazine	0.69	2.31
Sparteine	0.32	0.76	Trimecaine	0.48	1.42
STP	0.24	0.50	Trmipramine	0.88	2.90
Strychnine Sulfate	18.7		Trioxazine	1.39	
Tetrabenazine	2.26		Tripellenamine	0.51	1.52
Tetracaine	0.90	3.36	Tropicamide	1.63	
Tetrahydrozoline	0.45	1.32	Tryptamine	0.36	0.99
Tetramethylsuccinimide	0.17	0.28	Vinbarbital	0.32	0.82
Thebaine	3.12		Zylofuramine	0.24	0.54

TABLE XXI

VOLATILE SUBSTANCES RELATIVE RETENTION TIME TO ETHANOL

Minutes		Minutes	
0.19	petroleum ether	0.80	acrylonitrile
0.20	acetaldehyde	0.84	butanone
0.21	n-pentane	0.98	n-heptane
0.25	diethylether	0.98	1,1,1-trichloroethane
0.36	propionaldehyde	1.00	ethanol
0.38	methylacetate	1.01	carbon tetrachloride
0.40	acetone	1.14	propionitrile
0.40	carbon disulfide	1.22	benzene
0.41	acrolein	1.24	isopropanol
0.44	n-hexane	1.32	methyl cyclohexane
0.44	methyl iodide	1.39	allyl ether
0.47	isopropyl ether	1.40	butanol, tertiary
0.57	diethylamine	1.63	n-propyl acetate
0.60	methanol	1.64	chloroform
0.65	acetonitrile	1.69	allyl acetate
0.69	methylene chloride	1.72	1-chloro-3-methyl butane
0.71	ethyl acetate	1.80	trichlorethanol
0.72	cyclohexane	1.81	1,4-dioxane
0.78	tetrahydrofuran	1.84	ethylene dichloride

TABLE XXI — continued

Minutes		Minutes	
2.10	trichlorethylene	3.45	paraldehyde
2.40	n-octane	4.00	n-butylacetate
2.50	n-propanol	4.68	isobutanol
2.63	2,3-dichloropropane	5.95	n-nonane
2.75	methyl isobutyl ketone	6.08	pyridine
3.04	butanol, secondary	6.60	n-butanol
3.15	toluene	7.57	xylene

Finkle, Byron, Cherry, E.J., Taylor, D.M., *Journ Chrom Sci, 9:*393, 1971. F.I.D. Column 6' × 4" gloss, 5% Hallcomid — M-18, 5% Carbowax 600 on 40/60 Teflon 6 Hc. Column Temp. 50°C; Inlet Temp. 150°C; Detector Temp. 75°C; Carrier gas: Nitrogen 40 cc/min. operating sensitivity: ×30. Rt-ethanol 1.9 min ± 0.1 can also be performed with headspace (Dubowski).

TABLE XXII

Drug	Column Number with Corresponding Retention Time							
	1	2	3	4	5	6	7	8
metharbital	3.2							
barbital	4.2							
probarbital	4.7	5.6						
diallyl barbituric acid	5.5							
aprobarbital	6.5							
allyl barbituric acid	6.2							
butethal	6.8							
butabarbital	7.2							
methallatal	7.8							
butalbital	8.0							
amobarbital	8.4	10.9						
pentobarbital	8.8							
vinbarbital	9.3							
secobarbital	9.7	16.8						
thiopental	10.0							
hexobarbital	12.3							
cyclopal	13.6							
mephobarbital	14.0							
hexetal	14.3							
thiamylal	14.5							
phenobarbital	20.0	19.2						
cyclobarbital	21.3							
alphenol	24.8							
Placidyl		1.4						
phenethylamine		2.1						

TABLE XXII — continued

Drug	Column Number with Corresponding Retention Time							
	1	2	3	4	5	6	7	8
dibucaine		2.6						
amphetamine		2.4						
glutethimide		9.1						
meprobamate		10.4			5.4			
pheniramine		13.0						
chlorpromazine		9.7			5.7			
meclizine		6.2						
phenacetin		8.6						
Demerol		9.7						
Listica		11.3						
Benadryl		16.9						
Prominal		23.0						
methadone		12.1						
ambodryl		12.3						
Artane		16.4						
methamphetamine		3.0						
nicotine		6.7						
ephedrine		7.5						
ethinamate		9.5						
caffeine		14.7						
lidocaine		18.0						
antipyrine		20.0						
aminopyrine		12.0						
tripelennamine		14.7						
methapyrilene		14.8						
chlorpheniramine		16.3						
procaine		18.6						
propoxyphene		13.8						
atropine		14.0						
thonzylamine		14.7						
codeine		9.2						
chlorcyclizine		15.5			5.0			
tetracaine		17.2						
scopolamine		8.1						
ethylmorphine		10.7						
morphine		9.9						
cinchonine		13.6						
cinchonidine		14.6						
diacetylmorphine		6.4						
chloroquine		6.9						
quinidine		3.1						
d-desoxyephedrine			1.6					
amphetamine H_2SO_4			1.7					
phenethylamine			1.8					

TABLE XXII — continued

Drug	Column Number with Corresponding Retention Time							
	1	2	3	4	5	6	7	8
methoxyphenamine HCl			3.4					
ephedrine H$_2$SO$_4$			3.8					
ephedrine HCl salt			6.8					
pseudoephedrine HCl			3.4					
phenylpropanolamine HCl			4.6					
benzphetamine HCl			17.2					
methoxamine HCl			26.0					
1,4-pentane diamine			1.4					
1,5-pentane diamine			1.7					
chloroform				1.0		2.53	1.0	
methylene chloride				0.49			0.58	
dichloroethane				1.3			1.16	
carbon tetrachloride				0.59		1.61	1.39	
trichloroethylene				0.93		2.59	1.80	
perchloroethylene				1.11			4.0	
Stelazine					12.1			
Sparine					3.5			
Fluphenazine					6.6			
mepazine					7.3			
methoxypromazine					8.5			
prochlorperazine					2.9			
promethazine					7.3			
pyrathiazine					2.2			
triflupromazine					3.1			
adiphenine					5.2			
diphenylpyraline					3.2			
meclizine					16.8			
pipradrol					3.8			
piperilate					2.3			
carisoprodol					3.3			
mephenesin					1.3			
methocarbamol					6.1			
phenaglycodol					0.6			
ectylurea					1.0			
iproniazid					1.4			
phenelzine					3.3			
imipramine					5.0			
thonzylamine					2.7			
N-butyl alcohol						4.8		
paraldehyde						4.9		
amyl acetate						8.0		
xylene						8.5		
methyl alcohol						0.89		
ethyl alcohol						1.0		

TABLE XXII — continued

| Drug | Column Number with Corresponding Retention Time | | | | | | | |
	1	2	3	4	5	6	7	8
n-heptane						1.05		
isopropyl alcohol						1.19		
methyl ethyl ketone						1.44		
ethyl acetate						1.49		
benzene						2.08		
n-propanol						2.25		
propyl acetate						2.64		
ethylene dichloride						2.86		
isobutyl alcohol						3.53		
toluene						4.2		
ether						0.33		
acetaldehyde						0.33		
formaldehyde						0.56		
lindane								6.0
heptachlor								9.0
aldrin								12.0
heptachlorhepoxide								15.0
dieldrin								21.0
endrin								24.0
p, p-DDT								34.0
strychnine		8.7						
quinine		11.2						
anileridine		32.2						
meclizine		6.2						

1. Ionization (β-ray) (strontium 90) Detector. Column: borosilicated glass tube 4 foot × 5 mm i.d. Packed with SE-30, 5% by weight on firebrick 100/120 mesh, acid washed. Temperature, 180°C. Flow rate (argon), 28.6 ml per minute. Detector voltage, 1750 v (barbiturates) (Kirk, P., and Parker, K.D.: *Anal Chem, 33:*1378, 1961.)

2. Strontium 90 Argon Ionization Detector. Column: 6 foot × 4 mm i.d. Borosilicated glass, U shape. With 100/120 mesh Anakrom A.B.S. Coated with a liquid phase of siloxane polymer such as SE-30. Detector temperature, 75°C. Voltage, 1750 v. Column, 115 to 210°C. (U.S. Internal Revenue Service, Publ. No. 341, 1966.)

3. Ionization β-ray (strontium 90) Detector. Column: borosilicated glass tube, 4 foot × 5 mm i.d. with 5% Carbowax 20 m on 5% NaOH. Coated firebrick 100/120 mesh. Flow rate, 40 ml per minute. Detector voltage, 1750 v (Sympathomimetic amine). Column temperature, 190°C . (Parker, K.D.; Kirk, P.L., and Fontan, C.R.: *Anal Chem, 34:*1345, 1962.)

4. Flame Ionization Detector. Column: 8 foot × 3 mm i.d. with Carbowax 1540 on 75 gr of ST 116 Diatoport W (acid washed). Column temperature, 135° C. (F. and M. Scien. Corp.)

5. Strontium 90 Argon Ionization (β-ray) Detector. Column: 4 foot × 5 mm, borosilicated glass tube. With 60/80 mesh micro beads coated with SE-30 0.05%/w. Flow rate, 40 ml per minute. Parker, K.D.; Fontan, C.R., and Kirk, P.L.: *Anal Chem, 34:*757, 1962.

6. Beta Ionization (Ra 226) Microdetector. Column 6 foot × 3 mm i.d., borosilicated coiled glass tube. With 42/60 mesh, C22 firebrick impregnated with 28 gm of liquid to 100 gm of firebrick. Carrier gas, argon. Column temperature, 45°C. Detector temperature. 150°C. Voltage, 1.2 kv. (Goldbaum, L.R.; Domanski, T.J., and Schloegel, E.L.: *J Forensic Sci, 9:*1, 1964.)

7. Flame Ionization Detector. Column: 6 foot × 3 mm i.d. Stainless steel 20 gm Apiezor L. grease on 80 gm of Chromosorb (Perkin-Elmer Q). Column at 125°C. (F. and M. Scien. Corp.)

8. Electron Capture Detector. Column 6 foot × 4 mm i.d. Glass U shape. With 100/120 mesh coated with 10 wt% D.C. 200 (12,500 CSTK). Column temperature, 200°C. Carrier gas, nitrogen; flow rate 70 ml per minute. (*Gas Chromotography — Newsletter,* May 1968.)

Other References

1. Celeste, A.C. and Polito, M.V.: A rapid method for the quantitative determination of antihistamines and some related compounds by gas chromatography. *JAOAC, 49:*541, 1966.
2. Kazyak, L. and Knoblock, E. G.: Application of gas chromatography to analytical toxicology. *Anal Chem, 35:*1448-1452, 1963.
3. Nelson, D.F. and Kirk, P.L.: Identification of the pyrolyzates of substituted barbituric acids by gas chromatography. *Anal Chem, 36:*875-878, 1964.
4. Parker, K.S. *et al.:* Rapid gas chromatographic method for screening of toxicological extracts for alkaloids, barbiturates, sympathomimetic amines and tranquilizers. *Anal Chem, 35:*356-359, 1963.
5. Sunshine, I. *et al.:* Distribution and excretion of Methohexitone in man: A study using gas and thin layer chromatography. *Br J Anaesth, 38:*23-28, 1966.
6. Thompson, H.L. and Decker, W.J.: A simplified gas chromatography approach for toxicologic purposes. *Am J Clin Path, 49:*103-107, 1968. Strontium 90 Argon Ionization Detector. Column: 6 foot × ⅛ inch i.d. glass U shape. With 5% SE-30 silicone gum or acid washed Chromosorb W. Carrier gas, argon. Flow rate, 60 ml per minute. Injector heat, 250°C; detector, 290°C; column, 190°C.
7. Finkle *et al.: J Forensic Sci, 13:*236, 1968. Ethanol: 1.8 min. Flame Ionization Detector. Column: 6 foot × ¼ inch glass. With 5% Hallcomid-m-18 0.5% Carbowax 600 or 40/60 Teflon T-6. Column temperature, 55°C.
8. Radamski: *Med Surg, 34:*934, 1965. For dieldrin, DDT, other chlorinated hydrocarbon pesticides. Electron capture by tritium or nickel detector.
Temperature:
Inlet: 220°C;
Tritium detector: 220°C;
^{63}Ni detector: 270°C;
Transfer line: 225°C.
Nitrogen input pressure: 70 psi

Flow rate: 110 ml per minute for OV-1, QF-1
           90 ml per minute for QF-1

Columns: All glass, 6 foot × ¼ inch o.d. packed with high performance Chromosorb G, acid washed and DCMS-treated:

     1. 1.6% OV-1; 2.75% QF-1
     2. 2.75% QF-1

9. Cueto and Biros: Chlorinated hydrocarbons in human urine. *J Toxicol Appl Pharmacol, 10:*261; 1967.

Two (2) ml of urine in a 25 ml graduated cylinder is adjusted to PH 7 with either 2% NaOH or 0.5N H_3PO_4. Acetonitrile (4 ml) was added, plus 10 ml of water (previously washed with *n*-hexane). This entire solution was then extracted with *n*-hexane (3 × 2 ml portions) . The combined extracts are collected in a calibrated centrifuge tube and made up to 6 ml volume with *n*-hexane.

Add 0.2 gm of anhydrous Na_2SO_4 and gently shake to dry the *n*-hexane. A 5 ml aliquot (equivalent to 1.67 ml of the original urine) was pipetted into a 15 ml centrifuge tube which was then placed into a constant temperature bath maintained at 40°C. The *n*-hexane residue was picked up; 100 μl of hexane was saturated with methanol (3:1 v/v). A 10 μl aliquot (equivalent to 0.167 ml of the original urine) was inserted into GC apparatus.

Aluminum Tube Packed	Column I (6 foot × ¼ o.d.) 3% QF-1 on 70/80 mesh acid washed Chromosorb G.	Column II (4 foot × ¼ inch o.d.) 2% Dow 200 oil on 70/80 mesh di-methyldichlorosi-lane-treated Chromosorb G.	Column III (6 foot × ¼ inch o.d.) 3% diethylene gly-col succinate on 60/80 mesh acid washed Chromo-sorb G.
Conditions all were similar	Inlet and outlet blocks, 245°; column oven, 180°; electron cap-ture detector, 290°; carrier gas, 5% methane and 95% argon at 75 ml per minute power source; and pulse made of operation at 54 v.		
	Nickel-electron capture detector.		
BHC DDT Dieldrin			

10. Heagy, J. and Look, J.: U.S. Food and Drug Administration.

For detecting STP (2,5-dimethoxy-4-methyl amphetamine) in capsules of LSD (lysergic acid diethylamide). B.C. 5000 gas chromatograph with KCl thermionic detector.

Column temperature:	200°C
Injector temperature:	201°C
Detector temperature:	208°C
Nitrogen flow rate:	85 cc per minute
Hydrogen flow rate:	27 cc per minute

Air flow rate: 290 cc per minute
Sensitivity: 30×
Attenuation: 2

Column: 10% DC 200 on gas chromatrography Q 80/100 mesh.
Length: 6 foot
Diameter: 4 mm.

EVALUATION AND INTERPRETATION
OF ANALYTICAL RESULTS

CRITICAL consideration must be given to the items discussed below.

Sampling: Was the identified tablet or capsule responsible for the patient's symptoms? Were sufficient and proper body fluids analyzed? (Subsequent clear stomach washings obviously do not comprise the ideal specimen, nor are 5 ml of random urine.) Was there too long an interval (more than 24 hours) between exposure and examination? Some volatile gases cannot be found after several hours in many cases; very few organic compounds can be found after forty-eight hours; usually the metals are cumulative (a week at least).

Sensitivity of methods employed: The methods described in Section II under each poison will have a sensitivity sufficient to detect the quantities usually found in body fluids.

Specificity of tests: Some of the tests described may not be specific for the poison in question, such as the ferric chloride test for phenols. However, with the support of other suggested tests plus symptoms and additional facts, these will usually suffice for the purpose of emergency action. Other tests described will be sufficiently specific to support presumptive diagnosis.

Approximate estimation of quantity ingested and relative toxic evaluation: This is not a simple process. Too many variable factors are involved. However, a relative knowledge of toxicity of the agent will guide judgment of treatment and prognosis. Minimum lethal doses (MLD) will be given for each poison if such information is known. Some toxic agents are normally present in trace amounts in the human body, e.g. lead, arsenic, zinc.

Some compounds are very rapidly metabolized by the body, especially the alkaloids. It is fairly well established that approximately 75 percent of morphine, procaine, strychnine, chlorpromazine, and others is cleared from blood within several hours, therefore, *urine* is specimen of choice for analysis for these. Sometimes, the blood may be negative and the urine positive.

BLOOD LEVELS AND HALF-LIFE

Blood levels (plasma) will vary according to dose, whether acute or chronic, bioavailability, route of entry, sex, weight, body water balance, tissue binding, distribution, fat deposition, metabolism, detoxification and rate of elimination (pH of urine), disease state, synergism or antagonism of other drugs, and tolerance (congenital or acquired). Also of importance is the time of sampling (interval after dosing), the half-life of the drug or chemical, the normal or therapeutic levels found, the highest report level with recovery, and the approximate lethal level usually found. Also, consideration should be given to the type and method of analysis.

Half-life will vary between low blood levels and high blood levels (therapeutic versus toxic levels, and age and sex.)

TABLE XXIII

Compound	Blood level normal or therapeutic mg/dl		Lethal blood level mg/dl	Blood half life (hrs)
acetaminophen		2	40	5
acetone		3	50	5
acetohexamide		3	—	5
amitriptyline		0.02	1	—
aminopyrine		—	—	3
amphetamine	Blood	0.003	0.2	25
	Urine	0.01	0.5	
antipyrine		—	—	10
arsenic	Blood	0.01	0.2	Acute (up to
	Urine	0.1	—	10 days) Chronic (up to 3 months)
Barbiturates				
phenobarbital		2 (epileptic)	20	60

TABLE XXIII — continued

Compound	Blood level normal or therapeutic mg/dl		Lethal blood level mg/dl	Blood half life (hrs)
amylobarbital		0.3	4	30
pentobarbital		0.1	2	25
secobarbital		0.08	1	18
thiopental		1	5	—
benzene		—	0.1	—
beryllium	Blood	—	0.2	
	Urine	0.04	0.5	
boron		0.1	5	—
bromide		15	250	15 days
brompheniramine		0.002		
cadmium		0.0003	0.05	—
caffeine		0.5	10	4 hrs
carbon disulfide		—	0.02	—
carbon monoxide		2% (sat.)	40% (sat.)	3 hrs
carbon tetrachloride		—	0.1	—
chloral hydrate		1	10	6
chlordiazepoxide		0.2	3	24
chlorpromazine		0.05	0.5	—
chloroform		10	40	½ hr
chloroquin		—	4	5 days
cocaine		—	0.2	
cinchophen				4
codeine		0.003	0.5	5
copper		0.15	0.6	—
coumarin		0.5	—	30
cyanide		0.01	0.5	—
curare		0.07	—	1
DDT		0.001	0.5	1 year
desipramine		0.1	1	—
diazepam		0.1	2	10
dieldrin		0.0001	—	—
digitoxin		0.002	0.005	6 days
digoxin		0.0001	0.001	36 hrs
dinitro-o-cresol		—	7	—
diphenyl hydantoin (phenytoin)		1.5	8	24
diphenhydramine		0.1	1	5
doxepin		0.002	1	—
ethanol		—	450	20 mg/hr
ethchlorvynol		0.5	10	2 hr
ethyl ether		100	150	—
ethylene glycol		—	200	—
fluoride	Blood	0.005	0.3	—
	Urine	0.05	0.2	—
fluazepam		0.01	0.2	—

TABLE XXIII — continued

Compound		Blood level normal or therapeutic mg/dl	Lethal blood level mg/dl	Blood half life (hrs)
glutethimide		0.05	4	10
hydrogen sulfide		—	0.1	—
isopropanol		—	300	3
imipramine		0.02	0.2	4
iron salt	(Serum)	0.15	0.8	—
isoniazid		—	—	2
lead		0.04	0.150	months
lidocaine (Xylocaine)		0.2	1	—
LSD		—	0.0005	·3
marihuana		—	—	½ hr
meperidine		0.05	2	3
meprobamate		1	15	8
mercury	Urine	0.03	0.20	—
mescaline		—	—	6
methadone		0.05	0.5	—
methylene chloride		—	30	—
methanol		—	50 (3 days) 800 (rapid)	
methaqualone		0.3	3	3 hrs
methyprylon		1	10	4
morphine		0.01	0.1	4
nicotine		0.01	0.5	—
nitrobenzene		—	0.05	—
nortriptyline		0.02	1	20
oxalate		0.1	2	—
paraldehyde		5	50	6
pentazocine		0.02	0.3	—
phencyclidine		—	0.1	—
phenbutazone		10	—	50
phenmetrazine		—	0.4	8
procaine		0.5	—	0.3
procainamide		0.5	3	—
propoxophene		0.02	1	4
quinidine		0.5	4	—
quinine		0.2	2	15
salicylates		10	60	6
selenium		0.03	—	—
strychnine		—	0.5	5
theophylline		1.5	5	5
thioridazine		0.05	2	—
tolbutamide		—	—	5
toluene		—	1	
zinc		0.15	—	—

Therapeutic and toxic concentrations and half-life were approximated from

Evaluation and Interpretation

Evaluation and Interpretation

the following references (levels will vary widely due to many factors).

1. Winek, Charles L.: Tabulations of therapeutic, toxic and lethal concentrations of drugs and chemicals in blood. *Clin Chem, 22:*832, 1976.
2. Clarke, E.G.C.: *Isolation and Identification of Drugs.* London, Pharm Pr, 1969.
3. Hudson, R.P. and McBay, A.J.: Personal communications.
4. Dreisbach, R.H.: *Handbook of poisoning,* 9th ed. Los Altos, Cal., Lange Med Publ, 1977.
5. Baselt, R.C., Wright, J.A. and Crovely, R.H.: Therapeutic and toxic concentrations of drugs in blood. *Clin Chem, 21:*44, 1975.
6. Morrel, G. and Pribor, H.C.: *.Therapeutic Drug Monitoring, Lab. Mgment,* page 40, June 1977, quoting Koch-Weser.
7. Goldstein, A., Aronow, L. and Kolman, S.M.: *Principles of Drug Action.* New York, Har-Row, 1969.
8. Registry Human Toxicology (Fatal) AAFS (Rehling and Kazyak) 1970 and 1972.
9. Industrial Hygiene Services (quoting NIOSH).
10. NIOSH periodic reports (HEW).
11. Goodman, L.S. and Gilman, A.: *Pharmacological Basis of Therapeutics,* 5th ed. New York, Macmillan, 1975.
12. Sunshine, I. (Ed.): *Handbook of Analytical Toxicology.* Cleveland, CRC Press, 1969.
13. Vesell, E.S., and Passananti, G.T., Drug concentrations in biologic fluids, *Clin Chem, 17:*851, 1971.
14. Garriott ,J. (from Fisher and Petty).

SECTION II

ALPHABETICAL LISTING OF POISONS

ACETAMINOPHEN

Synonyms: N-acetyl-p-aminophenol, paracetamol; APAP; Actron; Tylenol; Tempra; p-hydroxyacetanilide, Panadol.

Uses: Nonnarcotic analgesiac and antipyretic.

Usual Dose: 0.3 gm per tablet; 2 tablets q.i.d.

MLD: Approximately 10 gms/70 kg person.

Approximate Blood Levels: Therapeutic, 2 mg/dl; lethal, 50 mg/dl; half-life, about 5 hours.

Remarks: Acetaminophen is the active metabolite of phenacetin and of acetanilid. Acetaminophen is excreted by the kidneys as the conjugated p-aminophenol.

Symptoms: Nausea, vomiting may occur. Early symptoms are *surprisingly* rare. Initial CNS stimulation including excitement, delirium, and convulsions may occur, followed by CNS depression, stupor, and coma. Liver damage within 12–72 hours with possible profound hypoglycemia, prolongation of prothrombin time and metabolic acidosis, and electrolyte and E.K.G. disturbances; kidney, cardiac, and cerebral damage are also possible.

Chronic Toxicity: May produce liver and kidney and myocardial damage. Protein deprivation, pre-existing liver damage or ingestion of microsomal-enzyme-inducing agents such as barbiturates and alcohol may compound the hepatic hazard. Reported to decrease liver glutathione.

Identification

Urine (10 ml) acidified with 1 ml of HCl and then hydrolyzed on a boiling water bath for 5 minutes will greatly increase yield and sensitivity.

Neutral chloroform extraction: Soluble in hot water, ethanol, or chloroform. Poorly soluble in ether. Mp 170°C.

1. UV: See Section I.

   In 0.5N H_2SO_4: maximum density, 243 nm; shoulder at 275–285 nm; $E_{1cm}^{1\%}$, 610; minimum density, none.

   In 0.5N NaOH: maximum density, 256 nm; $E_{1cm}^{1\%}$, 770; minimum density, none.

   In methanol: maximum density, 249 nm; $E_{1cm}^{1\%}$, 900.

2. TLC: See Section I.

   Developing solvent: chloroform:ethanol (99:1).

   Spray: $FeCl_3$ (5%).

   Rf: 65 (Fioresi).

3. 1 ml urine + 1 ml $FeCl_3$ (5%) → dark green.

4. Presumptive tests (2–5 days later).

   a. Prolongation of prothrombin time.

   b. Extreme elevation of serum enzyme levels of S.G.P.T. and S.G.O.T.

5. GLC: See Section I.

Treatment

Any "suspected" overdose must be treated with utmost seriousness because early symptoms are few and vague and misleading. Hospitalization is suggested because of the speed of absorption and onset of serious liver damage.

Immediate activated charcoal, emesis or gastric lavage, and cathartics are very helpful. Early gastric lavage has been reported to be more effective than emetics. Although electrolyte and water balance must be maintained, there may be water retention, so caution should be taken that fluids are not given in excess. It has been reported that forced diuresis and hemodialysis have not been proven effective in removing acetaminophen before liver damage can occur.

Not infrequently, after an initial period of malaise, the patient appears to improve on the second or third day. This may be a false interlude and patient later succumbs to liver necrosis; liver function tests should be normal for at least 24 hours.

Clinical or laboratory evidence of liver damage should institute all the usual measures for treatment. Metabolic acidosis should be treated with sodium bicarbonate; hypoglycemia with dextrose; vitamin K for prolonged prothrombin time. When food can be taken, it should consist of high carbohydrate, low fat diet.

Methionine (oral or IV) and IV cysteamine (mercaptamine) within twelve hours may be helpful.

Plasma levels can approximate the severity of poisoning:

	Necrosis unlikely	*Necrosis possible*	*Necrosis probable*
4 hours	120 μg	120–300 μg	300 μg
12 hours	50 μg	50–120 μg	120 μg

A plasma half-life in excess of 5 hours also suggests a high probability of necrosis (liver damage). Beyond the third day, rising levels of serum bilirubin, S.G.P.T., S.G.O.T., and continued lengthening of the prothrombin time provides concrete though belated evidence of hepatic damage.

Reference

Miles Laboratories Report, Oct. 24, 1975, Lyons et al: *N Eng J Med, 296*:174, 1977.

ACETANILIDE (C₈H₉NO)

ACETANILIDE (C_8H_9NO)

Synonyms: Antifebrin; acetylaminobenzene; acetylaniline.

Uses: Analgesic or antipyretic.

Properties: White crystalline, usually tablets. Mp 114°C. Neutral. Soluble in ether, chloroform, benzene, or ethanol.

MLD: Approximately 4 gm/70 kg person.

Remarks: Allergy and idiosyncrasy are not uncommon and may be severe. Cardiac patients are especially susceptible.

Symptoms

ACUTE: Nausea, vomiting, sweating, gastric irritation, chills, cold extremities, brown-black urine (*p*-aminophenol), tinnitus, fall in blood pressure, methemoglobinemia (chocolate-colored blood), cyanosis, oliguria, jaundice, convulsion, shock, collapse, death.

CHRONIC: Same as above, plus dizziness, irritability, muscular weakness, hemolytic anemia, shallow respiration, dyspnea, skin rash with possible ulceration, more kidney and liver damage, nephritis, anuria, severe jaundice, stupor, collapse.

Death may be sudden or delayed from circulatory and/or respiratory failure.

Identification

Acetanilid is eliminated partly unaltered in the urine, and also as the *p*-aminophenol metabolite within 2 hours and continues to be eliminated up to approximately 24 hours (depending upon quantity taken). Extracted with acid-ether procedure.

1. *Isonitrile test:* A few crystals are hydrolyzed with 1 ml of dilute hydrochloric acid (10%) by gently heating in a test tube. Then add 2 ml of 25% sodium hydroxide and 2 ml of chloroform and gently heat to boiling. The strong odor of isonitrile (skunk odor) is very characteristic, sharp, and pungent.

2. A few crystals are treated with 1 ml of concentrated hydrochloric acid and then diluted with 12 ml of water and gently heated to boiling. Cool and separate into four equal parts.

   a. To one portion, add 1 ml of 1% potassium permanganate → green.

   b. To another portion, layer with 1 ml of fresh aqueous calcium hypochlorite (run gently down the side of test tube) → blue color at interface (junction).

   c. To one portion, add a few drops of 5% sodium nitrite; then make alkaline to litmus with dilute sodium hydroxide (10%). Add a few drops of 5% β-naphathol in ethyl alcohol → red basic azo dye.

   d. *Indophenol test:* To one portion, add 1 ml of saturated aqueous solution of phenol. A freshly prepared solution of calcium hypochlorite is added drop by drop. A dirty red color appears on shaking. On adding ammonia, a deep blue color is produced. This test is also positive for phenacetin.

3. Purified extracted shiny leaflet crystals are white; Mp 110–114°C.

4. Phosphomolybdic acid gives a yellow precipitate with both acetanilide and phenacetin. To differentiate, heat precipitate → dissolves (acetanilide); undissolved (phenacetin).

5. Dissolve residue in hydrochloric acid (6N) ; gently boil; then add several drops of potassium bromate solution → purple color (phenacetin) . Acetanilide → no color.
6. Test for methemoglobin in blood. (Procedure described under aniline.)
7. Spectrophotometry: See Section I.
8. TLC: See Section I.

Treatment

Give milk or activated charcoal; gastric lavage or give emetics to remove as much as possible. Follow with saline cathartics (sodium sulfate, 30 gm) .

Keep patient warm and quiet and in a recumbent position; bed rest is essential. Maintain fluid, electrolyte, body heat, and respiratory balance. Give oxygen and/or artificial respiration to relieve cyanosis.

When methemoglobin is above 40 percent, give 1% methylene blue (5 to 20 ml, slowly IV) . If methylene blue is not available, give ascorbic acid (action is slower). Continue with oxygen therapy for several hours after giving methylene blue. See aniline.

Supportive measures for shock, liver, or kidney involvement.

Acetanilid may metabolize to acetaminophen and aniline.

ACETIC ACID ($C_2H_4O_2$)

Synonyms: Glacial acetic; strong vinegar.

Uses: Industry for synthesis and dyes.

Properties: Liquid, colorless, characteristic penetrating odor. Bp 118°C, volatile, soluble in water, ethanol, and water.

MLD: Approximately 10 ml/70 kg person.

Remarks: Strong characteristic odor. Powerful corrosive. May be produced from aged paraldehyde on standing.

Symptoms: Odor of vinegar identifies acetic acid. Burns on skin, mouth, esophagus. Severe gastrointestinal corrosion, abdominal pain, nausea, vomiting, thirst, difficult swallowing, rapid and weak pulse, slow and shallow breathing, twitching, convulsions, collapse, shock, death.

Identification

In stomach contents:

1. Strong odor of vinegar is characteristic.
2. Gently heat with ethyl alcohol plus 1 drop of sulfuric acid → fruity ethereal odor (of ethyl acetate) .
3. GLC (Porapak Q).
4. Two (2) ml is neutralized with NH_4OH; then add several drops of $FeCl_3$ (5%) → orange-red color. HCl or H_2SO_4 does not interfere.

Treatment

Do not use stomach tube or emetic if severe corrosion is evident. Dilute with water with caution. Neutralize with milk of magnesia, lime water, soap suds, Amphojel, Cremalin, or other mild antacid. *Do not use sodium bicarbonate* or other carbon dioxide forming compounds. Give milk, cream, or white of egg as a demulcent. Keep patient warm and quiet; give morphine for pain, sedatives, crushed ice to relieve thirst. If there are signs of asphyxia, tracheotomy may be indicated. Protect against esophageal obstruction, perforation, or stricture formations.

Guard against infection. Cortisone therapy has been recommended in persistent shock and to reduce esophageal stricture.

If burns are external, wash with plenty of water and then apply a paste of sodium bicarbonate.

ACETONE (C_3H_6O)

Synonyms: Dimethyl ketone; propanone.

Uses: Nail polish remover, solvent in industry.

Properties: Colorless, sweet-smelling liquid. Flammable. Bp, 56.5°C.

MLD: Approximately 100 ml/70 kg person (low toxicity) .

APPROXIMATE BLOOD LEVELS: Normal 3 mg/dl; lethal, 50 mg/dl.

Remarks: Can be absorbed through all portals.

Symptoms: Irritation of mucous membranes, possible kidney and liver involvement, headache, dizziness, dermatitis, fainting, hypoglycemia, CNS depression, bronchial irritation and pulmonary congestion, irregular respiration, weak pulse, lowered temperature, dyspnea, stupor, death by ketosis (acidosis) .

Identification

Steam-distillation separation: Acetone poisoning should not be confused with ketone bodies in the urine due to acidemia of other etiology. Metabolite of isopropanol.

1. Test stomach contents or urine:
    a. Take 10 ml of urine plus 3 gm of sodium hydroxide. To this mixture, add 20 drops of 10% alcoholic solution of salicylaldehyde. Gently warm to 70°C → intense purple-red ring at interface. See under Isopropanol.
    b. *Quick powder tests:* Acetest (Ames Co.) tablet: Several drops of urine → orange → dark red. Denco (Denver Chemical Co.): small pinch of powder; 2 drops of urine → light lavender to dark purple.
    c. To 5 ml of urine, add few drops of sodium nitroprusside solution (fresh) . Mix and add 1 gm of ammonium sulfate powder. Mix and stratify on this 2 ml of ammonium hydroxide. Allow to stand several minutes → purple ring at interface.
2. Stomach contents or urine is *gently* steam distilled. 5 ml distillate + 5 ml Deniges' reagent + gentle heat (for 5 minutes) → white fine precipitate.

Reagent: Deniges' (HgO + H_2SO_4): 2 gm of yellow mercuric oxide + 16 ml of water + 8 ml of sulfuric acid; stir and dissolve with addition of 16 ml more water. Also see under Isopropanol.

3. Stomach contents, urine, or blood filtrate is gently distilled into dilute (1:1) Nessler's solution → immediate precipitate.
4. Unknown sample is steam distilled. To 5 ml of distillate is added a few drops of sodium nitroprusside (fresh) plus a few drops of sodium hydroxide (10%) . Acidify with acetic acid (10%) → purplish red color.
5. GLC: See under GLC in Section I for ethanol.

Treatment

Remove by emesis or gastric lavage. Maintain respiratory exchange. If necessary, give glucose for hypoglycemia, sodium bicarbonate for acidosis; and oxygen therapy as needed.

Avoid fats or oils. Support against dangers of coma, hypoxia, pulmonary edema, or acidosis.

ACETYLSALICYLIC ACID ($C_9H_8O_4$)

Synonym: Aspirin.

Uses: Analgesic, antipyretic, antirheumatic.

Properties: Odorless. Bitter taste. White crystalline, Mp, 137°C, soluble in ethanol, chloroform, ether, or ethylene dichloride.

MLD: Approximately 15 gm/70 kg person.

Derivatives: Sodium salicylate: MLD, approximately 15 gm. Phenyl salicylate salol, (suntan lotion): MLD, 5 gm mp 42°C. Methyl salicylate (oil of wintergreen liniment mixture, Ben Gay): MLD, 10 ml. Salicylic acid (corn remover): MLD, 8 gm, mp, 157°C.

Remarks: Salicylates are rapidly absorbed and usually can be detected in the urine within 30 minutes. Serum half-life is about 10 hours. Allergy is not uncommon.

Symptoms: Nausea and vomiting may be early or delayed. Large doses first stimulate and then depress the central nervous system; initial excitement may be followed by convulsions and then followed by stupor and depression. Central stimulation may also produce hyperventilation (loss of carbon dioxide) and respiratory alkalosis; however, this is followed by a severe metabolic acidosis. Other possible manifestations are headache, fever, hypoglycemia, thirst, dizziness, irritability, cyanosis, *p*-aminophenol in urine (brown-black urine), diaphoresis, dehydration, gastritis with or without gastric hemorrhage, lowered prothrombin, disturbance of hearing and vision, tinnitus, peripheral vasodilatation, hyperpnea with dyspnea, renal and brain damage, weakness and fatigue, hypotension, delirium and confusion, coma; death from respiratory failure, cardiovascular collapse, or complications of electrolyte imbalance.

Identification

Separated by acid-ether extraction. Specimen must be strongly acid to allow a good extraction.

1. Presumptive (rapid) tests for salicylates:
   a. Add 1 ml of $FeCl_3$ (5%) to 2 ml of urine. An immediate persistent purple color is positive. Test is positive in urine after the ingestion of only several (0.3 gm) aspirin tablets (after $\frac{1}{2}$ hour).
   b. Add 1 ml of Trinder's reagent to 2 ml of urine. An immediate persistent purple color is positive (better test).
      Reagent: Trinder: 4 gm $HgCl_2$ in 85 ml of H_2O plus heat to dissolve; cool and add 12 ml of 1N HCl and 4 gm $Fe(NO)_3$; dissolve and then dilute to 100 ml with H_2O.
   c. Add 5 ml of Trinder's reagent to 1 ml of serum; mix, centrifuge → violet color → decant off supernatant and read in a spectrophotometer at 540 nm.

The finding of salicylates in the blood or urine in itself is of no great emergency unless the level is high. In all questions of doubt, there should be a determination of the alkaline reserve of the blood. It is of utmost importance to determine the degree (if any) of acidosis and to correct as necessary.

The simple ferric chloride or Trinder test is of great help whenever there is a doubt of ingestion. Children may sometimes have a delayed response and appear to be in better condition than they actually are. This test can alert to immediate action.

These tests are positive for salicylates and other derivatives of phenol.

Serum levels below 20 mg/dl are usually asymptomatic except perhaps with infants. It is usually above the 40 mg/dl (within 5 hours of ingestion) that symptoms will require treatment for toxicity. Blood half-life is about 10 hours.

2. Additional tests:
   a. Acidify 5 ml of serum by adding 0.2 ml of concentrated hydrochloric acid. Then extract with 10 ml of ethylene dichloride. Allow layers to settle and then separate. Discard upper blood layer and add 2 ml of 0.2% ferric nitrate

to the ethylene dichloride. A purple color results if salicylates are present. The color can be compared with standards similarly prepared or may be read in a spectrophotometer.

Reagent:

- *Standard:* Use 1 ml of water in a test tube (blank) and add 1 ml of 0.07N HNO_3. To another test tube, add 0.8 ml of water and 0.2 ml of salicylate standard and then 1 ml of Fe $(NO_3)_3$ reagent.

$$\frac{\text{absorbance unknown}}{\text{absorbance standard}} \times 25 = \text{mg of salicylate per 100 ml}$$

- *Salicylate standard:* 25 mg per 100 ml; 20 mg of sodium salicylate or 25 mg of salicylic acid per 100 ml of water.
- *Ferric nitrate:* 1% in 0.07N nitric acid.

b. Natelson: Put 0.01 ml of serum or urine on a white porcelain dish. One drop of 1% ferric nitrate (in 0.07N HNO_3) is added. A purple color is positive for salicylates. Report as negative, faint, moderate, or large amounts.

c. Quantitative: Measure 0.2 ml of serum or urine plus 0.8 ml of water into each of two small test tubes. To one test tube (which will be the reference blank), add 1 ml of 0.07N nitric acid; to the unknown, add 1 ml of Fe $(NO_3)_3$ reagent. Mix and allow to stand for about 5 minutes; read in a spectrophotometer at 540 nm.

Reagent: Nitric acid, 0.07N: 4.69 ml of HNO_3 (1.42) and 70.5% made up to 1 liter.

Small false readings of about 2 mg% may be produced by iron present. Since therapeutic levels of salicylates may be above 10 mg%, readings below 5 mg% are not significant.

Levels below 20 mg/dl may be considered nontoxic in adults; above 50 mg/dl may be lethal.

Thiocyanates will interfere if taken in large amonts.

3. Benedict's reagent is positive for sugar in urine.
4. Crystals extracted from urine can be differentiated with ferric chloride (5%) .

a. antipyrine + ferric chloride → red color

b. salicylate + ferric chloride → deep violet color

   c. aminopyrine (Pyramidon) + ferric chloride → fading light violet color

5. UV spectrophotometry: See Section I. To effect a good extraction, specimens must be strongly acidified. Use 5 ml of serum or tissue slurry plus 0.2 ml of concentrated hydrochloric acid. Gently extract with 25 ml of chloroform; re-extract with 0.9N NaOH and scan between 230 and 340 nm. Maximum density, 300 nm; minimum density, 265 nm. (Salicylic acid is the metabolite.)

6. Thin layer chromatography. See Section I.
   a. cyclohexane:$CHCl_3$:pyridine (20:60:5) (Gänshirt in Stahl)
      antipyrene 30 R f
      aspirin 10
      ethenzamidum 50
      acetaminophen 10
      phenacetin 67
      salicylamide 21
   b. cychohexane:ethanol (8:2) (Sunshine)
      aspirin 11
      Doriden 25
      meprobamate 16
      salicylic acid 22

All tests described above are for the salicylate radical. (salicylic acid metabolite).

Compound radicals such as methyl salicylate, aspirin, and salol must first be hydrolyzed if tests are done on tablets or original compounds.

Treatment

Activated charcoal, milk, and then gastric lavage with warm water; or 15 ml of syrup of ipecac to produce vomiting. Do not omit the lavage or emesis unless dose is known to be small or exposure was a very long time ago. Patient may appear deceptively well when first seen; signs and symptoms may be delayed.

Fluids (oral or parenteral) to increase urinary output and to correct dehydration due to vomiting and sweating. Maintain body heat, fluid, glucose, and electrolyte balance. Give alkaline drinks in mild cases.

Give sodium bicarbonate as needed to combat acidosis and sodium loss. Periodic blood determinations for alkaline reserve and electrolyte balance will estimate severity of poisoning and progress of treatment. Elimination of salicylates is more rapid if urine is kept alkaline. Supportive and symptomatic treatment.

Vitamin K_1 derivatives and ascorbic acid for low prothrombin (if necessary).

In severe poisoning, hemodialysis may be helpful.

ACONITINE ($C_{34}H_{49}NO_{11}$)

Synonyms: Aconite root, monkshood; Wolf's-bane.

Uses: No longer used medically.

Properties: White crystalline. Basic. Mp 198°C. Alkaloid.

MLD: Approximately 10 mg/70 kg person.

Remarks: Very toxic. Death may occur quickly. May be absorbed through all portals.

Symptoms: Nausea, vomiting, diarrhea, abdominal pain, salivation, sharp burning taste, numbness and tingling of mouth and throat extending to the rest of body—particularly to fingertips. Chills, restlessness, staggering, dizziness, convulsions, pupils first constricted then dilated, impaired vision, low temperature, shallow irregular respiration, bradycardia, syncope, great prostration, low blood pressure, collapse, coma, death from ventricular fibrillation or cardiac and/or respiratory paralysis.

Identification

Isolated by alkaline-chloroform extraction. Destroyed by heat: evaporate with electric fan in presence of several drops of dilute hydrochloric acid.

1. Residue is dissolved with 1 ml of 1% acetic acid. Use 1-drop aliquots for spot-precipitant tests; examine for characteristic crystals. See Alkaloids.
   a. Wagner's reagent → brown precipitate
   b. Mayer's reagent → white precipitate
   c. picric acid → yellow precipitate (only when aconitine is

present in large amounts)

    d. Na_2CO_3 (1%) → rosettes

    e. $KMnO_4$ (1%) → rosettes

2. Small aliquot portions of residue are transferred to spot plate and color reagents applied. See Alkaloids.

    a. sulfuric acid → colorless

    b. nitric acid → colorless → red-brown

    c. sulfuric acid + nitric acid → colorless → violet

    d. Fröhde's reagent → yellow → yellow-brown

    e. Mandelin's reagent → tan → orange

    f. Marquis' reagent → colorless

3. TLC: See Section I.

4. UV spectrophotometry: See Section I.

Treatment

Activated charcoal and then gastric lavage with dilute potassium permanganate (1:10,000) or milk.

Saline cathartics (sodium sulfate, 25 gm). Avoid emetics. Sedate and treat convulsions with short-acting barbiturates or Valium.

Keep patient quiet and warm in a recumbent position. Bed rest is especially essential. Guard against respiratory and cardiac depression. Symptomatic and supportive measures as needed: artificial respiration or oxygen therapy; atropine (1 mg) to improve pulse and to depress vagal stimulation.

Symptoms and treatment generally similar for veratrine, sparteine, delphinine, and larkspur.

ALKALIES

Synonyms: Sodium hydroxide (NaOH); potassium hydroxide (KOH); lye; caustic soda; caustic potash.

Uses: Soaps, industry, grease and oven cleaner, Drano, drain and pipe cleaner, sink and toilet flush, paint remover, cuticle remover.

Properties: Powerful corrosive. Solid, hygroscopic, slimy feeling to touch.

MLD: Approximately 5 gm/70 kg person.

Remarks: Very caustic, strongly alkaline.

Symptoms: Slimy, soapy taste; burns, severe gastrointestinal irritation and corrosion, nausea, vomiting, abdominal pains, scarrings of tissues (white eschars), alkalemia, pallor, weak slow pulse, swelling of throat, asphyxia, shock, death.

Identification

In stomach contents:
1. White solid slimy lump, flake, granule, or rod.
2. Turns litmus paper blue; becomes warm on addition of water.
3. If exposed to air, becomes moist and finally all dissolves.
4. Soapy or slimy persistent feeling when touched with fingers.
5. *Platinum wire flame test:* Touch platinum wire to unknown and then place wire in flame. Sodium gives an intense persistent yellow flame. (Caution: sodium is a common contaminant of most materials, including perspiration on fingers.) However, presence of large amounts of sodium is very yellow and very persistent in contrast to small amounts encountered as contaminants.

   Potassium gives a deep purple flame, which is easily seen through a cobalt glass filter.
6. Flame photometry.

Treatment

Carefully dilute with water or milk without delay; then neutralize with dilute vinegar or dilute (fresh or canned) lemon or lime juice. Milk, cream, white of egg, olive oil, or bismuth subnitrate as demulcent.

Keep patient warm and quiet. Give cracked ice to relieve thirst; morphine for pain and sedatives as necessary. If there are signs of asphyxia, tracheotomy is indicated. Protect against esophageal obstruction, perforation, or stricture formations with corticosteroids (for about 1 month or until healing is evident).

Esophagoscopy should be done as soon as possible (within 12 hours) so as to decide for future treatment. Therapy is aimed to prevent infection, to minimize stricture, and to relieve pain once the diagnosis is made. Esophageal stricture may develop even weeks later if corticosteroids are not given.

Therapy with liquid broad-spectrum antibiotics and corticosteroids is started. Bismuth subnitrate powder may provide sufficient local analgesia to manage pain.

If burns are external, wash with ample water and then wash with dilute vinegar or lemon or lime juice.

Other similar strong alkalies with the general symptoms and requiring the same general treatment are thioglycolate (permanent hair wave), sodium carbonate, sodium metasilicate, sodium perborate, sodium triphosphate, and sodium hexametaphosphate. Other caustics are Clorox, Drano, Saniflush, Ajax floor cleaner or bleach (E-Z bleach); Quicklime, calcium oxide, calcium carbonate.

Since phosphate preparations also deplete the body calcium, restore calcium with intravenous calcium gluconate.

ALKALOIDS

Members: Aconitine, atropine, cocaine, codeine, morphine, nicotine, quinine, scopolamine, strychnine, etc.; nicotine and coniine are liquid and are volatile with steam.

Uses: Medicinals, insecticides, rodenticides, narcotics, etc.

Properties: Names usually end in "ine." Effective in very small quantities (very toxic). All are basic (insoluble in free form); contain nitrogen. Soluble as the acid salt. Bitter taste.

MLD: These compounds are generally very toxic. (See under each compound listed. May be as low as 10 mg.)

Remarks: For specific particulars, see under individual alkaloid. Most alkaloids are rapidly removed from the blood, especially procaine, strychnine, morphine. Heat destroys morphine, cocaine, and aconitine; caution is necessary for isolation. Urine is the specimen of choice for detection. Add 1 drop of dilute hydrochloric acid prior to evaporation of solvent to prevent loss.

Identification

1. Alkaloids are isolated from tablets, capsules, blood, urine, gastric lavage, etc. by alkaline-ether or alkaline-chloroform extraction. The solvent is filtered, then evaporated, and the resi-

due is purified by re-extraction, chromatography, or microsublimation.

2. Alkaloids are precipitated by general precipitants. With careful technic and controlled comparisons with known alkaloids, the unknown can be identified by microscopic examination of typical crystals as to color, structure, and general appearance. Allow at least 1 hour for crystal formation. Prevent evaporation by a cover slip rimmed with Vaseline.

A small portion of the purified extract obtained by alkaline-chloroform extraction is dissolved in 1 ml of 2% acetic acid. One drop of this acidified extract is placed into each of several grooves of a spot plate and tested individually with the alkaloid reagents listed below. *(Caution:* Impure extract containing proteins may produce a false-positive test (precipitate), but this is amorphous and does not display typical crystals.)

a. alkaloid + Wagner's reagent → brown precipitate

Allow to stand; examine typical crystals under microscope. Compare with known alkaloid.

Reagent: Wagner's (modified): 2 gm of potassium iodide, 1 gm of iodine, 3 ml of hydrochloric acid, 100 ml of water. Mix, dissolve, allow to stand 15 minutes. Filter. Reagent is stable and is sensitive to approximately 0.005 mg of alkaloid.

b. Alkaloid + Mayer's reagent → white precipitate

Allow to stand; examine typical crystals under microscope. Compare with known alkaloid.

Reagent: Mayer's: 1.4 gm of mercuric chloride, 5 gm of potassium iodide, 100 ml of water; dissolve. Reagent is stable.

c. alkaloid plus picric acid → yellow precipitate

Allow to stand; examine typical crystals under microscope. Morphine does not precipitate with picric acid, whereas codeine and heroin do.

Reagent: Picric acid: Saturated picric acid in water.

d. Other reagents yielding typical crystals:

(1) *Dragendorff's reagent:* Saturate a 10% solution of potassium iodide with bismuth iodide

(2) *Mercuric chloride* (1:20)

(3) *Gold chloride* (1:20)

(4) *Platinic chloride* (1:20)

(5) *Phosphotungstic acid:* 1 part sodium tungstate + 3 parts water + $\frac{1}{2}$ part of 25% phosphoric acid

3. Many alkaloids give characteristic color changes with the various reagents described below. It is advisable to run several of these tests to differentiate one from another. Colors may vary slightly with those tabulated.

Take note of all sequences of color changes and of time intervals. Confirm all findings by color comparisons with known alkaloids. Use purified residue.

Place a small amount of alkaloidal residue on a porcelain plate or other similar white background plate. Add 1 small drop of reagent and note color changes. (*Caution:* Trace of impurities may produce color, usually yellow.)

a. *Sulfuric acid* (concentrated):

N-allylnormorphine → light brown

amitriptyline → orange

apomorphine → olive green

Atabrine → bright yellow

Benadryl → orange

berberine · SO_4 → bright yellow

Butamin → pale yellow

carbromal → white precipitate

cephaeline → light yellow

chlorcyclizine → light brown-yellow

cinchophen → light yellow

codeine → brown with violet hue → red (by heat)

colchicine → bright yellow

cortisone → orange

curarine → blue → red → light brown-yellow

delphinine → brown-orange

desoxyephedrine → pale orange-brown

Digalen → pale yellow

digitalon → red-brown → red (by heat)

digitonin → faint yellow → light orange

digitoxin → brown
dihydromorphinone → brick red
Diothane → brown
diphenhydramine → deep orange
emetine → red brown
ergotoxine → yellow → green → dark green
ethyl morphine → gray brown
Larocaine → strong orange-yellow
lobeline → red-brown
meconin → pale yellow
Mellaril → blue
meperidine → pale yellow
mephenesin → very pale pink
mescaline → yellow → brown → green-brown → orange
methadone → strong yellow + HNO_3 → red
methylparafynol → bright yellow
nicotine → brown-yellow
pamaquine → brown
phenothiazine → red
prednisone → yellow
procaine → pale yellow
procaine amide → pale bright orange
Pyribenzamine → green-yellow
Pyridium → bright red
pyrilamine → magenta
santonin → very pale yellow
solanine → yellow → orange
sparteine → brown
strophanthin → brown
terpin hydrate → yellow-orange
tetracycline → purple
thenylpyramine → orange → red-orange
Thonzylamine → magenta
Valmid → red
veratrine → yellow → orange → red → magenta
Xylocaine → brown
zolamine-HCl → magenta

b. *Nitric acid* (concentrated):
   aconitine →reddish brown
   apormorphine → violet → brown → orange
   brucine → blood red → orange-yellow
   codeine → orange → yellow
   curarine → purple
   Dilaudid → orange-red
   heroin → yellow, plus heat → green-blue → yellow
   methadone + △ → orange → green
   morphine → orange-red → red-yellow
   Numorphan → yellow → orange-red → yellow
   physostigmine → yellow → olive green → red
   strychnine → yellow (by heat)
   thebaine → yellow
   Valium → deep red
   yohimbine → yellow → orange-red (by heat)

c. *Fröhde's reagent* (5 mg of molybdic acid dissolved in 5 ml
   of sulfuric acid)—this reagent is not stable; it should be
   freshly made each time used:
   aconitine → yellow → yellow-brown
   N-allylnormorphine → magenta → gray-green
   amphetamine · HCl → pale red
   amphetamine base → bright yellow
   Antabuse → light green → green → gold
   antipyrine → very pale yellow with water
   apomorphine → blue → slate violet
   Atabrine → bright yellow
   berberine · SO_4 → yellow or green-brown
   brucine → colorless → rose → orange
   cephaeline → light red → yellow-brown → green-yellow
   chlorcyclizine → yellow
   cinchophen → pale yellow
   codeine → green → red-brown
   colchicine → bright yellow
   curarine → brownish magenta → light brown
   delphinine → red-brown
   Digalen → light brown → magenta casts

digitalon → light brown
digitonin → very pale brown-yellow
digitoxin → deep brown
Dilaudid → blue
dihydromorphinone → magenta (violet) → colorless
Dionin → green → blue
Diothane → brown, magenta casts
diphenhydramine → deep red-orange
DOM (STP) → yellow-green → green → blue
Dromoran → blue
emetine → red-brown → yellow-brown
ephedrine → pale brown
ethinamate → orange
ethyl morphine → brown → gray-green
heroin → magenta → gray-green
hydrastine → colorless → green
Larocaine → pale yellow
lobeline → red-brown → yellow-brown
LSD → gray green
meconin → very pale yellow
meperidine → very pale yellow
mephenesin → brown
mescaline → yellow → dark brown
methadone → orange-yellow → gray-green → green
methylparafynol → deep yellow → yellow-brown
metopon → magenta → purple → light green
morphine → deep magenta → blue → fades
α-naphthylthiourea → colorless → violet → yellow
nicotine → bright yellow
Pavatrine → yellow-brown
phenindamine → red-brown
phenylsalicylate → blue-violet →gray-blue → green
procaine → pale yellow
Pyribenzamine → pink → rust red
Pyridium → bright carmine
pyrilamine → light → deep magenta
quinine → pale yellow

salicylic acid → colorless → violet → colorless
solanine → bright yellow
sparteine → brown
strophanthin → brown
terpin hydrate → yellow → orange-yellow
thenylpyramine → orange → red → brown
thonzylamine → magenta →deep magenta
veratrine → yellow → orange → red → purple
Xylocaine → brown
yohimbine → blue → green → yellow
zolamine · HCl → magenta

d. *Mandelin's reagent* (5 mg of ammonium vanadate dissolved in 25 ml of sulfuric acid) :

aconitine → tan-orange
N-allynormorphine → pale brown → light violet
aminopyrine → very pale orange
amphetamine · SO_4 → orange → red → brown
Antabuse → very pale yellow
antihistamine (with thiophenyl) → blue → red
antipyrine → light green → blue-green
ANTU → magenta
apomorphine → dark blue
Atabrine → orange
Benzocaine → faint brown
berberine · SO_4 → dark brown
betaine · HCl → orange
Brucine → light orange
Butamin → faint violet with water
cephaeline → brown
cinchophen → green
codeine → green → blue
colchicine → blue-green → green → brown
curarine → brown
delphinine → red-brown
Digalen → brown → violet-brown
digitalon → red → brown
digitonin → colorless → pale brown

digitoxin → violet-brown
dihydromorphinone →brown → light magenta
Diothane → orange red → green → orange
diphenhydramine → brick red
Dromoran → green → gray-violet → violet
emetine → red-brown
ephedrine → light brown
ethyl morphine → brown → gray-violet
heroin → pale green
homatropine → colorless → light olive green
hydrastine → red → brown
meperidine → light brown
mephenesin → green → violet-brown → magenta
mescaline → green → brown
methadone → dark green → brown
metopon → pale magenta
morphine → brown → pale violet → slate
phenothiazines → blue → red
phenylbutazone → brown-red
phenylsalicylate → green → gray
pilocarpine → yellow → green → blue
Pyribenzamine → chocolate
Pyridium → green → purple
pyrilamine → brick red → carmine
quinidine → blue-green
salicylic acid → light green → gray
solanine → light red-brown
strychnine → blue → violet → red-orange
terpin hydrate → orange
thebaine → orange-red
thenylpyramine → red → purple
thonzylamine → brick red → carmine
veratrine → red-brown → red → red-purple
Xylocaine → red-brown
yohimbine → green → blue → brown

e. *Marquis Reagent* (5 drops of 40% formaldehyde in 5 ml of sulfuric acid) ; reagent must be prepared fresh:

acetanilide → red
N-allylnormorphine → deep magenta → purple
amphetamine · HCl → orange → red → brown
anileridine → orange-red
Antabuse → very pale yellow
antipyrine → salmon
ANTU → green
apomorphine → black → dark green
Atabrine → yellow → orange-yellow
Brucine → light red
cephaeline → brown-yellow
cinchophen → pale lemon yellow
codeine → blue-violet
colchicine → yellow
curarine → light yellow-brown
Darvon → violet
Decodid → yellow → orange → violet
delphinine → orange → brown-orange
dihydromorphinone → magenta → blue-violet
Dilaudid → red-violet → violet
Dionin → purple
diphenhydramine → orange → red → brown
Dromoran → brown
emetine → red-brown
ephedrine → brown → brown-orange
ethyl morphine → blue-violet
Eucodal → yellow → violet
heroin → magenta → violet
hydrastine → yellow → yellow-orange
Librium → yellow
lobeline → brown → red
meconin → purple
meperidine → yellow → light green
mephenesin → red
mescaline → green → dark brown → violet-brown
methadone → nothing
methylparafynol → yellow

metopon → magenta → violet
morphine → magenta → violet
nicotine → pale brown-orange
Nisentil → orange-red
Numorphan → purple
Pantopon → purple
papaverine → pink → blue
Paredrine → dark green
phenothiazines → purple
phenylsalicylate → colorless → pink → deep rose
procaine → pale yellow
Pyribenzamine → red → red-brown
Pyridium → deep red
pyrilamine → magenta → violet
salicylic acid → colorless → pink → rose
terpin hydrate → yellow-orange
thenylpyramine → red → carmine
Thonzylamine → deep carmine
trihexyphenidyl → yellow → orange → rose-orange
Valium → red-purple
Valmid → red
veratrine → yellow → orange → orange-brown
Wyamine → red-orange → red-brown → dark brown
yohimbine → green-gray → gray
zolamine → carmine
Note: This group is especially good for morphine and derivatives such as apomorphine, heroin, Dilaudid, codeine, Nalline.

f. *Oliver's test* (1 drop of copper sulfate [5%] plus 1 drop of hydrogen peroxide (3%) then 1 drop of ammonia):
apomorphine → red → quickly fades to brown
Dilaudid → yellow → brown
heroin → bright red which persists for $\frac{1}{2}$ hour
morphine → red → quickly fades to brown

g. *Mecke's reagent* (5 mg of selenious acid in 1 ml of sulfuric acid) :
N-allylnormorphine → blue → green

amphetamine → light rose

Antabuse → colorless → very pale yellow

apomorphine → violet

Benadryl → yellow →orange

berberine → yellow-brown → brown → violet-brown

brucine → colorless → light red → orange

cephaeline → brown-yellow

cinchophen → light yellow

codeine → blue

colchicine → yellow

curarine → light brown

Darvon → green

Dicodid → yellow → green

digitalon → brown

dihydromorphinone → blue → green

Dionin → dark green

DOM (STP) → green-yellow → orange

Dromoran → very pale yellow

emetine → yellow-brown

ephedrine → light brown

ethinamate → orange

ethyl morphine → green → blue

Eucodal → yellow → green

heroin → blue → green

meperidine → brown-orange

mephenesin → colorless → pale blue, gray-violet casts

mescaline → yellow → green → blue → brown

methadone → pink (10 minutes)

metopon → yellow → green → purple

morphine → blue → green

α-naphthylthiourea → pale yellow-green

nicotine → brown-yellow

pamaquine → brown

papaverine → green → blue

Paredrine → yellow-orange

Pavatrine → dark brown

phenindamine → red-brown

physostigmine → tan → red
Pyribenzamine → nut brown
Pyridium → deep red → orange-red
pyrilamine → pink → magenta
solanin → brown-yellow → red-brown
strophanthin → dark brown
terpin hydrate → yellow-orange
thenylpyramine → magenta → purple
thonzylamine → deep magenta
trihexyphenidyl → light brown
veratrine → yellow → orange → orange-brown
Xylocaine → brown
yohimbine → blue → green
zolamine → magenta

h. *Doper's Reagent* (Purex or chlorox laundry bleach, about 5.2% sodium hypochlorite, acts like Sanchez reagent for certain primary amines in the "-caine" group. *Reference:* Park Kaestner and Ferris Van Sickle: Reference Laboratory Notes DEA (6/4/74):
acetanilide → negative
m-amino benzoic acid → brown flaky
p-amino benzoic acid → brown flaky
amphetamine · SO_4 → negative
aspirin → negative
barbiturates → negative
Benzocaine → flaky chocolate-brown
boric acid → negative
caffeine → negative
carbromal → negative
chlordiazepoxide → negative
chloroprocaine → orange
cocaine-HCl → negative
cocaine base → negative
codeine PO_4 and base → negative
Demerol → negative
DET → orange → brown
dextrose → negative

diazepam → negative
dibucaine →negative
DMT → orange → brown
ephedrine · SO₄ → negative
heroin · HCl → negative
hexylcaine → negative
lactose → negative
lidocaine · HCl → orange-brown; oily drops floating
lidocaine · SO₄ → orange-brown; oily drops floating
LSD → negative
mannitol → negative
MDA · HCl → negative
mepivacaine → negative
mecaline · SO₄ negative
methadone · HCl → negative
methamphetamine · HCl → negative
methapyrilene.· HCl → light green flaky orange
morphine · SO₄ → brown flaky
oxytetracycline → green-yellow
PCP · HCl → negative
phenacetin → negative
phenylpropanolamine → negative
procaine → flaky chocolate-brown
propoxyphene → negative
quinine → negative
saccharine → negative
salicylamide → green-brown on standing
salicylic acid → brown on standing
starch → negative
stearic acid → negative
Stovaine · HCl → orange oily drops on standing
sulfadiazine → green-orange → green-yellow
sulfamerazine → green-orange → green-yellow
talcum powder → negative

i. *Vitali's test.* To a small aliquot of alkaloid residue, add 1 drop of fuming nitric acid. Evaporate to dryness on steam bath. Allow to cool. Add 1 drop of 10% potassium hydroxide in 95% alcohol:

atropine, hyoscyamine, Librium, LSD, scopolamine, strychnine → strong blue (violet)

j. *Sulfuric-dichromate test:* To a small aliquot of alkaloid residue, add 2 drops of sulfuric acid and then one small crystal of potassium dichromate is drawn through the solution:

strychnine → blue-violet → red-violet → red → orange → fades

yohimbine → blue → blue-violet → green

curare → red → violet

4. **Confirmation:** Many alkaloids show characteristic absorption bands as measured with a UV spectrophotometer. Extract is purified and is re-extracted with exactly 5 ml of 0.5N sulfuric acid. Absorption bands are plotted with this acid extract. When properly performed, this is a reliable and sensitive method to detect and quantitate most alkaloids. Morphine and derivatives, however, are not very sensitive.

5. Thin layer, gas, or paper chromatography should be used for confirmation. See Section I.

Treatment

Gastric lavage with potassium permanganate (1:10,000) or milk or activated charcoal. Give emetics to empty stomach; avoid apomorphine. Saline cathartics (30 gm of sodium sulfate in half a glass of warm water).

Use symptomatic and supportive measures. Support all vital functions.

See under specific alkaloid for details.

AMIDOPYRINE $(C_{13}H_{17}N_3O)$

Synonyms: Aminopyrine; Pyramidon.

Uses: Analgesic or antipyretic.

Properties: White crystalline. Mp 108°C. Neutral. Very soluble in $CHCl_3$ or ethanol.

MLD: Approximately 10 gm/70 kg person. Half-life about 3 hours.

Remarks: May produce agranulocytosis.

Symptoms

CHRONIC: Agranulocytosis, skin rash, malaise, severe inflammation of throat; fever, chills; anemia; urine is light red.

ACUTE: Vasodilatation, hypotension, excitement, delirium, tonic and clonic convulsions, followed by coma then death from respiratory arrest and cardiac and/or peripheral circulatory collapse.

Identification

Alkaline-chloroform extraction procedure:

1. Dissolve a small amount of residue in a small quantity of water; then add 0.5 ml of 10% ferric chloride → blue-violet color. Compare with standards similarly treated.
2. Dissolve a small amount of residue in a small quantity of water; then add 0.5 ml of 10% silver nitrate → blue → black (on standing). Antipyrine is negative.
3. To 5 ml of urine, add 5 ml of 20% ferric chloride; shake and then on this stratify with 2 ml of 10% iodine solution (tincture). Dilute by gently adding 10 ml of water and observe violet ring at interface, which may change to red-brown.
4. Fresh voided urine is light red color. This color may be extracted with ether. Urine, on standing, deposits red needlelike crystals.
5. Small amount of residue dissolved in 2 ml of 10% hydrochloric acid. Then add a trace of potassium nitrite → blue-violet → quickly fades.
6. Small amount of residue dissolved in 1 ml of 2% acetic acid. Place several 1-drop portions into a spot plate and then test with any of the following alkaloid reagents:
   a. Wagner's reagent → brown precipitate (typical crystals)
   b. Mayer's reagent → white precipitate (typical crystals)
   c. *Note:* Amidopyrine is not an alkaloid but does give positive reactions with the alkaloid precipitants. (See under Alkaloids for preparation of reagents.)
7. UV spectrophotometry. See Section I.
8. TLC: See Section I.
9. GLC: See Section I.

Treatment

Activated charcoal and milk, then gastric lavage; or emesis. Saline cathartics—30 gms Na_2SO_4. Control convulsions with Valium or short-acting barbiturates. Support all vital functions; guard against convulsions, respiratory or circulatory difficulties. Guard against secondary drug reactions.

AMINOPHYLLINE (THEOPHYLLINE: $C_7H_8N_4O_2$)

Synonyms: Diemethylxanthine; mixture of theophylline and ethylenediamine.

Uses: For asthma, heart disease, diuretic.

Properties: Mp 270°C; weak base; theophylline is soluble in ethanol or chloroform in neutral extraction.

MLD: Approximately 100 mg/70 kg person.

APPROXIMATE BLOOD LEVELS: Theophylline—Therapeutic, 1 mg/dl but should not exceed 2 mg/dl; lethal, about 10 mg/dl; serum half-life, about 5 hours.

Remarks: Therapeutic levels should be monitored for chronic use.

Symptoms: Gastrointestinal upset, nausea, vomiting, diarrhea, sycope, palpitations, dilated pupils, hyperventilation; alternate excitement and depression, hypotension, convulsions, hematuria, ventricular fibrillation, respiratory and circulatory failure (sudden collapse and death may occur from a few minutes to 1 hour).

Identification

Neutral chloroform extraction for theophylline:

1. Hydrolyze 1 ml of urine with 1 ml HCl in a boiling water bath for about 10 minutes. Transfer 0.1 ml of hydrolyzed urine to 10 ml of saturated *o*-cresol, then add 2 ml of 4N NH_4OH → deep blue (indophenol test).

   Reagent: Saturated *o*-cresol: 1 ml per 100 ml of water, then aged about 1 day.

2. UV spectra in absence of barbiturates: Extract 2.5 ml of serum with 25 ml of chloroform (neutral). Separate and filter chloro-

form and collect 20 ml. Re-extract with 2.5 ml of 0.5N NaOH. Scan UV absorption of the NaOH from 300 to 230 nm. Maximum density is at 275 nm. Parallel extraction of unknown with a standard and a control blank; or correct for extraction with factor 125×.

$$\left[\frac{100}{2.5} \times \frac{25}{20} \times \frac{2.5}{1} = 125 \right]$$

3. UV spectra in presence of barbiturates (Hicks): Proceed as above for first extraction, then collect 20 ml of filtered chloroform extract; re-extract this with 2.5 ml of (pH 9.0) bicarbonate/carbonate buffer. Transfer 2 ml of buffer extract and scan in UV as above. Record absorbance at 280 nm, even though maximum density is at 275 nm. Analysis at pH 9 avoids interference with barbiturates.

Reagent: Bicarbonate/carbonate buffer pH 9: 10 ml of 0.1M Na_2CO_3 (10.6 gm diluted to 1,000 ml) is added to 890 ml of $NaHCO_3$ (8.4 gm diluted to 1,000 ml).

4. TLC: See in Section I for theophylline.
5. GLC: See Section I.

Treatment

Maintain all vital signs, especially guard against fall in blood pressure and convulsions. Oxygen as needed, diazepam for convulsions, maintain blood pressure, and water balance (correct dehydration).

If overdose was rectally, enema may help partial removal.

AMMONIA (NH₄OH)

Synonyms: Ammonia water; ammonium hydroxide.

Uses: Refrigerant, cleaning and bleaching agent, widely used household cleanser, and to produce fertilizer.

Properties: Colorless liquid. Penetrating odor. Alkaline, caustic.

MLD: Approximately 10 ml/70 kg person.

Remarks: Powerful irritant and corrosive; strong odor.

Symptoms: Lacrimation, burning sensation, swelling of larynx, spasm of glottis, asphyxia, severe pulmonary and gastrointestinal irritation, nausea, vomiting, diarrhea, abdominal pains, cold and clammy skin, convulsions, collapse, coma, death. Milder exposure also may predispose to bronchopneumonia following a chemical pneumonitis.

Identification

In stomach contents:
1. Strong odor of ammonia—sharp penetrating odor.
2. Turns litmus paper blue (alkaline).
3. Place an open bottle of concentrated hydrochloric acid near unknown solution, stomach contents, or vomitus. This will produce white copious fumes of ammonium chloride.
4. plus chloroplatinic acid solution → typical crystals
5. plus Nessler's reagent → yellow-orange color
6. Distill into a known amount of hydrochloric acid and then titrate for residual hydrochloric acid.
7. Distill into a dilute solution of copper sulfate → blue.
8. By microdiffusion (Natelson): One (1) ml of blood in one pool is placed in outer chamber of a Conway diffusion dish. Place 1.5 ml of $N/100$ H_2SO_4 in the center chamber. Add 1 ml of potassium carbonate to the outer chamber on the opposite side of the dish where the pool of blood was placed. The cover is put on, and the dish is gently rotated to mix the blood and K_2CO_3 (40%). Allow to diffuse about 30 minutes and then add 1 ml of Nessler's reagent. Read and compare with standards in a spectrophotometer at 390 nm.

Treatment

Do not use stomach tube or emetics! Dilute with water with caution since heat may be generated. Neutralize with dilute vinegar or dilute lemon or lime juice. Give milk, cream, white of egg, or olive oil as demulcent. Keep patient warm and quiet. Give cracked ice to relieve thirst, morphine for pain, and sedatives as necessary. If there are signs of asphyxia, tracheotomy may be indicated. Protect against respiratory obstruction, perforation, or stricture formations.

Guard against secondary infection. Cortisone therapy has been recommended in persistent shock and as an antiinflammatory.

If burns are external, wash with ample water and then with dilute vinegar or lemon juice. See Alkalies.

AMPHETAMINE (C₉H₁₃N)

Synonyms

Benzedrine Sulfate: racemic *dl*-amphetamine sulfate; phenyl isopropylamine; methylphenethylamine sulfate; Alentol; Psychoton; Simpamina; "bennies," "Splash," "peaches."

Dexedrine Sulfate: *d*-amphetamine sulfate; *d*-α-methylphenethylamine sulfate; Afatin; Dexamphetamine; *d*-Amfetasul; Domafate; Obesedrin; Dexten; Maxiton; Sympamin; Simpamina-D; Albemap; Dadex; Amsustain; Betaferdrina; "dexies," "co-pilot," "oranges."

Methamphetamine Hydrochloride: *d*-desoxyephedrine hydrochloride; Adipex; Amphedroxyn; Isophen; Methedrine; Destim; Pervitin; Syndrox; "meth," "speed," "water," "crystal."

Uses: For hyperkinetic children; catalepsy; anorexic, to reduce appetite and weight. Antidepressant, combats fatigue. "Bennies for kicks" (for "speed"); alertness, excitation, mood elevator, feeling of well-being. "Doping" for athletes.

Properties: White crystalline; basic; soluble in ethanol, *n*-hexane, ethyl acetate, chloroform; partially soluble in ether.

MLD: Approximately 0.250 gm for a normal, 70 kg person, but a habitué can tolerate *very* large doses (2 gm).

Blood Levels: Therapeutic, 3 mcg/dl; Lethal, 0.2 mg/dl; half-life about 25 hours.

Remarks: Acts as a central nervous system stimulant (sympathomimetic); cerebral cortex is site of action. Dexedrine is two times more toxic than benzedrine; methamphetamine is more powerful than both.

Symptoms: Wakefulness, alertness, decreased sense of fatigue, elevation of mood; capacity for work may be increased with small dose, but this may be reversed with repeated dose.

MILD ADVERSE SYMPTOMS: Apprehensiveness, restlessness, anorexia, tremors, insomnia, talkativeness, tachycardia, flushed face, increased sweating, dilated pupils, dry mouth, chills, abdominal cramps, nausea, vomiting, cardiac arrhythmias, hypertension, glycosuria, hyperactive reflexes, analgesia, fever, belching, flatulence.

The presence of sweating and pupillary response to light differentiates amphetamine from atropine overdose.

MODERATE SYMPTOMS: All of the above but to a greater degree. Increased libido, anxiety, confusion, aggressiveness, delirium, hallucinations, panic state, profuse sweating, hypertension, extrasystoles, diarrhea or constipation. Powerful analeptic, hyperactive reflexes, stimulation followed by depression and fatigue, suicidal and homicidal tendencies, especially in mentally ill patients.

SEVERE SYMPTOMS: All of the above but more severe. Confusion, convulsions, high fever, chest pains, coma, circulatory collapse.

COMMENTS: The amphetamines as a group are often called "pep pills." This group of drugs may be useful when prescribed by a physician and used properly. Abusers, however, when attempting to combat fatigue in sports, or while driving on long trips, or trying to reach a feeling of exhilaration may get into trouble; these drugs may permit damaging exertion because the person may not sense (show signs or symptoms of) being overworked, and damage to the heart can occur.

Other dangers also occur with continuous use; a profound tolerance is developed. This tolerance is developed slowly and becomes very marked, but the margin between euphoria and toxic psychosis remains the same.

Although withdrawal symptoms following continuous use of large dosage are usually physically painless (psychic dependency), great discomfort is experienced, and severe depresssion sometimes leading to suicide may result.

Identification

Urine is the specimen of choice. Specimen must be made (NaOH) strongly alkaline prior to extraction or distillation to effect separation.

Amphetamine base is volatile; evaporate with care (with 5 drops H_2SO_4).

Slowly eliminated in the urine; up to 3 days or more.

Separation from urine is by (a) direct distillation with strong sodium hydroxide (best), (b) resin ion exchange (Amberlite), or (c) solvent extraction [chloroform:isopropanol (4.1); chloroform; *n*- hexane; or ethyl acetate.]

1. Stomach contents, or urine made strongly alkaline with sodium hydroxide, is extracted with three times volume of chloroform. Separate and filter the chloroform layer thru filter paper (to eliminate water droplets.). Add 2 drops of hydrochloric acid and then gently evaporate to barely dryness. Residue is picked up in 5 ml of 0.5N H_2SO_4 and the UV absorption curve is plotted. See next test.

2. Urine (100 ml) plus 4 gm sodium hydroxide (solution is now 1N NaOH). Gently distill (direct) and slowly collect about 90 ml into 10 ml of 6N sulfuric acid. Salting out with NaCl (during distillation) may increase recovery.

    Evaporate solution gently to almost dryness (1 ml). Dilute back to 5 ml with water. (Check pH; should be approximately 0.5N).

    Plot absorption curve with UV spectrophotometer between 220 and 310 nm.

    dl-amphetamine (Benzedrine) and *d*-amphetamine (Dexedrine) in 0.5N sulfuric acid have a maximum density at 258 nm $(E_{1cm}^{1\%}-14)$ and a minimum density at 230 nm.

    $$0.100 \text{ mg}/1 \text{ ml} - 74\% \text{ T} \text{ (den.} = 0.13)$$
    $$0.200 \text{ mg}/1 \text{ ml} - 55\% \text{ T}$$
    $$0.300 \text{ mg}/1 \text{ ml} - 40\% \text{ T}$$

    Tissue which is markedly decomposed may contain β-phenethylamine, tryptophane, or tyramine and will produce a "false" similar curve. These false levels will be usually *very high,* but this *is not* amphetamine and this artifact can be differentiated by GLC and/or TLC. See tests following.

    Some other drugs also give a similar curve with the same maximum density in the UV range. See Section I.

3. After performing test 2 above, the solution can be re-extracted, carefully concentrated, and then reconfirmed by TLC or GLC; or part of the same solution may be used for the following

color tests (see Alkaloids). Amphetamine does not react to yield crystals or a precipitate with Wagner's, Mayer's, Marme's, or picric acid reagent. Amphetamine base and its sulfate salt each give color reactions with the various alkaloidal reagents. Place small aliquot portions of residue into various grooves of a porcelain spot plate and test with fresh reagents:

a. *Sulfuric Acid:*
   salt → red-brown
   base → green-yellow
b. *Marquis reagent* (5 ml H_2SO_4 plus 5 drop formaldehyde 40%):
   salt → orange → red → brown
   base → orange → brown-orange
c. *Mandelin's reagent* (5 mg ammonium vanadate plus 5 ml H_2SO_4):
   salt → brick-red
   base → green, darkens rapidly
d. *Sulfuric acid/vanillin:*
   salt → brown-orange
e. *Frohde's reagent* (5 mg molybdic acid plus 5 ml H_2SO_4):
   salt → red (pale)
   base → brown-yellow

Frings-Queen-Foster method:

5 ml urine fixed at pH 5.5 with 2 ml of acetate buffer.

25 ml chloroform—extract for about 1–2 minutes.

Separate and transfer 5 ml of *aqueous* (upper) layer to a glass-stoppered test tube containing 2 ml of NaOH (2.5 mol/liter) and 25 ml of benzene and 0.5 ml of isoamyl alcohol; shake for 1 minute; centrifuge to separate.

Transfer 20 ml of benzene (upper) layer to a 50 ml tube containing 1 ml of methyl orange reagent. Shake for 1 minute; centrifuge layers.

Transfer 15 ml of the benzene (upper) layer to a 50 ml glass-stoppered centrifuge tube containing 3.5 ml of hydrochloric acid (1 mol/liter). Shake for 1 minute; centrifuge.

Aspirate and *discard* the benzene (upper) layer. Measure O.D. of acidic (lower) layer at 515 nm, against blank. Acidic layer to be measured is pink; color increases with concentration.

Conc	T
5γ	——
10γ	——
30γ	80
35γ	75
50γ	55T

Reagents:

- Acetate buffer (2 mol/liter, pH 5.5) : Dissolve 142 gm anhydrous NaAc in 800 ml H_2O. Adjust to pH 5.5 with glacial HAc. Dilute to 1 liter. Stable for 6 months.
- NaOH (2.5 mol/liter) : Dissolve 10.0 g NaOH in H_2O, to 100 ml. Stable in polyethylene bottle for 1 year.
- Working methyl orange reagent: Mix equal parts of stock methyl orange (dissolve 180 mg of sodium salt of methyl orange with heat) and saturated boric acid solution just before use. Should be used within 1 hour.
- Hydrochloric acid (1 mol/liter) : 83 ml of HCl diluted to 1 liter.

5. Tests to perform on tablets:
   a. Pulverize tablets (50 mg) with 5 ml of water. Allow to stand 15 minutes, then filter; add 1 ml of 10% sodium hydroxide; then add benzoyl chloride (0.5 ml) a little at a time until no further precipitation occurs. Filter; wash precipitate with 15 ml of cold water; recrystallize from dilute alcohol. Amphetamine benzoyl derivative: Mp 132 to 135°C.
   b. Tablet is ground; while grinding, add 2 ml of water. Filter and add 1 ml of 10% barium chloride to the filtrate. A white precipitate that is insoluble in nitric acid is positive for the sulfate radical.
   c. Tablet is ground; while grinding, add 5 ml of water. Transfer to test tube (Pyrex) and add two pellets of sodium hydroxide without touching the sides. Place a moist strip of red litmus paper across the test tube opening and then gently heat. The paper turns blue (ammonia) if a volatile primary amine is heated with a strong alkali.
   d. Tablet is ground; while grinding, add 10 ml of water.

Filter and add sodium bicarbonate until solution is saturated. Make sure the NaHCO$_3$ is in excess, then add 1 ml of acetic anhydride. Carbon dioxide is liberated; gently swirl to accelerate this liberation. Then add 0.5 ml of additional acetic anhydride. Swirl and allow to stand about 10 minutes. Add 25 ml of chloroform and extract the derivative. Separate and filter the chloroform to remove droplets of the aqueous phase; evaporate; add few drops of ether and re-crystallize. Examine the crystals. Melting points:

d-amphetamine: 119–122°C
dl-amphetamine: 98–100°C
Methamphetamine: 90–92°C

6. Thin layer chromatography (TLC):

Twenty-five (25) ml of urine plus 2 ml of 10N sodium hydroxide is gently extracted with 50 ml of chloroform: isopropanol (4:1). The organic solvent is filtered through filter paper into an evaporating dish, then gently evaporated to about 10 ml. At this time 2 drops of 0.5N hydrochloric acid is added and gentle evaporation is continued to dryness.

The residue is picked up with a *minimal* quantity of methanol. This is now analyzed by GLC and TLC, see Section I.

a. Method of Osorio:

Developing solvent: n-hexane:acetone:ammonium hydroxide (80:20:1).
Distance: 10 cm (which takes approximately 30 minutes).
Ninhydrin Solution Spray: 0.22 gm in 100 ml acetone. Prepare fresh each time.
Iodoplatinate Solution Spray: 0.25 gm platinic chloride in 10 ml of water is added to 5 gm potassium iodide in 50 ml of water. Mixture is diluted to 100 ml with water.

When developing solvent has traveled to premarked 10 cm distance, plate is removed, dried with current of air, and then heated to about 60°C for 5 minutes.

While plate is still hot, spray with ninhydrin and then place under UV light for 5 minutes. The pink spots due to amphetamine, dextroamphetamine and phenylpropanolamine are marked; hydroxyamphetamine is colored purple.

The plate now at room temperature is sprayed with iodoplatinate solution. This now yields a violet to brown spot for methamphetamine and benzphetamine.

Compound	Rf	Compound	Rf
amphetamine · HCl		ethoheptazine	
(Benzedrine)	38	(Zactane)	32
methamphetamine · HCl		phenelzine (Nardil)	34
(Methedrine)	23	methylphenidate	
phenylpropanolamine · HCl		(Ritalin)	40
(Propadrine)	51	mephenesin (Tolserol)	08
ephedrine · HCl	—	hydroxyzine (Atarax)	11
caffeine	06	benzactyzine (Suavitil)	14
hydroxyamphetamine		trihexyphenydil	
(Paredrine)	07	(Artane)	96
phenmetrazine (Preludin)	23	diethylpropion	
mephentermine		(Tenuate)	97
(Wyamine)	28		

Spot can be scraped off, re-extracted and confirmed by GLC.

b. Method of Repetto:

Developer: Petroleum ether: ether (4:1).

Urine (50 ml) or saliva (5 ml) is made alkaline with sodium hydroxide and then extracted with 50 ml of benzene: isoamyl alcohol (15:1) v/v.

Centrifuge to break emulsion; separate; and evaporate solvent to small volume. Spot this extract on a TLC plate with β-phenylisopropylamine as a marker. Add developing solvent for about 30 minutes. Then locate spot with a UV lamp (254); yellow fluorescence at Rf 0.40.

c. Method of Dole et al.:

Developer: Ethyl acetate:methanol: NH_4OH (85:10:5) (Davidow et al). Ninhydrin Spray: 0.4% ninhydrin in acetone, prepared within 30 minutes of use. Then irradiate plate with UV light for 15 minutes. Examine.

Iodoplatinate Spray: 3 ml of 10% platinum chloride plus 97 ml of water is mixed with 100 ml of 4% potassium iodide. Heat for about 30 minutes or allow to age 1 day.

Store in an amber bottle.

Compound	Rf	Ninhydrin and UV irradiation	Iodoplatinate
Amphetamine	0.57	red (sensitive to 0.5 μg)	yellow-purple (sensitive to 4 μg)

d. Method of Grant:

Developer: Acetonitrile:benzene:ethyl acetate:ammonium hydroxide (60:15:10:10).

Spray: Iodoplatinate.

Examine under UV light; dry: Be certain all ammonia is removed before spraying.

Compound	Rf	UV light	Iodoplatinate
Amphetamine HCl	0.40	Blue	Blue
methamphetamine HCl	0.34	Blue	Purple
phenylpropanolamine HCl	0.29	Blue	Tan-purple
ephedrine HCl	0.26	Blue	Tan with purple ring
caffeine	0.61	Dark blue	

e. Amphetamine by UV, Method of Wallace et al.:

Blood or urine (10 ml) is made alkaline with 5 ml of 1N sodium hydroxide and then extracted with 200 ml of n-hexane for about 3 minutes. Separate and record the recovered hexane. This is extracted with 10 ml of 0.8N hydrochloric acid for about 3 minutes. Separate and transfer 9 ml of the aqueous layer into a 250 ml round-bottomed flask that contains 1.5 gm anhydrous cerium sulfate and 50 ml of n-hexane (spectro quality). The contents are slowly refluxed with magnetic stirring for 30 minutes. Cool and remove the hexane, which is read in the (250–360 nm) UV range against the n-hexane as reference blank. Determine the absorbance at 287 nm. For trace quantities evaporate (concentrate) the hexane extract with a rotary vacuum evaporate to about 3 ml and read at 287 nm. Compare with standards prepared in a similar fashion.

This amphetamine derivative is almost twenty times

more sensitive to the UV than is amphetamine. Maximum density, 287 nm; $E_{1cm}^{1\%} = 220$; minimum density: 253 nm.

Other drugs containing the β-phenylethylamine group will also give a positive reaction with ceric sulfate. These may be differentiated by GLC, see Section I.

7. Gas liquid chromatography (GLC):

Extract used in the UV test above, or the isolated spraying spot on the TLC plate, may be scraped off and re-extracted and tested by GLC.

Inject 1-5 μl of the hexane extract. GLC column 10% SE 30, 6 × 35 mm on GC Q (100–200 mesh). Flame ionization detector. Column temperature 238°C, carrier gas N_2, 50 ml per minute.

a. Official Olympic Method (7):

Ten (10) ml of urine, then 1 ml of 20% sodium hydroxide are placed in a glass-stoppered tube. Extract with 2 × 5 ml of ether (salting with solid NaCl may improve extraction). The extract is concentrated to about 50 μl on a water bath at 40°C. Do not allow to dry; this will lead to loss. This extract is analyzed by TLC described above and also by GLC. Approximately 3–5 μl are injected into at least two different GLC systems.

b. Method of Lebish et al.:

Five (5) ml of urine plus 1 ml of *n*-propylamphetamine HCl (2.5 mg/100 ml H_2O) plus 0.1 ml HCl is shaken with 20 ml of chloroform. Shake for 1 minute and discard the lower chloroform layer. Add 1 ml KOH (60%) and extract with 25 ml of $CHCl_3$ (containing 0.1 mg/ml methyl laurate in $CHCl_3$). Separate and filter the $CHCl_3$ through a short glass tube packed with anhydrous calcium sulfate.

Collect one-half the extract into a 15 ml conical tube marked A. Collect the other one-half of the extract into a similar tube marked B. To tube A, add 0.2 ml redistilled acetic anhydride. To tube B, add 0.2 ml benzaldehyde reagent (0.1 ml in 5 ml $CHCl_3$). Evaporate the $CHCl_3$ in both tubes (gently) with a stream of filtered air. Redissolve the residue in each tube with 25 ml of $CHCl_3$. Inject

1.0 μl of tube A into OV-17 column at 140°C. Screen result of n-acetyl amphetamine:

Compound	Retention Time
methyl laurate	1.5 min
amphetamine	4.0
methamphetamine	5.5
N-propyl amphetamine	8.5

Inject 1.0 μl of tube B into OV-17 column at 165°C.

Compound	Retention Time
Amphetamine	3.5 min

To confirm the presence of benzyl derivatives (only amphetamine now appears). The presence of methamphetamine is confirmed by its metabolite amphetamine.

c. Method of Finkle:

Flame ionization detector and a 2 column system: S.E. 30 column temperature 130°C (6 ft. long and $\frac{1}{4}$ inch I.D.) and Alkaline carbowax column temperature 130°C (4 ft. long and $\frac{1}{4}$ inch I.D.).

If a positive response is obtained by either or both above columns, then add 5 μl of acetic anhydride to 5 μl of sample and mix. Inject 1 μl of this mixture, using the S.E. 30 column at 170°C.

Maximum urine concentration following a single dose (10 mg) of either amphetamine or methamphetamine is between 3 to 5 μg/ml and is achieved within 24 hours of ingestion. Detection is sensitive to about 0.5 μg/ml.

β-phenethylamine may occur in urine and can accumulate in vitro. Analyzing fresh sample and refrigeration is the best precaution in eliminating this interference.

Treatment

Patient should be isolated in a dark and quiet room; disturbance and manipulation must be kept at a minimum; control excitement and convulsion with diazepam (Valium). Chlorpromazine may also help to offset excitatory state.

Delay absorption with milk and/or activated charcoal, then remove by gastric lavage or emesis followed by cathartic. Maintain acid urine at approximately pH 5 with ammonium chloride; this will greatly hasten elimination from the body. Maintain patent airway and respiration; maintain body fluid and electrolyte balance. Artificial respiration if needed; control convulsions and blood pressure as required.

Barbiturates should not be given without deep consideration (of postexcitatory depression), and then only the short-acting ones (with caution).

References

1. Frings, C.S., Queen, C., and Foster, L.B.: *Clin Chem, 17:*1016, 1971.
2. Osorio, Raúl G.: *Toxicology of Amphetamines,* Thesis (MSc.), University of Puerto Rico, School of Medicine, 1970.
3. Repetto, M.J.: Amphetamine detection by TLC. *Inter Assoc Foren Toxicol, 3(3):* June, 1965.
4. Dole, V.P., Kim, M., and Eglitis, I.: Detection of narcotic drugs, tranquilizers, amphetamines and barbiturates in urine. *JAMA, 198:*115, 1966.
5. Grant, R.C.: Cited in Osorio (2).
6. Wallace, I.E., Biggs, J.A., and Ladd, S.L.: Determination of amphetamine by UV. *Anal Chem, 40:*2207, 1968.
7. Personal Communication with Official Olympic Committee, 1972.
8. Lebish, P., Finkle, B.S., and Brackett, J.W.: Determination of amphetamines in blood and urine by gas chromatography. *Clin Chem, 16:* 195, 1970.
9. Finkle, Bryan: Amphetamine and related phenethylamines. In Sunshine, I. (Ed): *Manual of Analytical Toxicology.* Cleveland, Ohio, The Chemical Rubber Co., 1971, pp. 24-27.
10. Davidow, B., Petri, N.L., and Quame, B.: Thin layer chromatography screening procedure for detecting drug abuse. *Am J Clin Path, 50:* 714, 1968.

ANILINE (C_6H_7N)

Synonyms: Aminobenzene; phenylamine; aniline oil.

Uses: Dyes, fat solvents, inks; aniline dyes in rubber stamp ink, paints, shoe polish, and colored crayons (as aniline dyes).

Properties: Yellow liquid. Unpleasant odor. Bp 184–186°C.

MLD: Approximately 5 gm/70 kg person.

Remarks: Eliminated in urine as *p*-aminophenol (dark-colored urine).   Can be absorbed by inhalation or through the skin (dye on diapers).   Symptoms appear within 1 to 3 hours.

Symptoms: Nausea, vomiting, abdominal pain, diarrhea, headache, dyspnea, anemia, weakness, mental confusion, skin irritation, mental excitement, restlessness, delirium, convulsions, depression, coma; marked *methemoglobinemia: Chocolate-colored blood* or cyanosis may be evident with blood levels at 20 percent. Liver and kidney damage may develop with jaundice, nephrosis, and anuria after a delayed period; *hemolysis* and red-colored urine are noted.   At levels of 60 percent of methemoglobinemia and above, there is extreme weakness due to oxygen lack.   Other effects of methemoglobinemia include tachycardia, headache, dizziness, mild confusion, dyspnea, salivation, ataxia, drowsiness, flushing of skin, palpitations, visual disturbances, fall in blood pressure, weak pulse, collapse, cerebral anoxia, respiratory and/or cardiac failure, convulsions before death.

Identification

Isolated by alkaline-steam distillation.

1. Extract residue, gastric lavage, or vomitus with 2 × volume of ether.   Separate and carefully evaporate solvent to near dryness; oily residue with a typical odor suggests aniline.

2. *Alkaline* steam distillation of gastric lavage or vomitus made alkaline with NaOH will distill and separate aniline.   Divide into several aliquot portions.

   a. Read in UV spectrophotometer; water reference blank: maximum density 280 nm; minimum density 260 nm.   See Section I.

      Nitrobenzene: maximum density, 270 nm; minimum density, 228 nm.

   b. To a 10 ml aliquot add 1 ml of bromine water → flesh colored precipitate (tribromo aniline) .

   c. Isonitrile test: To a 15 ml of aliquot add 1 ml of chloroform plus 5 ml of 20% NaOH and gently heat.   *Carefully* smell for characteristic skunk-like odor (isonitrile) , which is sharp and penetrating.

   d. To a 10 ml aliquot is added several drops of calcium hypochlorite (fresh). Blue-violet or purple-violet will appear, which changes to dirty red. Adding 1 ml of 10% phenol that contains a trace of ammonium hydroxide will again produce a blue color, which is stable.

3. See Section I (TLC).

   $CHCl_3$:ethanol (99:1).

4. Test for methemoglobin (modified from Jatlow and Horecher by Emma Rodriguez): Methemoglobin is converted to hemoglobin on standing at room temperature. If sample cannot be analyzed immediately then freeze it.*

   Blood should be heparinized or EDTA treated; all reagents should be reagent quality and freshly prepared.

   Place 25 ml of buffer solution into a centrifuge tube and then add 0.5 ml of specimen blood (1:50). Mix and allow to stand for 5 minutes.

   Centrifuge for 10 minutes and save the entire hemolysate. Measure the absorbance of hemolysate at 630 nm (A_1) using water as the reference blank; methemoglobin has a characteristic absorbance at 630 nm.

   To the same above hemolysate and reference blank add 1 drop of the cyanide solution to each cuvette (or TT for mixing).

   Mix and allow to stand for 2 minutes and then again determine the absorbance (A_2). NaCN converts methemoglobin to cyanomethemoglobin and the absorbance band at 630 nm is abolished.

   To another 10 ml hemolysate from above, add 0.5 ml of $K_3Fe(CN)_6$ solution; this will now convert all hemoglobin to methemoglobin. Mix and allow to stand 2 minutes. Measure absorbance (A_3) at 630 nm. All hemoglobin is converted to methemoglobin (100%).

   To this same solution now add 1 drop of cyanide solution. Mix and allow to stand for 2 minutes and then read absorbance

---

*Other drugs that can also produce methemoglobin: nitrobenzene, nitroglycerine, chlorates, amyl nitrite, sodium and potassium nitrites, and possibly nitrates in infants, which may convert to nitrites. Nitroaniline is more toxic than aniline.

at 630 nm (A_4), which will be 100% cyanomethemoglobin.

$$\% \text{ methemoglobin} = \frac{A_1 - A_2}{A_3 - A_4} \times 100$$

Normal blood contains less than 3% methemoglobin.
Levels of 30% methemoglobin (or less) revert to normal in about 3 days without treatment.

Note: Quantitative differences in the foregoing test are not too distinct, but reliable approximations may be made. These tests are easy to perform and are excellent for qualitative detection. Clinical signs and symptoms are very necessary and are even more reliable in determining degree of intoxication once the methemoglobin is positively established. Methemoglobin may be congenital or produced by some drugs or chemicals.

Reagents:

- Phosphate buffer: 1.2 gm Na_2HPO_4 in 500 ml of water; 1.1 gm KH_2PO_4 in 500 ml of water; add the Na_2HPO_4 solution to KH_2PO_4, until you get a pH of 6.6.
- NaCN neutralized solution: NaCN 10 gm in 100 ml water; 12 glacial acetic acid diluted to 100 ml with water; combine in a hood with great care (HCN) equal volumes of both solutions within 1 hour prior to use.
- $K_3Fe(CN)_6$ solution: 20 gm in 100 ml water.

References: Jatlow, P.; In Sunshine, I. (Ed.) : *Methodology for Analytical Toxicology,* Cleveland, CRC Press, 1975. Horecher and Brackett; *J Biochem, 152:*669, 1944.

5. Spectroscopic technic (most specific). With a spectroscope, absorption bands are seen:

α 630 nm
β 578
γ 540
Δ 500

Identify the band at 630 nm. If it is present, then add several crystals of potassium cyanide and the 630 band disappears.

Sulfhemoglobin has a band at 520 nm, and it does not disappear with cyanide.

Treatment

Avoid fats or oils or alcohol.

Use activated charcoal to slow up absorption and then gastric lavage and saline cathartics (sodium sulfate 30 gm). Wash skin with soap and water to fully remove exposure.

Oxygen therapy if cyanotic; methylene blue (1% IV) slowly for severe methemoglobinemia; or an exchange transfusion of whole blood. Ascorbic acid or sodium ascorbate or thionine have been reported to be of some help to hasten conversion to normal hemoglobin (but is slow acting).

Little treatment is required for methemoglobin if less than 30 percent and if the exposure has been removed. Normal conversion is about 0.5 gm per hour.

ANTIHISTAMINES

Members

antazoline (Antistine)
Antergan
brompheniramine maleate (Dimetane)
buclizine (Bucladin)
captodiamine HCl (Suvren)
carbetapentane (Rynatuss)
carbinoxamine maleate (Clistin)
chlorcyclizine (Perazyl)
chlorothen citrate (Tagathen)
Chlorpheniramine (Chlor-Trimeton)
chlorphenoxamine (Systiral)
clemizole (Allercur)
cyclizine (Marezine)
cyproheptadine HCl (Periactin)
dimenhydrinate (Dramamine)
dimethindene maleate (Forhistal)
diphenhydramine HCl (Benadryl)
diphenylpyraline (Diafen)
doxylamine (Decapryn) succinate
hydroxyzine (Atarax)
meclizine dihydrochloride (Bonine; Antivert)

methaphenilene (Diatrin)
methapyrilene (Dozar; Histadyl; Nods; Nytol; Triohistine; Thenylene; Semikon)
methdilazine HCl (Tacaryl)
phenindamine (Thephorin)
pheniramine (Trimeton; Inhiston)
promethazine HCl (Phenergan)
pyrathiazine HCl (Pyrrolazote)
pyrilamine (Antamine; Antihist; Diamidide; Neo-Antergan; Renstamin; Thylogen)
pyrrobutamine (Pyronil)
thenalidine (Sandostene)
thenyldiamine (Thenfadil)
thonzylamine HCl (Anahist; Neohetrimine, HCl; Resistab)
trimethobenzamide HCl (Tigan)
tripelennamine (Pyribenzamine)
triprolidine HCl monohydrate (Actidil)

Uses: Allergies, colds, sedation, motion sickness, aid to sleep. To block histamine receptors.

DURATION OF ACTION (THERAPEUTIC) : About 4–6 hours.

MLD: Varies with drug from about 250 mg upwards, for 70 kg person.

Symptoms

OVERDOSE: May vary between drugs and even between patients; convulsions and coma are most frequently seen with severe poisoning. Anticholinergic action and generally resembles atropine overdose (see atropine).

GENERALIZED: May produce convulsions in children and depression in adults. Onset may be slow. Nausea, vomiting, ataxia, impaired coordination, excitement, disorientation, drowsiness, hyperpyrexia, dry mouth, irritability, headache, dilated pupils, hallucinations, tachycardia, generalized depression, urine retension, convulsions, stupor, coma, respiratory failure.

Identification

Urine is best, Acid hydrolysis for 5 minutes; neutralize with strong sodium hydroxide and fix pH at 11. Direct extraction with chloroform or ether, whichever is best as indicated below in test 1.

Direct extraction is not effective for diphenhydramine where you must use ion exchange (Amberlite) or steam distillation for in vivo recoveries. Chlorpheniramine is recoverable in vivo by steam distillation and direct extraction but is not recoverable by ion exchange.

All *others* listed above are *not* recoverable by steam distillation.

1. UV Spectrophotometry: See Table XXIV.

TABLE XXIV
UV SPECTROPHOTOMETRY*

	H_2SO_4 (0.5N) Max den	$E \frac{1\%}{1cm}$	Min den	Best extraction *solvent* at pH 11 except: **
antazoline	241	553	273	chloroform
	291	65		
azatadine	283	173	257	chloroform
brompheniramine	264	271	245	chloroform
chlorothen	237	585	271	chloroform
	312	267		
chlorpheniramine	264	280	242	chloroform
cycliramine	239	392	240	ethyl ether
	295	129		
cyproheptadine	224	1204	263	ethyl ether
	285	367		
dexbrompheniramine	265	284	245	ethyl ether
dexchlorpheniramine	264	292	242	chloroform
dimenhydrinate	276	300	246	**
dimethindene	258	620	232	chloroform
diphenhydramine	258	20	243	**
shoulder	252	17		
methapyrilene	237	643	263	chloroform
	312	284		
methdilazine	252	1000	274	ethyl ether
	302	110		
phenindamine	259	300	241	ethyl ether
promethazine	249	959	270	ethyl ether
	300	105		
tripelennamine	239	482	238	chloroform
	312	284		
tripolidine	290	300	240	chloroform
zolamine	227	420	244	chloroform
	265	469		

*From Narvaez, V.: *Toxicology.* Thesis (M.Sc.), University of Puerto Rico, Medical Sciences Campus, 1975.

2. TLC: See Table XXV.

TABLE XXV

DEVELOPING SOLVENT SYSTEMS AND THE RECORDED RF VALUES FOR EACH DRUG*

Antihistamine	1	2	3	4	5	6	7	8	9	10	11	I.A.S.
antazoline hydrochloride	.55	.35	.86	.21	.26	.24	.20	.06	.06	.28	.72	d.b.‡
azatadine maleate	.80	.42	.65	.25	.25	.43	.42	.13	.05	.31	.25	d.b.
brompheniramine maleate	.80	.74	.71	.14	.23	.76	.38	.24	.10	.73	.49	d.b.
chlorothen citrate	.90	.92	.78	.33	.32	.84	.53	.63	.45	.96	.39	d.b.
chlorpheniramine maleate	.84	.68	.74	.36	.55	.79	.57	.47	.13	.80	.39	d.b.
cycliramine maleate	.87	.56	.71	.24	.27	.59	.44	.17	.09	.49	.27	d.b.
cyproheptadine hydrochloride	.92	.94	.86	.40	.43	.89	.57	.59	.44	.95	.64	d.b.
dexbrompheniramine maleate	.83	.67	.77	.24	.55	.75	.43	.37	.11	.75	.43	d.b.
dexchlorpheniramine maleate	.82	.65	.75	.23	.35	.73	.43	.35	.10	.70	.40	d.b.
dimenhydrinate	.92	.92	.85	.44	.46	.90	.55	.75	.38	.82	.56	d.b.
dimethindene maleate	.84	.70	.63	.17	.23	.75	.30	.27	.10	.73	.25	d.b.
diphenhydramine hydrochloride	.80	.90	.87	.52	.54	.93	.63	.69	.45	.97	.74	d.b.
methapyrilene hydrochloride	.33	.92	.81	.47	.57	.89	.57	.68	.36	.57	.54	d.b.
methdilazine	.78	.77	.85	.26	.29	.82	.36	.45	.20	.84	.51	d.b.
methdilazine hydrochloride	.77	.77	.85	.15	.19	.78	.29	.32	.21	.82	.51	d.b.
promethazine hydrochloride	.92	.96	.90	.41	.46	.87	.63	.77	.52	.97	.78	d.b.
phenidamine tartrate	.98	.97	.90	.58	.56	.94	.70	.80	.56	Front	.60	d.b.
tripelennamine citrate	.93	.94	.68	.33	.35	.92	.45	.50	.40	.97	.38	d.b.
tripelennamine hydrochloride	.94	.96	.77	.32	.34	.93	.49	.61	.37	.84	.42	d.b.
triprolidine hydrochloride	.91	.83	.84	.37	.42	.84	.41	.30	.16	.93	.74	d.b
zolamine hydrochloride	.96	.96	.78	.47	.55	.78	.64	.62	.37	.96	.55	d.b.

*From Narváez, V: Toxicology, Thesis (M.Sc.), University of Puerto Rico, Medical Science Campus, 1975.

†*Developing Solvents:*
1. Strong ammonia solution: methanol (1.5:100) (Sunshine, 1963).
2. Strong ammonia solution: benzene: dioxane (5:60:35) (Colchin & Daly, 1963).
3. Acetic acid (glacial): ethanol: Water (30:50:20) (Colchin & Daly, 1963).
4. 95% ethanol (100 ml) (Sunshine, Fike, Landesman, 1966).
5. n-Butanol: methanol (40:60).
6. Cyclohexane: benzene:diethylamine (75:15:10).
7. Methanol (100 ml).
8. Acetone (100 ml).
9. Benzene: acetone: ammonium hydroxide (100:20:6).
10. Basic developing solvent: (100 ml ethyl ether: 25 ml ammonium hydroxide (shake, mix allow to settle, and separate and discard aqueous).
11. Acidic developing solvent: Methylene chloride: 95% ethanol: acetic acid (shake, mix allow to settle, and separate and discard aqueous).

I.A.S.: Iodoplatinic Acid Spray

‡d.b. = Dark brown

TLC SPRAYS

• Iodoplatinic acid: 0.25 gm of platinic chloride and 5 gm KI in 100 ml of water plus 2 ml of HCl. Adding the HCl before spraying will increase stability of stock reagent.
Spray produces a dark brown stain.

• Dragendorff: Mix (a) 0.2 gm bismuth subnitrate in 10 ml H_2O plus 0.25 ml of glacid acetic acid, (b) 0.4 gm KI in 10 ml H_2O, and (c) 20 ml of glacial acetic acid plus 100 ml of H_2O → Spray produces an orange yellow stain.

• $KMnO_4$ 1% → yellow stain

• H_2SO_4 60% → pink or white

• H_2SO_4 5% → pink or white

OTHER SYSTEMS FOR TLC:

Developer: S-1 acetone:methyl alcohol:isopropylamine (85:15:1)

Developer: S-2 acetic acid:ethanol:water (30:50:20)

Spray: Acid-iodoplatinate reagent.

	S-1 (Rf)	S-2 (Rf)
Phenergan	78	74
Benadryl	76	75
Chlor-trimeton	46	57
Thorazine	78	77
Tofranil	72	75
Elavil	71	77
Compazine	65	63
Stelazine	67	69

For other TLC systems, see Section I.

3. Color and crystal tests, see Alkaloids.
KCN; Na_2CO_3; PbI_2 (1% in acetic acid solution) may also give crystals for some.

4. Gas chromatography (GLC):
Varian Aerograph 200; column 4 feet by $\frac{1}{4}$ inch o.d., glass 2% SE-30, 2% carbowax, 20M on 80–100 mesh diatoport S. Column temperature 220°C; injection port temperature 240°C. Detector temperature 245°C; carries gas nitrogen. 26 ml/minutes;

hydrogen flow 38 ml/minute; air flow 230 ml/minute; Detector: flame ionization.

Also see Section I.

Treatment

Control convulsions with Valium; activated charcoal. Then follow with gastric lavage and catharsis (saline) ; or induce vomiting. Ipecac syrup may still be effective in spite of a possible antiemetic action of the antihistaminic drug. Maintain all vital functions, especially respiratory exchange with a patent airway. Maintain water, heat, electrolyte balance, and blood pressure. Do not use stimulants.

Treat hyperpyrexia with tepid water sponging. Physostigmine salicylate (with caution) may help to alleviate the anticholinergic (atropinelike) symptoms. Continue to treat symptomatically and supportive (*see* atropine).

ANTIMONY (Sb)

Derivatives: Tartar emetic; stibnite; antimony trichloride; stibine.

Uses: Alloys, plating, pigments, mordants, batteries, ant paste, matches.

Properties: Corrosive.

MLD: Approximately 1 gm/70 kg person.

Remarks: Similar to arsenic in properties and treatment; cumulative. Stibine (SbH_3) gas is especially toxic and may be generated when antimony is present in battery plates.

Symptoms: Metallic taste, gastrointestinal irritation, nausea, vomiting, diarrhea, rice-water stool, increased capillary permeability, dermatitis, conjunctivitis; spasm of fingers, arms, and legs; abdominal pain, depression, salivation, slow shallow respiration, cyanosis, cold sweat, great thirst, subnormal temperature, liver and kidney damage, collapse, coma, death from cardiac failure.

Identification

1. Solution of antimony strongly acidified with hydrochloric acid and saturated with hydrogen sulfide gas produces an orange

precipitate, which is insoluble in ammonia but soluble in ammonium sulfide solution.

2. Twenty (20) ml of urine, stomach contents, etc., is placed in a small Erlenmeyer flask. Hydrochloric acid (4 ml) and a small copper strip (5 × 5 mm) or copper spiral are added. (The copper spiral is prepared by winding a length of 20 gauge copper wire tightly and closely around a glass rod and then cutting it into $\frac{1}{4}$ inch lengths.) The contents of the flask are gently heated for approximately 1 hour, after which time the spiral is removed and examined. A dark purple sheen deposit will indicate the presence of antimony. This deposition is sensitive to 0.020 mg per 20 ml of solution. The intensity of deposit is directly proportional to concentration and can be compared with standards similarly prepared.

3. Further confirmation and determination: The antimony deposit on the copper spiral prepared in test 2 above is immediately placed into a modified Gutzeit apparatus (described and illustrated under arsenic) but, when testing for antimony, it is preferable to impregnate the disc of filter paper with a 5% solution of silver nitrate instead of the mercuric bromide as suggested for arsenic, because antimony will not react with mercuric bromide if present in less than 100 μg.

If antimony is present, it is converted in the Gutzeit test into stibine, which stain the silver nitrate paper a light gray to dark black. The intensity of this stain is proportional to the quantity of stibine produced. This color stain is matched with a series of standards similarly prepared—values ranging from 0.01 to 0.10 mg of antimony. These standard stains are stable if stored in the dark. Since arsenic may act similarly, to confirm further, place stained disc over bottle of hydrochloric acid. The hydrochloric acid fumes will completely fade the stain due to antimony (in 15 minutes), whereas if due to arsenic the stain remains unchanged.

This test is specific for antimony.

To test for mercury, bismuth, sulfur, selenium, and tellurium, refer to Section I.

4. Atomic absorption is best, if available.

Treatment

Activated charcoal and gastric lavage, or give emetics. Use demulcents such as raw eggs, cream, or milk; saline cathartics (sodium sulfate, 25 gm).

Keep patient warm and quiet. Morphine for pain.

SPECIFIC TREATMENT: BAL (dimercaprol), follow package insert directions. Guard against shock, dehydration, and pulmonary edema.

Maintain body heat, fluid, and electrolyte balance. Oxygen and/or artificial respiration as needed. Support against possible liver damage. See under Arsenic.

ANTIPYRINE ($C_{11}H_{12}N_2O$)

Synonyms: Sedatine; pyrazolons.

Uses: Anodyne, analgesic.

Properties: White crystalline. Mp 110–113°C. Neutral compound. Very soluble in chloroform or ethanol.

MLD: Approximately 5 gm/70 kg person.

Remarks: Similar to acetanilide in symptoms.

Symptoms: Hypopyrexia, methemoglobinemia, cyanosis, excitement, muscular twitching, weakness, drowsiness, dyspnea, cold perspiration, pallor, anemia, skin eruption, agranulocytosis, rapid and feeble pulse, diminished urine volume, delirium, convulsions; kidney, liver, and brain changes; respiratory failure, death.

Identification

Alkaline-chloroform group extraction.
1. Urine is light red (if urine is acid).
2. urine (10 ml) + 10% ferric chloride (2 ml) → blue
3. urine (10 ml) + glacial acetic acid (1 ml) + 5 drops of alkaloidal reagent:
    a. Wagner's reagent → brown precipitate
    b. Mayer's reagent → white precipitate.
    c. Picric acid (saturated) → yellow precipitate (Mp 188°C)
4. residue + drop of bromine water → violet → rapidly changes → pink → yellow

5. residue + drop of Mandelin's reagent → brown → olive green → green

6. Both antipyrine and amidopyrine yield alkaloidal precipitates. To differentiate:
   a. silver nitrate → purple (amidopyrine)
                    → nothing (antipyrine)
   b. ferric chloride → blue-violet (amidopyrine)
                     → blood red (antipyrine)
   c. Dissolve in dilute sulfuric acid and a trace of sodium nitrite
      → blue-violet → quickly fades (amidopyrine).
      →intense green color (antipyrine).

7. UV: See Section I.
8. TLC: See Section I.
9. GLC: See Section I.

Treatment

Gastric lavage and/or emetics. Saline cathartics (25 gm of sodium sulfate). Keep patient warm and quiet. Counteract stimulation with Valium; symptomatic treatment for cardiac and respiratory distress; artificial respiration and oxygen therapy, and other supportive measures, as needed.

ANTU ($C_{11}H_{10}N_2S$)

Synonym: Alpha-naphthylthiourea.

Use: Rodenticide.

Properties: Odorless. Bitter taste. Neutral white crystalline. Mp 198°C. Soluble in propylene glycol, dioxane, or acetone; relatively insoluble in water, ether, ethyl alcohol (cold).

MLD: Approximately 5 gm/70 kg person.

Remarks: Relatively low toxicity for chickens, man, and rabbit. Much more toxic for dogs and cats, and especially Norway rats.

Symptoms: Massive pulmonary edema and pleural effusion; acts as a mild emetic; dyspnea, hypopyrexia; affects hair growth and skin pigmentation; hyperglycemia (three times normal in 3 hours).

Identification

ANTU is a neutral compound and can therefore be extracted in either acid- or alkaline-chloroform group.

Extract the acidified solution of powder, stomach contents, etc., with three times its volume of ether. Evaporate the ether layer and perform the following tests (see under alkaloids).

1. ANTU is precipitated by alkaloidal reagents. Small residue is acidified with 1 drop of 2% acetic acid. See Alkaloids.
   a. one drop of Wagner's reagent → brown precipitate (typical crystals) (50 μg/ml)
   b. one drop of Mayer's reagent → white precipitate (typical crystals)
2. The following alkaloidal reagents produce characteristic colors. A small trace of ANTU extract is placed into groove of a porcelain spot plate. See Alkaloids.
   a. add 1 drop of concentrated sulfuric acid → no color → heat → no color
   b. add 1 drop of Marquis' reagent → green → heat → gray
   c. add 1 drop of Fröhde's reagent → violet → heat → green-blue
   d. add 1 drop of concentrated nitric acid → red → heat → yellow
   e. add 1 drop of Mandelin's reagent → violet
3. Dissolve a minute amount of residue in chloroform, plus a few drops of bromine water. Shake for $\frac{1}{2}$ minute. Add excess sodium hydroxide and shake again. Chloroform layer becomes blue or blue-violet. Color persists even when chloroform layer is separated and shaken with 60% sulfuric acid. Sensitive to 0.050 mg of ANTU in 1 ml of chloroform (specific).

Treatment

Gastric lavage, or emetics, cathartics.

Quiet and rest, in recumbent position. Bed rest is essential. Withhold fluids until edema subsides. Treat hyperglycemia. Oxygen inhalation for anoxia; cysteine appears to diminish toxicity; supportive and symptomatic treatment as required.

ARSENIC (As)

Derivatives: Fowler's solution; lead arsenate; arsenical soaps; arsenic oxide; organic arsenicals; copper arsenite (Paris green); Triox; cocodylates; iron arsenate; arsenic iodide; Donovan's solution; many herbicides, insecticides, and rodenticides; arsine; calcium arsenate.

Uses: Rodenticides, paints, tanning, fly killer, insecticide, weed and tree killer, cattle dip, fungicide, wood and taxidermy preservative. The fact that it is very effective and relatively inexpensive makes it easily available in many homes.

Properties: Odorless, tasteless compounds usually are white, with the exception of copper or sulfur compounds. Arsenic combines with tissue sulfhydryl. All portals of entry, even by cigarette smoke; radiopaque; carcinogenic (chronic).

MLD: Approximately 100 mg/70 kg person, as As_2O_3; trivalent is more toxic than pentavalent; organic compounds are less toxic. Arsine is the most toxic derivative.

Remarks: So-called tolerance is unlikely, but some *degree of effect* may be due to altered rate of absorption, cumulation, and rate of elimination. Arsenic can kill very quickly—within 1 hour; or within several hours, within 24 hours, within 5 days; or can be delayed 1 week, 1 month, or even 1 year.

It was the poison of choice of the "professional poisoners" because chronic small doses may produce confusing progressive debilitation prior to a delayed death and because small doses are tasteless, odorless, and colorless. Chronic poisoning may be easily obscured. Therefore, all sudden unexplained gastrointestinal upsets *should* be investigated chemically.

Symptoms

ACUTE: Sudden and explosive gastroenteritis (may be delayed about $\frac{1}{2}$ hour or more). Metallic taste, constriction of throat (dysphagia), hoarse voice, nausea, persistent vomiting, rice-water stools developing into bloody diarrhea, blisters of epithelium and sloughing of parts, severe abdominal pain, garlic odor of breath, salivation, thirst, oliguria, capillary oozing (increased permeability), shredded stomach lining, bloody vomitus (looks like cholera), distended stomach, pallor, hyperpyrexia, moist skin, tremors, convulsions; shock via loss of fluids, electrolytes and proteins; hypotension. Death usually in less than 15 hours due to circulatory collapse.

Delayed acute symptoms: Loss of hair (which grows back with recovery), brittle fingernails, and deformities. "Mees" lines start to form when nail bed is in contact with blood circulation (time of arsenic exposure). Hoarse voice, cough, motor paralysis, and neurologic pain.

CHRONIC (small continuous exposure): Insidious general weakness, anorexia, nausea, vomiting, nose bleed and bleeding gums, conjunctivitis, "Mees" lines, thirst, coryza, hoarseness, coughing, dermatitis, severe skin exfoliation, low-grade fever, weight loss, stomatitis, salivation, hyperkeratosis of palms and soles, brittle nails, edema of ankles and lower eyelids, progressive vague weakness. Increased pigmentation known as "arsenic melanosis" seen on neck, eyelids, or nipple; garlic odor to breath, renal damage, anuria, hepatic damage and degeneration, jaundice, motor paralysis, tingling of skin of extremities, peripheral neuritis, extremities more involved, foot drop, wrist drop, loss of hair, tremors, colitis, severe pain, anoxic convulsions, spinal-cord involvement, and ataxia.

Identification

Vomitus, gastric lavage, urine, blood, powder, tablets, residues, hair, or fingernails.

1. Approximately 20 ml of gastric lavage, vomitus, urine (or powders, tablets, or residues dissolved or suspended in 20 ml of water) is placed in a small Erlenmeyer flask. Hydrochloric acid (4 ml) is added. A small copper strip (5 × 5 mm) is washed and then introduced into the flask (if copper sheet is not available, a small copper wire coil may be used). Solution is *gently* heated for about an hour; then the copper is removed and examined. A silver deposit may indicate mercury; a dark deposit may indicate arsenic, bismuth, antimony, sulfur, selenium, or tellurium. (See scheme for differentiating the latter

compounds, Section I.) The black arsenic deposit is very sensitive and is visible to as low as 0.010 mg of arsenic. An estimation may be made by comparison with standards prepared in a similar fashion:

arsenic → dull black; sensitive to 0.010 mg.

bismuth → shiny black; sensitive to 0.020 mg.

antimony → dark purple sheen; sensitive to 0.020 mg.

a. The arsenic black deposit is confirmed by placing the copper and deposit into 2 ml of 10% potassium cyanide. If the black deposit is due to arsenic, it will dissolve. The black deposit, if due to bismuth or antimony, will persist.

b. Black deposit is gently sublimed in a small test tube (with heat). Test tube is covered with a watch glass cooled by ice. Arsenic crystals are white and octahedral when microscopically observed on watch glass. Very sensitive.

Arsenic may still be found in the urine up to several months following an exposure (especially a chronic exposure).

2. A fresh copper strip with the arsenic deposit is prepared as described in test 1 above.

This copper (black deposit) is placed into a modified Gutzeit apparatus (Fig. 2).

The rubber stopper in the flask supports a small drying tube trap into which is plugged some cotton moistened with lead acetate solution. Above this tube is attached a set of flanges,* between which is placed a disc of "mercuric bromide-sensitized" filter paper (prepared by cutting a round disc of Whatman No. 40 filter paper impregnated with 5% mercuric bromide in 95% alcohol for about 3 minutes. After drying the droplets, the disc is fastened between the flanges with a rubber band.

The apparatus is charged with a few small pieces of mossy zinc (arsenic-free), and 2 drops of 40% stannous chloride (prepared in 50% hydrochloric acid), and 2 drops of 20% potassium iodide and 15 ml of 10% sulfuric acid. The generation of hydrogen and arsine (AsH_3) is then allowed to proceed for

*Manufactured by Eck and Krebb.

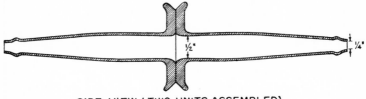

SIDE VIEW (TWO UNITS ASSEMBLED)

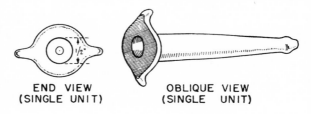

END VIEW
(SINGLE UNIT)

OBLIQUE VIEW
(SINGLE UNIT)

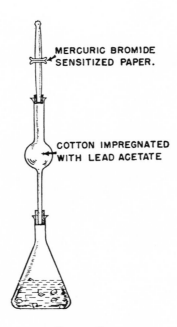

MERCURIC BROMIDE
SENSITIZED PAPER.

COTTON IMPREGNATED
WITH LEAD ACETATE

FIGURE 2.

about 1 hour. Do not allow gas to generate too rapidly. If too rapid, cool in an ice bath and again allow to proceed more slowly. If sulfuric acid is above 10%, H_2S may be generated. This is shown by the cotton pledget in the trap turning dark black.

The liberated hydrogen forms arsine on reacting with the deposited arsenic. Arsine travels upward, and any impurity of hydrogen sulfide is removed by passing through the "lead acetate-moistened" cotton. The arsine, when contacting the mercuric bromide paper, turns it a canary yellow to orange-brown color. The yellow is very sensitive and is directly proportional to the arsine liberated.

This test is specific for arsenic and is sensitive to 0.005 mg. However, since only approximately 50 percent of the arsenic present can be recovered by this deposition method, it is suggested that a factor of two $(2\times)$ be used to compensate for the partial recovery. The best ranges for comparison are standards made by similarly treating, with the Gutzeit, varying concentrations between 0.005 and 0.040 mg of arsenic.

3. One hundred (100) ml of urine, 10 ml of blood, or several grams of hair, or finger- and toenails (or vomitus, powders, residues, etc.) is digested with nitric acid—sulfuric acid—perchloric acid. (See Section I.)

Make certain that all the nitric and perchloric acid is removed by heating. The digest is cooled and residual sulfuric acid volume is estimated; then, sufficient water is added to make the final solution approximately 10% sulfuric acid (tenfold dilution). A measured aliquot (no more than 15 ml) is added to a Gutzeit apparatus described in test 2 above. This test is sensitive to 0.0005 mg of arsenic. There is a well-defined increase in yellow intensity that is directly proportional to the concentration of arsenic up to about 0.015 mg when the disc turns orange to brown. These yellow discs should be compared with standards similarly prepared.

4. Arsenic (trivalent form) can be isolated and separated by distillation with concentrated hydrochloric acid. The volatile arsenic distillate is caught into sodium hydroxide. This is acidified and is estimated by tests above.

INTERPRETATIONS: Normally, there are small traces of arsenic in blood, urine, hair and finger- and toenails, but these are very low and will not be detected with the tests described above and using the sample size suggested. Frequent analysis of all reagents is necessary to rule out contamination.

Normal arsenic in urine is less than 0.01 mg/dl; in hair or fingernails, less than 0.001 mg per 1 gm. Scalp hair growth is approximately $\frac{1}{4}$ to $\frac{1}{2}$ inches per month. Fingernail growth is about $\frac{1}{8}$ to $\frac{1}{4}$ inches per month.

Note: Stomach contents should be examined for crystals and color. Green is suggestive of Paris green; yellow of arsenic sulfide; white of the trioxide. Arsenic trioxide is the most common.

Sudden onset of severe gastroenteritis may sometimes suggest arsenic. Levels above normal should be further studied.

Treatment

Gastric lavage with warm milk and water followed by sodium sulfate (30 gm) cathartic. Keep bowels open. Keep patient warm and quiet; maintain body heat, fluids, and electrolyte balance. Sedation and morphine for pain; combat shock and dehydration.

Diet high in glucose and low in fat for possible liver damage; also calcium gluconate, methionine, and B complex vitamins. Artificial respiration, oxygen therapy, whole blood, or fluids as needed. Supportive measures for anuria, pulmonary edema, dehydration, or liver involvement as needed.

SPECIFIC TREATMENT: BAL (dimercaprol) by intramuscular injection. Consult the literature accompanying the vial for doseage; since BAL sometimes produces side reactions, 50 mg of Benadryl given prior appears to eliminate this. BAL effectively hastens removal of arsenic from cellular sulfhydryl and is more rapidly eliminated from the body.

Test urine or blood periodically to determine rate of arsenic elimination. This will help check effectiveness of treatment and can be correlated with clinical impressions. Blood arsenic levels will become relatively low, whereas urine levels may be high for at least 10 days. In chronic exposure, urine may be positive for months.

BAL is not effective for arsine poisoning. An early exchange transfusion may be of some value (for the hemolysis). Treat arsine poisoning also for possible jaundice and nephritis.

Signs, symptoms, and treatment for selenium are generally similar to arsenic. Soluble selenium compounds are highly toxic, whereas insoluble selenium sulfide is less toxic. Tellurium is less toxic than selenium.

ASPIDIUM

Synonyms: Oleoresin; male fern.

Uses: Anthelmintic.

Properties: Green liquid plant extract.

MLD: Approximately 20 ml/70 kg person.

Remarks: Death may occur in from 5 to 15 hours. Agent is not to be used in debilitated patients, cases of gastric ulcers, pregnancy, etc.

Symptoms: Gastrointestinal irritation, nausea, vomiting, diarrhea, colic, initial excitement followed by depression of central nervous system and heart, dyspnea, somnolence, headache, fever, muscular twitching, confusion, convulsions, vertigo, yellow vision, blindness (blindness may be temporary or permanent), glycosuria, albuminuria, collapse, coma, death by respiratory failure.

Identification

Extracted by acid ether. Filicic acid is the chief constituent and can be hydrolyzed to phloroglucinol and butyric acid.
1. filicic acid + ferric chloride (10%) → red color
2. butyric acid → foul odor
3. phloroglucinol + pine wood splint (moistened with hydrochloric acid) → red color (*see* Sulfanilamide).

Treatment

Gastric lavage with activated charcoal. Emetics to evacuate stomach; cathartics. Mucilaginous substances as demulcents. Avoid fats and oils. Short-acting barbiturates or Valium to control convulsions.

Recovery slow; may leave permanent blindness (rare). Manic psychosis may develop. Treat symptomatically; oxygen and artificial respiration as necessary.

ATROPINE *(Belladonna Group)* $(C_{17}H_{23}NO_3)$

Synonyms or Derivatives: Scopolamine (hyoscine) ; hyoscyamine; deadly nightshade; Datura stramonium; Angel's trumpet (compana); Jimson weed.

Uses: Dilatation of pupils, diminution of secretions, night sweats. Antidote for parasympathomimetic poisons (organic phosphate esters).

Properties: Basic white crystalline. Mp 116°C. Very soluble in chloroform. Anticholinergic. See list for synthetic derivatives, section I.

MLD: Approximately 75 mg/70 kg person.

Remarks: Alkaloid, parasympatholytic; death usually occurs within 15 hours.

Symptoms: Decreased secretions, dry mouth, difficult swallowing, thirst, dry flushed skin (red face and neck), lack of sweating, dilatation of pupils, loss of accommodation and light reflex, persistent cycloplegia, slurred speech, cerebral excitement, talkativeness, hallucinations, confusion, possible quarrelsomeness, muscular and peristalic relaxation, great excitation, occasionally convulsions followed by a marked depression, tachycardia, rise in temperature, delirium, rapid pulse, urine retention, coma, anoxia, rapid respiration that becomes slow and shallow, respiratory failure within 10 hours.

Identification

Separated by alkaline-ether extraction group. Chloroform or amyl alcohol are especially good solvents. Unstable with heat. Add 1 drop HCl, then evaporate gently with stream of air.

1. Residue is dissolved with 1 ml of 2% acetic acid. Use 1-drop portions for spot-precipitant tests.
   a. Wagner's reagent → red triangular plates or rods
   b. Mayer's reagent → white precipitate
   c. Picric acid → yellow precipitate

d. Compound	Wagner's Reagent	Picric Acid Reagent	Gold Chloride Reagent
atropine	crystals	crystals	oil drop
hyoscyamine	crystals	crystals	crystals
hyoscine	oil drop	oil drop	crystals

See under Alkaloids.

2. Small trace aliquot portions of residue are transferred to a spot plate and color reagents applied:
   a. Mandelin's reagent → red → yellow
   b. Marquis' reagent → brown → brown-green (by heat)
   c. Vitali's test → violet
   d. *p*-dimethylaminobenzaldehyde → red-violet
3. Physiologic tests:
   a. Inject 5 to 15 mg of methacholine; failure to produce moistening of mouth, lacrimation, or sweating may help confirm impression of overdosage of atropinelike drug.
   b. Place 1 drop of extract or urine in kitten's eye → pupillary dilatation. (Dog or rabbit not satisfactory.)
4. UV spectrophotometry, paper chromatography, TLC, GLC: See Section I.

Treatment

Activated charcoal and/or milk; then remove by gastric lavage or (ipecac) emetic, followed by 30 gm Na_2SO_4 (cathartic). Keep patient quiet in darkened room. Sedate excitement or mania with Valium, control convulsions with ether or Valium. Treat fever with sponge baths with water or alcohol. Physostigmine salicylate to offset some peripheral and central anticholinergic effects. Maintain fluid balance. Catheterization for urine retention. Keep mouth moist with chips of ice. Monitor all vital signs. Avoid morphine.

Symptoms and treatment are generally similar for all the natural and synthetic derivatives of the belladonna group.

BARBITURATES AND DERIVATIVES

Synonyms: Sleeping pills; goof balls; yellow jackets (Nembutal); red devils (Seconal); blue heaven (Amytal); urea malonate.

Uses: Sedative, hypnotic, anticonvulsant, subhypnotic, pre-anesthetic (basal), anesthetic, "truth serum" (narcolepsy), antidote for convulsants.

Properties: White crystalline powder. Odorless, bitter, weakly acid. Water-soluble as the sodium salt; soluble in chloroform, ether, or alcohol.

Compound	R_1	R_2
barbital	ethyl	ethyl
phenobarbital	ethyl	phenyl
amobarbital	ethyl	isoamyl
allobarbital	allyl	allyl
pentobarbital	ethyl	1-methyl butyl
secobarbital	allyl	1-methyl butyl
thiopental	ethyl	1-methyl butyl sulfur substitutes for oxygen; thiourea instead of urea

Generally as the R_1 and R_2 radical increases in length or complexity (up to six carbons), the potency increases. Also the presence of a double bond or of sulfur will usually increase potency.

MLD: Varies for a 70 kg person from about 1 to 5 gm, depending upon the derivative potency. Short-acting members (rapid onset) usually are more potent; longer-acting members (slow onset) are usually less potent. For example, the MLD for secobarbital is about 1 gm; the MLD for phenobarbital is about 5 gm/70 kg person.

ADVANTAGES OF THERAPEUTIC USE: Sedation, depression, sleep (to any degree, by choosing the specific derivative and varying the dose to suit the situation or as needed). Many in group to choose from. Produces calmness, relieve tensions. Margin of safety is wide. Sedation is about one-third of the hypnotic dose. Antidote for strychnine and other convulsants.

DISADVANTAGES: Hangover is possible. Easily crosses placental barrier. Too easily obtained; widespread use for suicides. No analgesia until near coma (not like aspirin or morphine). Fast-acting derivatives are contraindicated with liver damage. Possible addiction (compulsion to use; withdrawal symptoms). Contraindicated for the very old and very young. Synergism with many other depressant drugs; even with fatal outcome.

Symptoms

ACUTE: Lethargy, depression, ataxia, sleep to deep coma, lowered body temperature, depressed circulation, marked fall in blood pressure, respiratory depression, anoxia, cyanosis, flaccid limbs; retention of urine common; usually constriction of pupils but dilatation of pupils may occur later; corneal and other reflexes may be absent; deep coma, shock, cold extremities; death due to respiratory arrest, frequently associated with marked cardiovascular collapse or pneumonia.

CHRONIC: Skin rash, slurred speech, cyanosis, amnesia, anorexia, emotional instability, ataxia, constipation.

Remarks: The barbiturate derivatives are powerful depressants. In the presence of any other depressants, this effect is even more powerful; at least additive action. This is especially so with alcohols, morphine derivatives, reserpine, tranquilizers, etc. Great precaution or avoidance of these combinations is urged so as not to promote a crisis by combined action.

Identification

1. Gently shake 5 ml of chloroform plus 0.5 ml of blood for about 1 minute and then filter through Whatman #31 paper into a test tube, completely wetting the paper.

   To this chloroform filtrate, add 0.5 ml of buffer (pH 8); shake and mix for 15 seconds and filter through small filter paper (Whatman #31) into a small test tube.

   Transfer 2.5 of filtrate into a 10 mm cuvette; add 0.5 ml of diphenylcarbazone; mix and wait 2 minutes. Blank is light pink; barbiturates yield a darker pink-lilac.

   Read in a spectrophotometer at 550 nm with a reference blank containing 2.5 ml of chloroform and 0.5 ml of diphenylcarbazone.

   Compare with each known standard for an approximation since the color and molar "absorbity" are not the same for each

TABLE XXVI

Compound	MLD (gms)	Therapeutic Blood Level	Lethal Blood Level	Half-life (hours)	Approximate duration of therapeutic action
phenobarbital (Luminal)	5	2 mg/dl	20 mg/dl	60	(long) 18 hr.
amylobarbital (Amytal)	3	0.3 mg/dl	4 mg/dl	30	(moderate) 10 hr.
pentobarbital (Nembutal)	2	0.1 mg/dl	3 mg/dl	25	8 hr.
secobarbital (Seconal)	1.5	0.08 mg/dl	2 mg/dl	18	(short) 6 hr.
pentothal (Thiopental)	1	0.5 mg/dl	5 mg/dl	—	(ultrashort) ½ hr.

barbiturate derivative.

Hydantoins, Dilantin, and Doriden interfere; check reagents for contamination by substituting water for blood and follow through procedure. Resulting solution should have same reading as the blank.

Confirm if possible by UV spectrophotometry and/or TLC. See later tests 4 and 6.

Reagents:

• pH 8 Buffer: Add 2 ml of saturated Hg $(NO_3)_2$ solution [1 gm Hg $(NO_3)_2$ and 0.2 ml HNO_3 and 50 ml of water] to 100 ml of the pH 8 buffer [95.5 ml of 0.15M Na_2HPO_4, i.e. 5.3 gm per 100 ml, and 5.5 ml of 0.15M KH_2PO_4, i.e. 2.0 gm per 100 ml; check with pH meter and adjust if necessary]. Filter if turbid. This is stable at room temperature.

• Standard secobarbital: 1–10 mg/99 ml of water plus 1 ml of 0.5N NaOH.

• Diphenylcarbazone: Add 100 mg of "S diphenylcarbazone" to 100 ml of chloroform. Allow to stand (age) for 2 to 3 days in a flask in a light room. Then store in a dark bottle in the refrigerator. Solution is stable for many months.

Reference: Baer: Rapid detection and estimation in blood. *Am J Clin Path, 44*:11, 1965.

Metabolism and Elimination	Approximate blood Levels for impending coma— awaken.	Type of action	Other similar-acting Members
Kidney; may be in urine up to six days.	8 mg. %	weak sedation and delayed.	Barbital, Mebaral, Pyrictal, Gemonil, Mysoline, Kutonal.
Kidney and liver.	2 mg. %	hypnotic, moderate, long, mild.	Dial, Alurate, Butisol, Pernoston, Ipral, Neonal, Lotusate, Delvinal, Noctal.
mostly liver	1.5 mg. %	hypnotic, moderate, short.	Ortal, Sandoptal, Phanodorn Medomin, Sombucaps, Transithal, Cyclopal.
almost all by liver, rapid destruction.	1 mg %	hypnotic, moderate, short.	
Storage in fat; and all by liver.	0.2 mg. %	Anesthetic, ultrashort, potent.	Evipal, Surital, Brevital, Hexobarbital.

2. Presumptive test (Koppanyi) : Put 50 to 100 ml of urine or stomach contents into a large separatory funnel and test with litmus paper. If alkaline, barely acidify (dropwise) with dilute sulfuric acid.

Add 2 × volume of ether (100–200 ml) and gently shake for several minutes. Allow layers to stand for several minutes to effect good separation. The barbiturate is in the ether. Discard the lower aqueous layer.

Pass the ether through filter paper to remove droplets of water; collect in a beaker or Pyrex evaporating dish.

Water inhibits color production of the test, so the ether now must be dry. *Carefully* evaporate to dryness on a water bath. (No open flame or high heat.) The residue must be dry and not too yellow-brown. If it is brown, dissolve it in about 10 ml of methanol and add a pinch of activated decolorizing charcoal and stir. Filter through Whatman #42 filter paper and collect the clear methanol extract in a small container. Gently evaporate to a final small volume (1–2 ml) .

Transfer a few drops to a white porcelain spot plate. Add 1 drop of cobalt acetate (1% in absolute methyl alcohol) and then 2 drops of isopropyl amine (5% in absolute methyl alcohol) or lithium hydroxide (5% in methanol) .

A purple to lilac color is positive for a barbiturate derivative. Test is sensitive to about 0.050 mg.

Report as negative, trace, moderate, or large amounts.

Note: Presence of water, even in traces, inhibits color production. Cobalt acetate should be kept in a light-resistant bottle; when the cobalt pink color is faded, renew the reagent. To check efficacy of reagents and for quality control, parallel a negative blank (a drop of pure chloroform) and positive controls (standards of a known barbiturate) at the same time of testing unknown. (To prepare a 1 ml = 1 mg standard, dissolve a 100 mg capsule of a barbiturate in 100 ml of chloroform.)

This test will be positive in urine even days later when the barbiturate is a long-acting one (phenobarbital), but will be positive for only a very short time with a short-acting barbiturate such as secobaribtal.

Phenobarbital requires both cobalt acetate and isopropyl amine to give a color, *whereas* the other barbiturates turn blue on addition of only cobalt acetate, which however intensifies on addition of the isopropyl amine, which turns it lilac. They can differentiate phenobarbital from the others, especially in tablets.

Other similar drugs may also give a color: ureides, hydantoins, Bromural, Dilantin, and glutethimide.

3. Since urine is an excellent vehicle for most drugs and since a drug is usually found in the greatest concentration here, look for the presence of crystals in the test 2 extraction. Purification by solvents or microsublimation would yield typical structures to be microscopically studied and compared with the known barbiturate crystals. Secobarbital is difficult to crystallize from tissue, but time and effort may yield some crystals. Barbiturates are insoluble in petroleum ether at 40 to 60°C (good way to get rid of fats and oils).

Melting point is an excellent confirmation for the identities of characteristic crystals. See Table XXVII.

4. UV spectrophotometry: To 25 ml of redistilled chloroform in

TABLE XXVII

TRADE NAME	CHEMICAL STRUCTURE position 5	M.P.°C
Alurate (aprobarbital)	allyl, — isopropyl	140–142
Amytal (amobarbital)	ethyl, — isoamyl	152–155
Brevital (methohexital sodium)*	allyl, — 1-methyl-2-pentyl	
Butisol (butabarbital)	ethyl, — 1-methyl propyl	168–170
Cyclopal (cyclopen)	allyl, — cyclopentenyl	140–143
Delvinal (vinbarbital)	ethyl, — 1-methyl, 1-butyl	162–163
Dial (allobarbital)	allyl, — allyl	171–173
Evipal (hexobarbital sodium)*	methyl, — cyclohexenyl	143–145
Gemonil (metharbital)*‡	ethyl, — ethyl	154–155
Ipral (probarbital Ca or Na)	ethyl, — isopropyl	200–203
Kutonal	methyl, — phenyl	200–223
Lotusate (talbutal)	allyl, — 1-methyl propyl	108–110
Luminal (phenobarbital)	ethyl, — phenyl	173–174
Mebaral (mephobarbital)*§	ethyl, — phenyl	176
Mysoline (primidone)//	ethyl, — phenyl	281–282
Medomin (heptabarbital)	ethyl, — cycloheptenyl	174
Nembutal (pentobarbital)	ethyl, — 1-methyl butyl	127–130
Neonal	ethyl, — butyl	127–130
Nostal; Noctal (Propallylonal)	isopropyl, — 2-bromoallyl	177–179
Ortal	ethyl, — hexyl	122–125
Pentothal (thiopental sodium)†	ethyl, — 1-methyl-butyl	159–160
Pernoston (butallylonal)	1-methyl-propyl, — 2Br-allyl	130–133
Phanodorn (cyclobarbital)	ethyl, — cyclohexenyl	171–173
Pyrictal (N-phenyl barbital)¶	ethyl, — ethyl	
Sandoptal (butalbital)	allyl, — isobutyl	138–139
Seconal (secobarbital)	allyl, — 1-methyl-butyl	100
Sombucaps (hexobarbital)*	methyl, — cyclohexenyl	144–147
Surital (thiamylal sodium)†	allyl, — 1-methyl-butyl	
Transithal (buthalital)†	allyl, — isobutyl	
Veronal (barbital)	ethyl, — ethyl	188–191

COMBINATIONS OF BARBITURATES. —

Fiorinal	Sandoptal, aspirin, phenacetin, caffeine.
Ethobral	Secobarbital, butobarbital, phenobarbital.
Tuinal	Sodium secobarbital, sodium amobarbital.
Carbrital	Pentobarbital sodium, carbromal.
Flexinal	Barbital, phenobarbital, sandoptal.

* Methyl substitutes for Hydrogen in position #3.
† Sulfur substitutes for Oxygen in position 2.
‡ Metabolizes to barbital.
§ Metabolizes to phenobarbital.
// Di-hydrogen substitutes for oxygen in position #2.
¶ Phenyl substitutes for hydrogen in position #1.

a 125 ml separatory funnel, add 5 ml of blood, urine, or ground tissue.

Gently shake with swirling motion for several minutes. Emulsions sometimes form with brain or tissue. Several drops of petroleum ether or isopropyl alcohol, centrifuging, or the addition of a little more chloroform usually corrects this. Allow to stand, to separate layers. The lower chloroform is carefully filtered into another separatory funnel through coarse filter paper to remove water droplets. To this clear chloroform extract, add 5 ml of 0.5N sodium hydroxide (3 ml of saturated NaOH diluted to 110 ml with water).

Gently shake by swirling for several minutes; allow to stand. Pour off the lower chloroform; drain off last drop. Transfer the sodium hydroxide extract to a centrifuge tube and spin down any suspended chloroform droplets.

Transfer one-half to a silica cuvette (1 cm light path) and scan in the UV range of the spectrophotometer. Phenobarbital, amylobarbital, pentobarbital, and secobarbital will show characteristic absorption spectra with a maximum density at 255 nm and a minimum at 235 nm. This test is sensitive to about 1 μg per 5 ml of blood. See Figure 3.

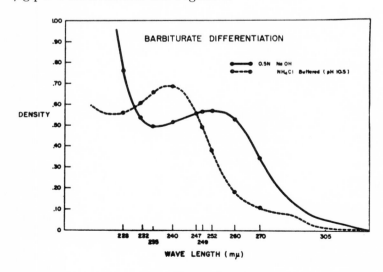

FIGURE 3.

Pentothal shows a maximum density at 305 nm and a minimum at 246 nm. Evipal and Mebaral show maxima at 242 and 244 nm and minima at 229 and 230 nm, respectively.

To estimate the quantity of barbiturate present, the absorbance at the maximum density is recorded; this is compared with a standard graph. See Figure 4; and then determine the microgram quantity present in the 1 cm light path of 5 ml of sodium hydroxide that was extracted from 5 ml of blood with 25 ml of $CHCl_3$ (20 ml of which was recovered). To correct for losses and convert to percent, multiply above reading of graph by $125 = \mu g/dl$ (when original sample was 5 ml).

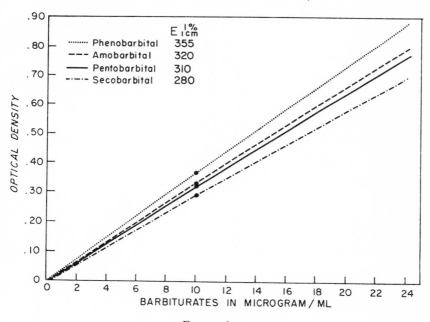

FIGURE 4.

Salicylates interfere with this test for barbiturates. To determine if salicylates are present: To 1 ml of urine, add 5 drops of $FeCl_3$ (10%). If salicylates are positive, even in traces, there will be a purple color produced.

It is necessary to remove this salicylate first to allow this test for barbiturates. To 50 ml of purified chloroform, add 5 ml of blood, urine, or liver slurry, and then gently extract by swirling for several minutes. Separate layers. The salicylates are removed from the chloroform by extraction-washing with 10 ml of freshly prepared 1% $NaHCO_3$. Discard this $NaHCO_3$ washing. Only barbiturate remains. Extract now with 5 ml of 0.5N sodium hydroxide and scan in the UV as above.

To further confirm presence of barbiturates, take 3.0 ml of *original* 0.5N NaOH extract and shift pH to 10.5 with the addition of 0.5 ml of 16% NH_4Cl. The slope changes and the maximum density is now shifted from 255 nm to 240 nm. See Figure 3.

5. Barbiturate and neutral separation: Three (3) ml of blood + 25 ml $CHCl_3$; shake in a 60 ml glass—stoppered bottle. Separate and filter; the blood stays on the filter.

Extract filtered $CHCl_3$ with 5 ml 0.5N NaOH. Read NaOH in UV for barbiturates (see above test). The $CHCl_3$ *still* has the *neutral drugs* (save).

The 5 ml of 0.5N NaOH (above, after UV scanning) is made slightly acid with HCl; then extract with 25 ml $CHCl_3$. Evaporate the $CHCl_3$. Residue is picked up in methanol. Do TLC for barbiturate; $CHCl_3$: acetone (9:1). See Section I.

Gently evaporate the $CHCl_3$ that was saved (above) *almost* to dryness. Pick up residue in methanol (minimal). Do TLC for neutral drugs. See Section I. *Dilantin, meprobamate, Doriden, caffeine, Valium, and Librium* will be found in this fraction.

DIFFERENTIATION: It is not sufficient just to know that a barbiturate is present in blood, even if the exact level is determined. One must also know which one. For example, a report reads "Barbiturates: Positive (3 mg/dl)."
In this case, if it were
(a) secobarbital, it would be fatal;
(b) pentobarbital, fatal or at least in deep coma;
(c) amylorbarbital, coma;
(d) phenobarbital, an average therapeutic level for epilepsy (ambulatory).

Note: During survival time between ingestion and death, the barbiturates are being metabolized and eliminated from the blood. Secobarbital is eliminated rapidly (within several hours), whereas phenobarbital much more slowly (even up to 1 week). Survival time is therefore an important factor in evaluating a blood level of the particular barbiturate derivative in question.

The UV spectrophotometric methods provide a very sensitive technic for detection of barbiturates (about 1 μg). However, this is limited because the forms of the absorption curves (255 nm maximum density and 235 nm minimum density) are quite similar for the common members.

6. Thin layer chromatography (TLC) is the method of choice to differentiate the barbiturates. This technic is rapid (about 1 hour). Many determinations can be performed on the same plate at the same time with minimal streaking and, because of increased sensitivity and being a means of further differentiation between the various barbiturates, this is the technic of choice. Semiquantitative estimations may be made by varying intensities of colors and area. See Section I.

Coat several glass plates (20 × 20 cm) with silica gel G in usual manner (250 μ layer thick). Dry in a ventilated oven at 100°C for 20 minutes. Store at room temperature for future use. Prior to analysis, make parallel vertical lines with a ruler $\frac{1}{2}$ inch apart to act as guide for many concurrent sample analyses at one time. Twelve to fourteen may be made. Prepared plates may be purchased.

Several drops of a chloroform or methanol extract of each sample are carefully placed with a Pasteur disposable micropipette (in the smallest possible area) at a point 1 inch from the bottom of the plate and in the middle of a column. These spots are air dried and the plates then placed in a rectangular jar with a ground glass cover containing 110 ml of the 9:1 chloroform-acetone mixture. The jar space should be saturated with this vapor prior to placing of plates. Jar and solution can be reused for about 2 days.

With this solvent system, the solvent front will rise 10 cm

in about 30 minutes. Remove plate and mark the solvent front immediately with a horizontal scratch. Air dry at room temperature and, when dry, the plate is first sprayed with the $HgSO_4$, allowed to partially dry, and sprayed with an excess of diphenylcarbazone. In each position, note the area size, position (Rf), and color intensity of each spot. After an excess of diphenylcarbazone, the colored background will slowly fade and the purple-violet spots will remain to permit reliable measurement of Rf values.

Alkaline fluorescein is also helpful when sprayed on the plate initially and then viewed under a 254 nm light. Barbiturates give a purple spot against a yellow-green background.

$KMnO_4$ spray gives a yellow spot against a purple background with *unsaturated* barbiturate derivatives and also with the *thio*-derivatives.

Since multiple samples (12 to 14) can be run simultaneously, include the common barbiturates as standard for comparison. Since there are variances in physical conditions between each run, the absolute Rf may vary slightly. To improve reproducibility, each entire run is always compared with the Rf of phenobarbital, which is included in every run. Ratio of Rf to the Rf of phenobarbital is reproducible.

PREPARATION OF BIOLOGIC SPECIMENS: Specimens of blood or urine or ground tissue are directly extracted by chloroform. No pH adjustment is necessary. Use 5 ml of specimen per 50 ml of $CHCl_3$.

Or, continue with sample from above test 4 and 5. The 5 ml of 0.5N NaOH after UV scanning is made slightly acid with HCl; then extract with 25 ml of $CHCl_3$. Evaporate the $CHCl_3$, and the residue is picked up with several drops of methanol. Spot onto a TLC plate.

Reagents:
* Chloroform:acetone (9:1) v/v (Sunshine).
* $HgSO_4$ spray: Add 5 gm HgO to 100 ml of water and, while mixing and suspending, slowly add 20 ml of sulfuric acid. After it dissolves, cool and dilute to 250 ml with water.
* Diphenylcarbazone spray: Dissolve 5 mg in 50 ml of chloro-

form. Store in dark bottle and in a cool place.
* Fluorescein spray: Add 20 gm of sodium hydroxide to 500 ml of water and then add 20 mg of sodium fluorescein.
* $KMnO_4$ spray—0.1% aqueous solution.
* Silica gel G—according to Stahl.
* Standard barbiturates: 10 mg per 100 ml $CHCl_3$.

Comments: It is desirable to include, with the internal standard of phenobarbital, a standard of amylobarbital, pentobarbital, and secobarbital. These are the most common and could be compared with the unknown for Rf, intensity, and hue of color under identical set of conditions, on the same plates.

Compound	Approximate Rf	Color of Spot Developed
phenobarbital	0.45	lilac
amylobarbital	0.60	lilac
pentobarbital	0.55	lilac
butabarbital	0.53	lilac
secobarbital	0.70	light blue

(Sensitive to less than 5 μg.)

Other suitable TLC developing solvents for barbiturates:
* $CHCl_3$:ethanol   (90:10) Machata
* $CHCl_3$ethanol   (80:20) Machata
* $CHCl_3$:ether   (85:15) Machata
* Ethyl acetate:benezne (10:20)
* 2-propanol:$CHCl_3$:25% ammonia (9:9:2)
* Iso-octane:acetic acid (100:7)
* $CHCl_3$:diethylamine (9:1) Waldi in Stahl

    amobarbital 31
    butalbarbital 27
    meprobamate 41
    pentobarbital 47
    phenobarbital 19
    secobarbital 53

Spray with $HgSO_4$ reagent and note position of spots; allow to partially air dry, and then spray with diphenylcarbazone reagent in slight excess and note position of spots. All are violet *except* secobarbital, which is blue (diphenylhydantoin also is blue) . The colored background will slowly fade.

Compare color, intensity, position (Rf) , area size, and presence of metabolites with parallel standards.

View under ultraviolet radiation at 350 and 254 nm. Look for absorbance or fluorescence.

7. Barbiturate differentiation by GC: 4 foot column SE-30, 5% on 100–120 firebrick packing; 180°C argon carrier gas. Retention time 3–24 minutes differentiates various common barbiturate derivatives.

Other GLC: See Section I.

Reference: Kirk and Parker: *Anal Chem, 33:*1378, 1961.

Treatment

Carefully evaluate all reflexes (especially corneal and patellar). This is an excellent guide to depth of depression. At all times, maintain adequate respiratory exchange. Keep air passages open; prevent aspiration. Give artificial respiration, or oxygen (if indicated) , using endotracheal tube if needed.

Remove as much of the drug *as soon as possible* by gastric lavage, taking every precaution to avoid aspiration. Avoid emetics if patient is depressed. Saline cathartic (sodium sulfate, 30 gm) could help to minimize further absorption of drug.

Maintain adequate circulation and blood pressure with fluids or plasma, or plasma expanders. Avoid unnecessary drugs.

Carefully evaluate all reflexes, respiratory pattern, skin color, response to pain stimuli, at frequent intervals to guide further therapy.

Place patient on his side so as to minimize dangers of aspiration. Turn him at regular intervals to prevent hypostatic pneumonitis.

Maintain fluids, electrolyte balance, blood pressure, and body heat; catheterize as necessary to prevent urine retention.

To combat *respiratory difficulties,* artificial respiration or oxygen therapy should be used. The use of picrotoxin, Metrazole, amphetamine, or other strong analeptics is believed ineffective and *perhaps dangerous* for patients in deep depression and unnecessary for mild cases. Use mild analeptics (if you must) such as Emivan, Megimide, or Ritalin to just maintain reflexes and keep E.E.G. active. These should not be used in an attempt "to wake" the patient.

Give supportive measures as indicated; careful monitoring.

Intensive nursing care is vital, especially during the acute phase.

Coma may persist for days with the long-acting barbiturates. Guard against pulmonary and cerebral edema. Prognosis is good if you can prevent anoxia and pneumonia.

If the blood-drug level is high and the drug is a long-acting barbiturate, hemodialysis may be used to advantage.

The foregoing suggestions are for the markedly depressed. If, however, the depression or overdosage is mild, then treatment also should be "mild." If respiration is normal, color is good, and twitching and corneal reflexes are present, it may suffice to let the patient "sleep it off," carefully watching to prevent aspiration and any possible later development of respiratory difficulties, or secondary infection. Supportive.

BARIUM (Ba)

Derivatives: Barium sulfate, sulfide, chloride, or carbonate, etc.

Uses: Rodenticides, gastrointestinal x-rays, depilatory, fireworks, insecticides, golf balls ($BaSO_4$ + ZnS + fish oils), Lithopone ($BaSO_4$ + ZnS).

Properties: White crystalline salt.

MLD: Approximately 1 gm of soluble salt for a 70 kg person.

Remarks: Death may be sudden or delayed several days. Cumulative. Barium sulfate is insoluble and nontoxic; barium sulfide and chloride are soluble and very toxic; barium carbonate is soluble in the stomach and is therefore toxic. Barium sulfide will also produce symptoms of H_2S (see under Sulfides).

Symptoms: Metallic taste, nausea, vomiting, diarrhea, severe abdominal pain, salivation, convulsions, great rise in blood pressure, extrasystoles, palpitation of the heart, digitalis like effect on heart, paralysis of extremities, death from cardiac arrest, consciousness until death.

Identification

Digestion with sulfuric acid—nitric acid—perchloric acid.
1. Flame test. Burns with green flame on platinum wire.
2. sulfuric acid (10%) → barium sulfate ↓ white precipitate, which is insoluble in nitric or hydrochloric acid
3. sodium carbonate → barium carbonate ↓ white precipitate
4. Spectrographic analysis or atomic absorption.

Treatment

Emetics to induce vomiting. Sodium sulfate solution orally to precipitate barium. Gastric lavage; charcoal. Cathartics: sodium sulfate orally, 25 gm (keep bowels open). Valium or short-acting barbiturates to counteract convulsions (with great caution).

Oxygen and artificial respiration as needed. Morphine for pain. Quinidine sulfate as needed. Demulcents. Keep patient warm and quiet. Symptomatic treatment for cardiovascular symptoms. Maintain fluid and electrolyte balance; monitor respiratory and cardiac signs.

BENADRYL ($C_{17}H_{22}Cl\ NO$)

Synonyms: Diphenhydramine; Amidryl.

Uses: Antihistaminic (see Antihistamines).

Properties: White crystalline basic, mp 168°C.

MLD: Approximately 1 gm/70 kg. person.

Approximate Blood Levels: Therapeutic, 0.1 mg/dl; lethal, 1 mg/dl; half-life, 5 hours.

Remarks: Parasympatholytic. Central nervous system excitant (atropinelike) and depressant.

Symptoms: Drowsiness, dizziness, weakness, nausea, vertigo, dry mouth, confusion, muscular twitching, tachycardia, irritability, fever, hallucinations, dilatation of pupils, narcolepsy, palpitation, malaise, disturbed vision after signs of initial central nervous system depression; this may be followed by convulsions, collapse, death.

Identification

Alkaline-ether or chloroform group separation.
1. A small portion of residue is dissolved with 1 ml of acetic acid

(2%). Use 1-drop portions in a spot plate and, with micro-technic, do alkaloid precipitant tests. (Technic and reagents described under Alkaloids.) Examine for typical crystals.

a. chloroplatinic acid (5%) → granular orange precipitate (leaflike crystals)
b. phosphotungstic acid (1:20) → amorphous white precipitate
c. phosphomolybdic acid (10%) → amorphous greenish precipitate
d. Mayer's reagent → granular yellow precipitate
e. Wagner's reagent → granular brown precipitate
f. picric acid → yellow precipitate (mp 131°C) (pyribenzamine also gives similar precipitates)

2. Small aliquot portions of residue are transferred to a spot plate and, with microtechnic, do color tests (see Alkaloids).
a. Mandelin's reagent → red with oily red globules
b. Marquis' reagent → canary yellow → reddish orange → chocolate brown
c. Mecke's reagent → canary yellow → reddish orange
d. Fröhde's reagent → canary yellow → orange → orange-red
e. sulfuric acid → orange
f. resorcinol and concentrated sulfuric acid → orange → reddish orange → wine color on dilution with water
g. furfural (1%), overlay sulfuric acid → orange-brown → yellow-green on shaking
h. chromic acid (5%) → orange-red precipitate

Refer to section on Alkaloids and antihistamines

3. Spectrophotometry.
4. Paper chromatography, TLC.

Treatment

Withdrawal of drug. Activated charcoal. Gastric lavage with potassium permanganate (1:10,000). Emetics, cathartics, ice packs.

To counteract convulsions, give Valium in *small doses*. However, this is to be given with caution and careful observation for secondary respiratory depression. Give oxygen and artificial respiration, fluids as needed.

Symptomatic treatment. DO NOT GIVE STIMULANTS!

Effects disappear within 48 hours after withdrawal of drug.

Treatment is generally similar for other antihistaminic and atropinelike agents.

BENZENE (C_6H_6)

Synonyms: Benzol; coal naphtha; benzole; phenyl hydride; coal tar derivative.

HOMOLOGUES: Toluene, xylene.

Uses: In the manufacture of drugs, chemicals, insecticides, glues, degreaser, adhesives, varnishes, stains, dyes, paints, explosives, art glass, batteries, detergents, polishes, inks; lithography, printing, type cleaners, oil cloth, pencils, perfumes, pesticides; "dry cleaning"; refining of coke and gas fuels; photography; putty; tires and rubber manufacture and products; wax production; cork, linoleum, and plastic workers; wire insulation and various coverings; a common solvent in clinical and chemical laboratories.

Properties: Clear, colorless, noncorrosive, highly inflammable, with a strong and rather pleasant odor, relatively low boiling point and a high vapor pressure to give off vapors to the atmosphere. Boiling point 81°C. Soluble in acetone, ether, or ethanol.

MLD: Approximately 25 ml/70 kg person. Approximately 1500 ppm within 15 minutes. Maximum allowable concentration (MAC) 1 ppm in 8 hour TWA; with a ceiling of 5 ppm for any 15 minute period (OSHA).

APPROXIMATE LETHAL BLOOD LEVELS 0.1 mg/dl.

Remarks: Most of (USA) benzene is produced by the petrochemical and petroleum refining industries. Benzene can be absorbed thru all portals.

Symptoms

ACUTE: Strong CNS depressant, dizziness, weakness, euphoria, headache, irritability, nausea, vomiting, ataxia, staggering, anorexia, flatulence, tightness in chest, rapid irregular pulse, shallow and rapid respiration, ventricular irregularities, excitement, restlessness, delirium, blurred visual blindness, tremors, paralysis, coma, convulsions, massive hemorrhage of lungs, congestive gastritis, marked cerebral edema and kidney involvement. Death by cardiac and/or respiratory failure.

LATE EFFECTS: Severe skin rash, capillary permeability, petechial hemorrhages, decreased coagulation, severe anemias.

CHRONIC (VAPORS) : Signs and symptoms similar to above and including depression of the hematopoietic system and damage to bone marrow. Chromosomal changes are also possible. Symptoms may be early or delayed months. Loss of appetite, drowsiness, euphoria which can develop into emotional instability, and tremulousness. Severe anemia, skin rash; fatty degeneration of heart, liver, or adrenals. Blood dyscracias have been common with chronic benzene exposure and include agranulocytosis, thrombocytopenia, aplastic anemia, hemolytic anemia and even leukemia. Chronic exposure has now clearly incriminated benzene in producing leukemia (OSHA, 1977) .

Identification

Benzene is eliminated unchanged through the lungs and in smaller amounts in the urine. The urine will also eliminate higher than normal total sulfates and appreciable amounts of phenol as metabolite. About 40 percent of the retained benzene is excreted in the urine as phenol (complete within 24–48 hours).

Normal urinary phenols: Below 20 mg/liter. (Benzene) urinary phenols: Above 75 mg/liter. (Doctor and Zielhuis, *Ann Occup Hyg, 10:*317-326)

Steam distillation; or carbon tetrachloride extraction.

1. Test for phenol in urine:
   a. urine (5 ml) plus 1 ml $FeCl_3$ (10%) → purple
   b. urine (20 ml) steam distilled and collect 10 ml distillate:
      (1). Read in UV spectrophotometer for phenol.
      (2). Test for phenols: See Phenols.
   c. Urine or serum (5 ml) made slightly acid with 1 drop of 10% HCl is extracted with 35 ml of ether or chloroform. Separate and then re-extract with 5 ml 0.5N NaOH and read in UV (very sensitive) .

2. Test for benzene in acute exposure (gastric lavages or blood): Steam distill into (ice packed) receptacle and collect 10 ml.

a. Read in UV spectrophotometer for benzene; then extract (concentrate) with 5 ml of *n*-hexane (spectral) and read again in UV. Read in ethanol:maximum density, 255 nm.
b. Shake with 5 ml CCl_4 (spectral grade) and read in NIR.
c. Benzene in CCl_4 (in above test) plus 1 ml H_2SO_4 + 1 ml HNO_3 (keep temperature below 60°C during adding and mixing). Then heat at 60°C for 1 hour → nitrobenzene (shoe polish odor) ; bp 206°C.

3. Screening test for benzene, toluene, xylene, kerosene, benzine.
    a. Conway microdiffusion (Hensel) ; see Section I.
        Marquis reagent → red
            14 drops H_2SO_4, outer chamber
            14 drops H_2SO_4, inner chamber
    b.   1 drop of formaldehyde, inner chamber (Marquis's reagent)
            1 ml H_2SO_4 for sealing well (outer rim)
            2 ml of urine + 2 ml of ether + 2 gm $(NH_4)_2SO_4$
        Shake and separate; then centrifuge and transfer the ether layer to another tube containing Na_2SO_4 (anhydrous) and quickly shake again, separate, and centrifuge. Transfer the ether *very quickly* to outer chamber Conway cell and close lid; twist gently to liquid seal.
        Ether is soluble in H_2SO_4, and vapor tension is reduced so that only kerosene, benzene, toluene, and gasoline diffuse. Allow to diffuse for 1 hour at room temperature (30°C).
        Red color positive for all (Marquis' reagent in inner chamber). Can make a semiquantitative estimate by comparison with standards. Very sensitive reaction.
    b. Gerarde Test (Marquis') very rapid and sensitive: See Kerosene.
    c. To differentiate benzine (petroleum) from benzene: Benzine + Picric acid → does *not* dissolve (colorless). Benzene + Picric acid → dissolves (yellow).

4. Benzene or toluene (Feldstein) : Fifty (50) ml of urine, blood, or tissue homogenate is made acid with dilute H_2SO_4 and is steam distilled. Collect 100 ml of distillate in an ice-packed receptacle.

The distillate (100 ml) is made acid with dilute H_2SO_4 and is redistilled in a fractionating column until 10 ml of distillate is collected. Transfer 3 ml into a silica cuvette (1 cm) and read in UV range of spectrophotometer (340 nm to 220 nm).

Benzene: Maximum density, *254*, 261, 249, 243 nm; Sensitive to 10 μg.

Toluene: Maximum density, *262*, 268 nm; Sensitive to 10 μg.

5. GLC. See Section I

6. Blood and bone marrow studies may be suggestive of blood dyscrasias due to benzene.

Treatment

If ingested, treatment and precautions are the same as for Kerosene. If gastric lavage is used, great care should be exercised to avoid aspiration. Bed rest until respiratory process is normal. Avoid epinephrine and related drugs. Saline cathartics.

Guard against hemotopoietic, respiratory, renal and hepatic complications.

Workers (in benzene industry) should have *periodic* check-up including *careful* blood studies. Urine should be screened for elevated total urinary sulfates and for elevated phenols.

Symptomatic and supportive measures may include iron therapy, whole blood transfusions as indicated. Maintain fluid and electrolyte balance. Guard against cardiac and respiratory difficulties. Guard against secondary infections.

Symptoms and treatment are similar for toluene and xylene; these are more toxic (acute) but less toxic (chronic) and do not produce leukemia. Severe exposure to xylene may produce neurologic, cardiac, hepatic, and renal damage.

Benzene is rapidly metabolized and is eliminated in about 2 days: as unchanged benzene, about 1 percent; glucuronate conjugate, about 10 percent; and ethereal sulfate, about 10 percent.

BENZINE

Synonyms: Petroleum ether; naphtha. Also known as petroleum spirits; mineral spirits; benzoline; petrol; ligroin. Consists mainly of hexanes, heptanes, and some pentane, octane, and other aromatic and aliphatic hydrocarbons; mixture varies widely with source and processing.

Uses: Lighter fluid, charcoal ignitor, paint thinner and remover, standard solvent, automobile spirits, cleaning spirits, varnish spirits, gasoline fuel, rubber solvent, adhesive solvent, engine operation, paints and varnishes, glue manufacturing, leather processing, color solvent and type cleaner (printing), plus many other uses in industry and at home.

Properties: Highly volatile, inflammable, colorless, aromatic. Insoluble in water. Bp 35–80°C. Soluble in ether, chloroform, or carbon tetrachloride. Temperature mixtures with Bp 80-150° C are apt to be used as gasoline fuel. Above 150°C apt to be used as kerosene oil.

MLD: Approximately 100 ml/70 kg person.

Remarks: Kerosene, gasoline, and naphtha show the same general symptoms and require the same treatment. Absorbed through all portals.

Symptoms: Burning and pain in mouth, throat, and stomach; headache, nausea, vomiting, inebriation, giddiness, cold skin, thirst, tremors, diarrhea, flushed face, feeble pulse, dyspnea, convulsions, cyanosis, narcosis, anorexia, dilated pupils, mental confusion, ataxia, delirium progressing to coma. Pulmonary edema (chemical pneumonitis) may result from aspiration with rapid fatal outcome.

Death by respiratory failure or by complication with pneumonia.

Identification

Steam-distillation separation.
1. Characteristic odor.
2. Flammable; burns with smoky flame.
3. a. Kerosene: Bp, 150–300°C. Moisten a sheet of paper and hold it to light → translucent.
   b. Gasoline: Bp 30–200°C.
4. Characteristic UV spectrophotometric curve in chloroform. Maximum density: 243, 249, 255, 261 nm (see Section I).

5. Distill into CCl₄ and scan in NIR: See Section I.
6. GC: See Section I.
7. See under Kerosene for Gerarde test.

Treatment

Gastric lavage with caution, saline cathartics (25 gm of sodium sulfate), morphine (15 mg for pain). Prevent aspiration into lungs.

Short-acting barbiturates with caution, or Valium (preferably), for irritability or convulsions. Keep patient warm and quiet; maintain body fluid balance. Artificial respiration and oxygen therapy. Wash skin with soap and water. See Kerosene. Supportive

BENZODIAZEPINE GROUP

	Librium (chlordiazapoxide)	Valium (diazepam)	Serax (oxazepam)	Dalmane (flurazepam)	Tranxene (clorazepate)
Members					
Uses	antianxiety tension irritability agitation	antianxiety spasm convulsions	antianxiety tension irritability agitation	hypnotic	antianxiety antidepressant
MLD/70 kg person	2 gm	2 gm	7 gm		0.5 gm
Therapeutic Plasma Level	0.3 mg/dl	0.2 mg/dl	0.1 mg/dl	0.01 mg/dl	0.03 mg/dl
Lethal Plasma Level	2 mg/dl	2 mg/dl		0.2 mg/dl	
Plasma Half-Life	24 hours	24 hours			24 hours

Properties: In general, basic, soluble in ether (best) or chloroform in neutral or very weakly basic pH. Also found in quick screening *in the solvent after* the 0.5N NaOH extraction of the *neutral* ether or $CHCl_3$ extraction.

Remarks: Low toxicity; death to overdose is *rare*, except when in combination with other CNS depressants or with tricyclic antidepressants or amino oxidase inhibitors. Especially dangerous with ethanol or barbiturates; can be fatal.

Symptoms: Nausea, vomiting, diarrhea, overly sedated, drowsiness, ataxia, vertigo, CNS depression (appears like drunk), incoordination; hypotension, hyperexcitability, tremors; hallucinations and rage reaction are also possible; coma, respiratory or cardiovascular difficulties, cyanosis.

Identification

Ammonium hydroxide—ether extraction.

1. Five (5) ml of blood is hydrolyzed with 2 ml HCl (30% v/v) on a H_2O bath for about 5 minutes. Cool. Make alkaline with NH_4OH; extract with 25 ml ether. Separate and filter the ether; collect and re-extract with 5 ml H_2SO_4 (0.5N). Save the ether layer and evaporate and test for neutral drugs if required. Scan the H_2SO_4 extract in UV spectrophotometer.

	Max den	$E_{1cm}^{1\%}$	*Min den*
Librium	245 nm	1100	290 nm
	301	300	
Valium	240	1300	260
	285	700	
Serax	236		262
	282	170	
Dalmane	238		263
	285	190	
Tranxene	235		256
	275		318

2. Confirm by GC: See Section I.
3. Thin layer chromatography (TLC) (See Section I): Extract as above through the ether extraction; gently evaporate the

solvent.   Reconstitute with methanol or chloroform or re-extract the 0.5N H_2SO_4 extract above with $CHCl_3$ after making it barely alkaline with NH_4OH.

	(1)	(2)	(3)	(4)
Librium	64	100	13	15
Valium	65	96	61	80
Serax	57	78	11	30
Dalmane	60	72	28	10-20
Tranxene	—	—	—	—
Tessalon	53	—	34	
Soma	63	100	36	
Meprobamate	54	73	—	
Elavil	46	47	36	

(Dalmane and Valium metabolize to Serax.)

Developing solvents:
- Methanol: NH_4OH (100:1.5) — (1) above
- Ethyl acetate:methanol:NH_4OH:H_2O (85:13.5:0.5:1) — (2) above
- Benzene:acetone:NH_4OH (100:20:6) — (3) above
- chloroform:acetone (9:1) — (4) above

Spray:
- Iodoplatinate.
- Mercuric sulfate.

Treatment

Activated charcoal or milk to slow absorption, gastric lavage. Ipecac for emesis (if charcoal *was not* given) . Saline cathartics, maintain patent airway, maintain all vital signs; especially guard against respiratory difficulties and hypotension.

Do not use barbiturates or any other depressant for hyper-excitability. Symptomatic treatment and general support as for depression described under Barbiturates. Hyperexcitability may occur during recovery phase. Guard against specific action of other drugs that may also be present.

Dialysis is of limited value.

Physostigmine salicylate reported of value for cardiac arrythmias and CNS toxic effects produced by Diazepam overdose (Arena).

Reference: Hoffman, La Roche Inc.

BERYLLIUM (Be)

Derivatives: Beryllium sulfate, fluoride, or oxide.

Uses: Used in fluorescent lamps, in industry.

Properties: Gaseous form is most toxic.

MLD: Approximately 100 mg per cubic meter.

Remarks: Poorly absorbed orally; storage is chiefly in the bones. Cumulative.

Symptoms: Metallic taste. Delayed onset may be acute or chronic. Pulmonary symptoms, granulomatous lesions of the skin and lungs, cough, blood-stained sputum, cyanosis, intense dyspnea, anorexia, marked loss in weight. Conjunctivitis. Pneumonitis with cough may be delayed and prolonged.

When in contact with skin (intact or broken), may produce symptoms such as contact dermatitis (delayed wound healing).

Identification

Atomic absorption spectrophotometry.

Treatment

Removal from exposure. Symptomatic treatment for dermatitis or ulcers.

Oxygen therapy during acute phase. Treat pneumonitis symptomatically. Rest and good diet. Corticosteroids have been reported effective.

BISMUTH (Bi)

Derivatives: Subnitrate; subcarbonate; subsalicylate.

Uses: Medicinals, dressings, antiluetic treatment, gastrointestinal demulcent.

Properties: Compounds are usually white or yellow.

MLD: Approximately 15 gm/70 kg person.

Remarks: Relatively nontoxic. Cumulative.

Symptoms: Metallic taste, black feces, black gum line (Burton), ulcerative colitis, nausea, vomiting, abdominal pain, diarrhea, salivation, swelling of the gums, sore throat and tongue, possible liver damage, collapse, death.

Identification
1. On the original salt:
   a. potassium iodide → brown precipitate, dissolves in excess)
   b. ammonium carbonate → white precipitate
2. Place 20 ml of urine or stomach contents, or 20 gm of tissue or fluids, in small Erlenmeyer flask and add 4 ml of hydrochloric acid. Place into the solution a tightly wound copper spiral* (20 gauge wire) and gently boil 2 hours. Maintain volume with 10% hydrochloric acid. A black deposit may indicate arsenic, antimony, selenium, tellurium, sulfur, or bismuth. Remove copper spiral; wash with water, and place in small test tube. Add 1 ml of sodium sulfite (10%) and 1 ml of 15% nitric acid. Bismuth will dissolve. The other metals will not be affected. To the sodium sulfite-nitric acid solution, add 1 ml of quinine-potassium iodide reagent. If bismuth is present, an orange suspension develops that is directly proportional to the concentration.
   Reagent: Quinine-potassium iodide reagent: 1 gm of quinine sulfate dissolved in 100 ml of 0.5% nitric acid, and then 2 gm of potassium iodide is added and allowed to dissolve.
3. Bismuth solution slightly acidified with hydrochloric acid and then saturated with hydrogen sulfide gas produces a black precipitate of bismuth sulfide.
4. Acid digestion: Do dithizone titration at pH 3. See Lead.
5. Acid digestion: Do Gutzeit as for Antimony (with AgNO₃ stain and flanges). Bismuthine gives a black stain with AgNO₃ that also fades with HCl fumes. Arsenic black does not fade; antimony does. See Arsenic.

Treatment
Activated charcoal and then remove by gastric lavage. Milk and then remove by ipecac. Saline cathartics (Na₂SO₄—30 gms).

*Or copper strip 5 by 5 mm.

Maintain water and electrolyte balance. Guard against dehydration, pulmonary edema, shock, kidney and liver damage.

SPECIFIC TREATMENT: Dimercaprol (BAL) ; see under Arsenic.

BORIC ACID (H_3BO_3)

Derivatives: Borax; sodium borate; boracic acid; borates.

Uses: Medicinals, water softener, industry, roach killer, dance floor wax, antiseptic, eye solution, foot powder, douche powder, denture cleaner and adhesive.

Properties: White crystalline material.

MLD: Approximately 12 gm/70 kg person. Infants are especially susceptible.

APPROXIMATE BLOOD LEVELS: Therapeutic, below 0.1 mg/dl; lethal, above 3 mg/dl.

Remarks: Boric acid gives weak acid reaction. Sodium borate is alkaline. Symptoms may come on slowly (several hours later), and death may occur 2 to 3 days later. Cumulative. May be absorbed through skin (diaper).

Symptoms: Acute gastroenteritis, nausea, vomiting, diarrhea (may be bloody), restlessness, headache; early raw erythematous rash on exposed areas, face, and on palms and soles. Severe dermatitis ("boiled lobster") , conjunctiva may be red. Enterocolitis, dysphagia, cold sweats, fatty degeneration of liver, jaundice, nephrosis, oliguria, albuminuria, acidosis, cerebral edema, pyrexia, cardiac weakness, depressed circulation. Convulsions may develop. Shock, coma.

Identification

1. Urine acidified with hydrochloric acid will color turmeric paper brownish red when positive for borates. Drying the turmeric paper will intensify the color; moisten with ammonia and the color changes to green-black.
2. Boron in tissue or urine (Cohn, Rieders, Rieders) :
   Two (2) ml (1 + 3 homogenate) plus 5 ml $(NH_4)_2SO_4$ (4%) . Vortex—let stand at least 1 hour with shaking. Heat in boiling H_2O bath for 10 minutes with shaking. Centrifuge at 4500 rpm for 15 minutes.

1 ml clear supernatant + 10 ml H_2SO_4 → charr blank. Vortex carefully; stopper, and let stand 5 hours. Read at 620 nm versus H_2O blank = A_1.

1 ml clear supernatant + 5 ml H_2SO_4. Vortex carefully. Add 5 ml Quinalizarine (0.0045% in H_2SO_4). Vortex carefully; stopper; let stand 5 hours for complete color development. Read at 620 nm versus reagent blank = A_2.

$A_2 - A_1 = A$ (boron/ml sample. Example: 0.1 mcg Boron /ml = 0.03 AU

	Toxic above
plasma (adult male)	0.5 mg/dl
serum	0.2
whole blood	0.5
urine	0.5
liver, gm drained wet weight	8
brain, gm drained wet weight	3
kidney, gm drained wet weight	2

Remarks: Antimony, iron, copper and oxidizing acids interfere.

A_1 (blank) step can be omitted on serum or plasma. If levels are high, take a small aliquot.

Powders or ointment placed on damaged skin may produce eventual toxicity (Fisher and Freimuth).

Treatment

Gastric lavage with milk. Emetics, cathartics, alkaline fluids if agent was boric acid. Maintain body heat, water, and electrolyte balance. Correct acidosis with sodium bicarbonate. Protect against liver damage with low-fat, high-carbohydrate intake, and B complex vitamins. Exchange transfusion may be beneficial (especially in children). Supportive

Hemodialysis may hasten elimination and support against anuria. Control convulsions with Valium or short-acting barbiturates. Guard against respiratory or circulatory depression.

BROMIDES (Br)

Derivatives: Triple bromides; sodium, potassium, or ammonium bromides.

Uses: Medicinals, sedatives, photography.

Properties: White, crystalline, inorganic.

MLD: Not known (large amounts).

APPROXIMATE BLOOD LEVELS: Therapeutic, 15 mg/dl; lethal, 250 mg/dl; half-life, 15 days.

Remarks: Rarely acute or fatal. Cumulative. Slowly eliminated. Serum level above 150 mg/dl is intoxication, as NaBr.

Symptoms: Salty taste, mental dullness, lassitude, slow thoughts, foul breath, conjunctivitis, coryza, drowsiness, indistinct memory, depressed reflexes, low sodium chloride retention, skin rash (with ulceration and difficult healing), nausea, vomiting, anorexia, amnesia, slurred speech, peculiar gait, tremors, coma, death.

Identification

1. Two (2) ml of serum is shaken with 8 ml of 10% TCA (trichloracetic acid). Allow to stand 5 minutes and then filter.

   Five (5) ml of clear filtrate plus 1 ml of gold chloride (0.5%) produces a yellow to orange color with bromides. Read color intensity at 440 mμ with a Beckman DU 1 cm cuvette (reference blank, 5 ml of TCA + AuCl$_2$).

Mg NaBr(%)	Transmission
50	64
100	42
150	28

2. Dissolve a small amount of crystalline material or residue in 15 ml of water. Divide into three portions.

   a. To one portion, add 1 ml of silver nitrate → silver bromide (yellow precipitate), which is insoluble in nitric acid and slightly soluble in ammonia.

   b. Shake second portion with chlorine water to liberate free bromine from the bromide. Now shake with 3 ml of chloroform. The heavy chloroform layer will absorb the free bromine and will give a yellow color. If the silver nitrate test was positive (precipitate), the foregoing test will differentiate between chloride, bromide, or iodide.

Chloride → no color in chloroform.

Bromide → yellow color in chloroform.

Iodide → violet color in chloroform.

c. To third portion, add several crystals of $KMnO_4$ + 3 drops H_2SO_4. Suspend fluorescein test paper into tube (strip of filter paper soaked in saturated fluorescein in acetic acid 60%). Yellow → pink.

Treatment

Discontinue exposure. Gastric lavage and/or emetics in acute cases. Cathartics. Sodium chloride, daily intake 8–12 gm, to replace chloride loss. Supportive measures

Maintain body heat, fluids, and electrolyte balance. Recovery is long and slow. Hemodialysis will hasten elimination.

BUTAZOLIDIN (PHENYLBUTAZONE) ($C_{19}H_{20}N_2O_2$)

Identification

1. Steentoft: Urine (50 ml) is slightly acidified and extracted with three times 50 ml of ethylene dichloride. Combine all extracts and filter. Both phenylbutazone and its metabolite (oxyphenbutazone) are extracted. The metabolite is removed from the solvent by extraction with a phosphate buffer pH 8; then the metabolite is re-extracted back into fresh ethylene dichloride at acid pH.

Re-extract each extract with 2.5N NaOH and read each in UV spectrophotometer.

Phenylbutazone: Maximum density, 265 nm.

Oxyphenbutazone: Maximum density, 255 nm.

2. TLC: See Section I.

3. Do alkaloidal color tests: Mandelin's test and Vitali's test (see Alkaloids).

4. UV spectrophotometry: See Section I.

5. GLC: See Section I.

CADMIUM (Cd)

Derivatives: Cadmium metal; cadmium acetate.
Uses: Welding, plating, alloys, paints and pigments.
Properties: White metallic salt, mp 320°C.
MLD: Approximately 1 gm/70 kg person.
Remarks: Acutely toxic, cumulative.

Symptoms: Metallic taste, nausea, vomiting, diarrhea, severe GI irritation, abdominal pains, dizziness, salivation, loss of appetite, loss of weight, headache, rapid pulse, liver and kidney damage, convulsions. When inhaled: dryness in throat, tight chest, dyspnea, pulmonary edema, shock, collapse, death.

Identification

Dialyze gastric lavage or acid digest as described under metals in Section I.

1. Unknown is slightly acidulated with hydrochloric acid plus hydrogen sulfide (H_2S) gas → yellow precipitate.
2. Cadmium salt is made neutral to litmus; then add 1 ml of an alcoholic solution of diphenylcarbazide → red-violet or a red-violet precipitate. (Copper, lead, mercury also give positive results.)
3. ammonium carbonate → white precipitate
4. Atomic absorption.

Treatment

Charcoal, milk, or albumin, then gastric lavage. Cathartics, emetics; demulcents for irritation.

Maintain body heat; fluids, and electrolyte balance. Artificial respiration and oxygen as needed. Support against liver and kidney damage. Symptomatic treatment and supportive measures. Edatate reported of some use.

BAL is contraindicated; BAL and cadmium combination is nephrotoxic.

CAFFEINE ($C_8H_{10}N_4O_2$)

Synonyms: Methyl theobromine; xanthine chemical group; trimethyl xanthine. Theophylline and theobromine are related xanthines that are pharmacologically similar to caffeine.

OCCURRENCES Coffee *(coffee arabica)*—about 100 mg of caffeine per cup. Tea *(thea sinensis)*—about 75 mg of caffeine per cup (caffeine plus theophylline). Cocoa *(thio broma cocoa)*—about 200 mg of theobromine per cup. "Cola" drinks *(cola acumento)*—about 60 mg of caffeine per cup.

Uses: Caffeine is a powerful CNS stimulant and a mild diuretic; it has been used as a mild antidepressant. It maintains wakefulness (antihypnoid), decreases drowsiness and fatigue, while increasing clearness of the mental process, acting as a cortical stimulant. It is incorporated in "cold treatment or pain tablets" such as APC and others.

Caffeine is most commonly used in the form of coffee as a "pick up" mental stimulant, since it decreases the feeling of sleepiness, especially at breakfast, and also the feeling of boredom or tiredness at midmorning and midafternoon. Many millions of cups of coffee are consumed daily at the customary "coffee breaks."

Properties: Caffeine is a white crystalline and shiny, powder with a melting point of 236°C and is a weak base.

MLD: Very few deaths have been reported by its use and probably only when used in excess of 10 grams.

APPROXIMATE BLOOD LEVELS: Therapeutic, 0.5 mg/dl; lethal, 15 mg/dl; half-life, about 4 hours.

Remarks: No deaths have been reported by an overdose of drinking coffee, but an overdose of coffee of more than five cups per day may have a direct dose-related effect on the central nervous system and may affect the heart and its rhythm, blood vessel diameter, coronary circulation; may increase blood pressure, urine volume, and gastric secretions. These effects are capable of producing bizarre signs and symptoms that are very baffling, i.e. high fever or low grade fever unresponsive to persistent antibiotic treatment, psychoneurosis (anxiety) unresponsive to diazepam, and paraxysmal atrial tachycardia.

Heavy coffee drinkers report tolerance, including cross tolerance with other xanthine-containing beverages. Physical dependence with mild withdrawal symptoms such as headache, "craving," irritability, nervousness, restlessness, lethargy, and inability to work effectively may occur on abstinence.

Coffee can have a more profound effect on the old and on the very young. Limited amounts may be allowed to the old; but we should question the practice of feeding coffee to the infant (or child) as is the practice in Puerto Rico and other Latin-American countries.

Symptoms: The symptoms vary with acquired or inborn tolerance, but in general the patients may complain of light-headedness, dizziness, breathlessness, chest discomfort, nervousness, irritability, tremulousness, muscle twitching, tension headache, insomnia (difficulty in getting to sleep or staying asleep), psychoneurosis (anxiety), lack of appetite, loss of weight, restlessness, silliness, elation, euphoria, confusion, disorientation, excitation; even violent behavior with wild, manic screaming, kicking, and biting; progressing to semistupor. Heart palpitations, extra systoles, tachycardia, and arrhythmias may be present. Increased gastric secretions and gut motility, nausea, vomiting, diarrhea, epigastric pain may be produced, and elevated plasma levels of fatty acids and diuresis may be found.

The symptoms intensify with increased dose, which now may produce high fever, dehydration, convulsions, severe cerebral edema, hypotension, circulatory failure, respiratory failure, and death.

Identification

Soluble in dilute acid, chloroform, or benzene; insoluble in ether.

1. UV Spectrophotometry (see Section I). Five (5) ml of serum or 10 ml of urine is alkalinized with NH_4OH and then extracted with 30 ml of chloroform.

   a. The chloroform is separated and is extracted with 5 ml of $0.5N$ H_2SO_4. This is read in an UV spectrophotometer. Maximum density, 272 nm; $E_{1cm}^{1\%}$ 540; minimum density, 243 nm.

   b. The same maximum and minimum o.d. and the same $E_{1cm}^{1\%}$ in $0.5N$ NaOH are shown.

   c. In ethanol: maximum density, 275 nm, $E_{1cm}^{1\%}$ 160. See Aminophylline.

2. To 2 ml of serum or urine and to a 2 ml H_2O blank is added 1.5 g of NaCl and 0.5 ml of 0.1N NaOH; each is then extracted with 10 ml of benzene in a 15 ml glass-stoppered centrifuge tube. Mix and shake for about 15 minutes on a horizontal mechanical shaker.

Centrifuge for about 5 minutes and then transfer 8 ml of the benzene layer to another tube containing 4.0 ml of 6N HCl. Shake the tubes for 5 minutes; centrifuge for about 5 minutes.

Remove the benzene by careful aspiration; transfer the aqueous and remove any dissolved benzene by passing through air using a fine-tipped glass tube; place a 3 ml aliquot of this aqueous to a cuvette and read in an UV spectrophotometer. Determine the absorbance at 237 nm using the H_2O reference extracted in parallel.

One cup of strong coffee (about 150 mg caffeine) will show about 3–6 $\mu g/ml$ *of caffeine* in serum (1–1.5 hours) and in urine in 2–3 hours. (Routh)

3. Thin layer chromatography (TLC).

Developing solvent:
- Methanol:acetone:triethanolamine (1:1:0.03).
  Rf 0.70 (Fiorisi)
- Methanol:ammonium hydroxide (100:1.5).
  Rf 0.63
- Ethyl acetate:methanol:NH_4OH (85:10:5)
  Rf 0.80—caffeine
     0.80—same for pure heroin
     0.90—nicotine (cigarette)
     0.32—morphine
- Ethanol:acetone (9:1) plus trace of NH_4OH (just to saturate)
  Rf 0.89—caffeine → brown
     0.51—theobromine → brownish blue
     0.21—theophylline → violet blue
- Chloroform:ethanol (9:1)
- Methanol:chloroform:NH_4OH (200:18:2.5). Rf 65
- *n*-Butanol saturated with 5N ammonium hydroxide

Spray:
- Locate by UV light.

•Strongly acid iodoplatinic.
- 10% chloramine T in HCl; then expose to NH_3 gas (NH_4OH head space) → red color
- Iodine (0.1N) in HCl 25% v/v and ethanol (1:1)

4. Gas chromatography (GC).
The aqueous from above test 1 is alkalinized with NH_4OH and is then extracted with chloroform. The chloroform is evaporated to dryness; the residue is reconstituted with 50 μl of chloroform and an aliquot is injected into a gas chromatograph (flame ionization detector).
Column 6 feet by 2 mm i.d.; coiled glass; 2.5 % SE-30 on 80-100 mesh
Chromosorb G (AW/DMCS)—temperature 180°C
Temperature: inject port—200°C; detector—300°C.
Gas flow: N_2—30 ml/minute; H_2—30 ml/minute; air—140 ml/minute.

Treatment

Coffee *over indulgence* many times is overlooked because the bizarre symptoms may resemble and masquerade as an organic or mental disease.

Remove the daily intake of coffee and if the above symptoms were due to caffeinism, the symptoms would go away *dramatically* within 36 hours. If the patient again takes *excess* coffee, (challenged) symptoms may reappear. Supportive as necessary.

CAMPHOR ($C_{10}H_{16}O$)

Derivatives: Camphorated oil; spirit of camphor.

Uses: In industry and medicine, formerly used as a stimulant for central nervous system; rubefacient, a liniment.

Properties: Strong odor, white crystalline. Gummy translucent mass soluble in alcohol, ether or chloroform. Mp 176°C.

MLD: Approximately 2 gm/70 kg person.

Remarks: The synthetic is more toxic than the natural product. Recovery may be delayed several days to several weeks.

Absinthe is similar in symptoms and treatment.

Symptoms: Characteristic odor of breath and urine (strong bitter odor). Burning throat and mouth, nausea, vomiting, abdominal pain, diarrhea, headache, dizziness, disturbed vision, delirium, epileptiform convulsion, weak pulse, hyperpyrexia, mental excitement, delirium, narcosis, tinnitus, hallucinations, loss of consciousness, blue lips, lockjaw, pallor, cold moist skin, kidney damage, anuria, collapse (circulatory), coma.

Identification

Steam-distillation separation.

1. Steam distill. Shake out distillate with ether; separate and evaporate distillate on water bath. A crystalline residue is left, which may be identified by the following physical properties:
   White, translucent, tough masses or granules.
   Characteristic penetrating odor, aromatic taste.
   Soluble in

    800 parts water
    1 part alcohol
    0.5 parts chloroform
    1 part ether
    carbon disulfide (freely)

   Melts at 174–177°C.

2. Spectrophotometry in *n*-hexane: Maximum density 290 nm.

Treatment

Charcoal or give water to precipitate the camphor; gastric lavage. Demulcents such as egg white or milk.

Saline purgative (sodium sulfate, 25 gm). Valium to keep patient sedated. It is essential to control convulsions (carefully).

Avoid opiates. Maintain body heat, fluids, and electrolyte balance. Support against possible kidney damage. Artificial respiration and oxygen therapy as needed.

Avoid alcohol and fats and oils, which hasten absorption.

CANTHARIDES ($C_{10}N_{12}O_4$)

Synonyms: Spanish fly or Russian fly; cantharidin (pure).
Uses: Aphrodisiac in animals, local skin irritant, hair tonics.

Properties: White or yellow powder extract from flies. Mp 218°C. Soluble in acid, chloroform, or alcohol; insoluble in ether.

MLD: Approximately 30 mg/70 kg person, as cantharidin.

Remarks: Highly toxic and irritating. Has no aphrodisiacal effect in humans. Death may be delayed several days.

Symptoms: Burning sensation in mouth and throat, thirst, salivation, gastrointestinal irritation, blisters on skin, nausea, vomiting, bloody diarrhea, abdominal pain, renal damage, anuria, hematuria, syncope, tetanic convulsions, chills, slow and feeble pulse, delirium, collapse, death.

Identification

Acid-chloroform extraction group.
1. Residue plus few drops of hot almond oil to dissolve it; then apply 1 drop to forearm. It irritates and reddens the skin.
2. Extract from weak acid (H_2SO_4) solution with 40 ml of chloroform. Filter chloroform layer; add 7 drops of fuming nitric acid; evaporate to dryness. To warmed residue, add 5 drops of reagent (1 part vanillin + 100 parts hydrochloric acid). Heat on water bath → orange-red to brownish red.
3. To the extact, add 1 drop of formaldehyde (10%) plus 4 to 5 ml of sulfuric acid. Heat with shaking → brown color that changes to black as temperature is increased.

Treatment

Gastric lavage with much water (not used if extensive corrosion is evident). Demulcents such as egg whites, milk, cream. (Avoid oils.)

Valium, ether, or short-acting barbiturates, with caution, for convulsions. Maintain body heat and fluid balance.

Treatment is symptomatic and supportive for circulatory failure, shock, or renal impairment.

CARBAMATES

Derivatives: Aldicarb; Allyxcarb; Baygon; carbachol carbaryl (1-naphthyl *N*-methylcarbamate; Sevin); carbofuran (Furadan)

Dimeton; Diacarb; ethinamate; Formetanate; Landrin; Metacil; Methylpetynol; metomyl; Oxamyl; promecarb; pyrolan; styramate; and urethane.

Used as insecticides.

Properties and MLD will vary with derivative.

Symptoms: In general, similar to the organic phosphate ester pesticides. They also depress the cholinesterase activity in blood, (see Parathion.) In this case, it is reversible and the activity of the enzyme comes back to normal within 15 hours.

Identification

Benzene:isopropanol (2:1) or methylene chloride extraction.
(1) Development of TLC: see pages 76 & 118 also
   • 2% methanol in CHCL₃
   • CHCl₃:nitromethane (1:1)
   • CHCl₃:benzene (1:1)
   • Ethyl ether:*n*-hexane (1:1)
   • Chloroform
(2) UV in hexane — see page 106

Treatment

In general, treatment is also the same as for the organic phosphate esters, *except* that 2-PAM and other oximes are *contraindicated* (may even be harmful); see Parathion.

Reference: Hayes, W.: *Clinical Handbook on Economic Poison.* Washington, D.C., E.P.A. 1971.

CARBON DISULFIDE (CS₂)

Synonyms: Carbon bisulfide; dithio, carbonic anhydride.

Uses: Rubber vulcanization, artificial silks, rayons, solvent, cellophane, defatting, insecticide, rodenticide, millerfume.

Properties: Colorless or yellow, odorous, flammable liquid. Bp 46–47°C. Will dissolve sulfur. Soluble in ether, CHCl₃, or CCl₄.

MLD: Approximately 10 ml/70 kg person.

APPROXIMATE LETHAL BLOOD LEVEL: 0.02 mg/dl.

Remarks: Exposure usually by inhalation; absorbed through all portals. Exposure may produce permanent nervous and mental disorders, psychoses.

Symptoms: Nausea, irritant, vomiting, diarrhea, abdominal pain, pulmonary edema, convulsions, collapse, coma, death. CHRONIC: dizziness, weakness, vertigo, visual disturbances, hysteria, nervous disorders, pains in limbs, paralysis with tremors, psychoses.

Identification

Separated by steam distillation; second fraction contains most; first distillate gives poor yield.
1. Add Fehling's solution to 10 ml of urine and boil → gray precipitate.
2. To 10 ml (second distillate), add 5 drops of formaldehyde, 7 drops of 30% KOH, then 3 drops of 10% lead acetate → creamy to black color or precipitate. Sensitive to 0.1 mg per 10 ml.
3. Gently heat 10 ml of distillate plus 2 ml of ammonia and 2 ml of alcohol. Add 3 ml of hydrochloric acid and 1 ml of ferric chloride (10%) → red color.
4. Alcoholic potassium hydroxide → neutralize with acetic acid → add copper sulfate (10%) → yellow precipitate (copper xanthate).
5. Gas liquid chromatography: See Section I.

Treatment

Remove from the exposure; emesis and gastric lavage if ingested. Administer oxygen as necessary; artificial respiration if needed. Treat pulmonary edema.

Keep patient warm and quiet. Valium or short-acting barbiturates (with caution) for sedation. Blood transfusion if indicated. Fluid therapy (carefully) and other supportive measures.

CARBON MONOXIDE (CO)

Sources: Illuminating gas, synthetic gas, automobile exhaust fumes, fire combustion (smoke), furnace gas, heavy auto traffic, garages, and refineries. Commercial or synthetic gas contains approximately 25 percent carbon monoxide; natural gases contain no carbon monoxide, nor does "bottled gas." Carbon monoxide, however, may be produced readily from bottled gas or natural gas as a result of incomplete combustion, improper burning and back-fire, or carbon deposits on combustion parts. (Gas refrigerators or ranges, if not periodically serviced or adjusted, may be a slow but constant source.)

Uses: Fuel, illuminating gas (synthetic).

Properties: Pure carbon monoxide is an odorless, colorless, tasteless gas. However, as we encounter it, it likely will have impurities due to products of combustion that will impart a garlic or aldehyde odor. It is lighter than air and is readily diffusible. It has an affinity for combining with hemoglobin more than 200 times greater than oxygen. This is the basis for its sinister toxicity; it prevents the normal transportation and supply of oxygen to the cells. The brain and heart are especially sensitive to this reduction in oxygen supply. Persons with anemia or an increased metabolic rate (children) are more susceptible.

MLD: The fatal concentration in the blood usually ranges between 40 and 80 percent carboxyhemoglobin saturation. The normal carbon monoxide level in humans may vary from 0 to about 5 percent (smokers), and even higher.

Remarks

Strong affinity for blood to form toxic carboxyhemoglobin, which is bright cherry red and usually prevents clotting. Carbon monoxide combines more readily with hemoglobin in increased concentrations, humidity, temperature, or exercise. Symptoms are emphasized in the very young and in persons with heart disease, anemia, asthma, or hypermetabolic diseases.

The most common exposure is from the exhaust of gasoline engines in an enclosed space (closed garage). Strange as it may seem, there have even been deaths resulting from exposures in open-canopy cruisers at sea during a calm.

Following too closely (tailgating) behind a truck or bus in traffic can easily raise the driver's blood-carbon monoxide level above 10 percent carboxyhemoglobin (series of unpublished data by author).

Breathing vapors of "paint remover" or "paint thinner," such as methylene chloride or ethylene chloride or other similar chlorinated hydrocarbons (and "dry cleaner" solvents), also can produce carboxyhemoglobin in the blood.

Accidental exposure and suicide are the two most frequent means of death due to carbon monoxide.

Carbon monoxide is ubiquitous and is a serious pollutant in our modern society. The smog in Los Angeles and in Brooklyn is known to be "loaded" with carbon monoxide from automobiles and industry.

Since carbon monoxide (carboxyhemoglobin) may produce (anemic anoxia) hypoxia by *reducing* (1) the oxygen-carrying capacity of the blood, (2) the normal dissociation of the oxyhemoglobin available at cell level, and (3) the uptake and utilization of oxygen at cell level by depressing the respiratory enzymes; and since the heart among other sites will suffer during a hypoxic episode, it will be of no surprise that, on close investigation, there is an increase in the incidence of myocardial infarction, especially in those persons predisposed with a cardiac or pulmonary complication.

Response is more rapid at high altitudes, at high temperature and in high humidity. Children are more susceptible to carbon monoxide because they have less hemoglobin and a greater metabolic rate, which requires a higher oxygen demand, as also are persons with an abnormally low hemoglobin (anemia), heart disease, asthma, or hypermetabolic diseases. Symptoms are magnified by exercise (rapid and deeper breathing) because of the increased CO intake and the extra oxygen demand. Factors involving relative toxicity to adults and children can be of great importance, especially in questions of who was the last survivor.

Minimal and maximal limits of concentration of carbon monoxide in the atmosphere were suggested by Henderson and Haggard (see Table XXVIII). Since the time factor had to be considered, an index of monoxide concentration in parts per million (ppm) and time (t) represents the length of exposure in hours (see Table XXIX).

TABLE XXVIII
PHYSIOLOGICAL RESPONSE TO VARYING CONCENTRATIONS*

Concentration of Carbon Monoxide in ppm	Effect†
100 (0.01%)	Allowable for only several hours
400 (0.04%)	Allowable for only one hour
600 (0.06%	Noticeable effect after one hour
1000 (0.10%)	Unpleasant but sublethal effects for only one hour
2000 (0.20%)	Unconscious and dangerous in one hour
3000 (0.30%)	Unconscious and dangerous in thirty minutes
6000 (0.60%)	Unconscious and dangerous in ten to fifteen minutes
10,000 (1.0%)	Unconscious and dangerous in one to five minutes

*From Henderson, Y., Haggard, H.W., Teague, M.C., Prince, A.L., and Wunderlick, R.M., *J Indus Hyg. 137,* 1921.

†A person doing moderate exercise will breathe about twice as much air as when at rest and consequently will absorb twice as much carbon monoxide.

TABLE XXIX
INDEX OF TOXICITY OF CARBON MONOXIDE

$c \times t = 300$	No perceptible effect
$c \times t = 600$	Barely perceptible
$c \times t = 900$	Headache and nausea
$c \times t = 1500$	Dangerous levels

Reference: Henderson, Y. and Haggard, H.W.: *Noxious gases.* New York, Chemical Catalogue Co., Inc., 1927.

Symptoms

Weakness, vertigo, severe headache, nausea, vomiting, apprehension, air hunger, sleepiness, ataxia, great weakness in legs, delirium, tightness around forehead, disturbed vision, clonic and tonic spasms and convulsions, cyanosis, anemic anoxia, paralysis of respiratory center, coma. Heart often continues to beat for a short time after death. Bright cherry red blood, pink discoloration of skin surface.

SYMPTOMS AT VARIOUS BLOOD LEVELS:

Less than 10 percent: Usually no symptoms.

Below 20 percent: Very mild symptoms (if any)—slight headache, shortness of breath during exercise.

Above 20 percent: Moderate to severe symptoms—severe headache, vertigo, tightness around forehead, easily fatigued, diplopia, constriction in chest, sleepiness, noise in ears, cherry red (pink) coloring to blood and skin (this is characteristic).

Above 40 percent: Coma, convulsions, death by respiratory arrest.

SYMPTOMS RELATED TO TYPE OF EXPOSURE:

Sudden exposure to large amounts of carbon monoxide: drowsiness, dizziness, loss of muscular movement, coma, respiratory failure, death very quickly (10 minutes).

Prolonged exposure to small amounts of carbon monoxide: severe headache, vertigo, tightness around forehead, loss of appetite, fatigue, flushing face, diplopia, blurred vision, noises in ears; cherry red blotches on face, neck, and chest; mental depression, lethargy, speech difficulty (may act drunk), difficult breathing, nausea, vomiting, convulsions prior to death.

AFTEREFFECTS

Subtoxic exposure is not cumulative since the carbon monoxide is rapidly removed from the blood.   After 3 hours of ordinary breathing, the blood level is reduced by about one-half of the original level.   If patient is given oxygen therapy, this 50 percent reduction (half-life) is produced in about 30 minutes.   Any permanent aftereffect as described below is usually preceded by a period of depression.   This is due to oxygen starvation, the nerve cells being most sensitive to this lack, the midbrain undergoing irreversible degeneration.   Carbon monoxide per se has no direct irritating effect or lasting action on tissue.

Residual or late effects of acute poisoning: Most mild cases go unrecognized with an uneventful recovery.   However, there may be *aftereffects* following recovery from a marked depression (coma).   Anoxia for several minutes may result in *permanent brain damage,* which may later show up as amnesia, psychoses, excitement or depression, convulsions; difficulty in walking, talking, hearing, or seeing; generalized weakness and fatigue, pain in extremities, frequent headaches with nausea and vomiting.

A person surviving several hours after an exposure has already eliminated a major percentage of carbon monoxide from his body. If death is delayed 10 hours, terminal concentrations may then be negligible.

Identification

1. Take a small porcelain spot plate. Into one groove, place 1 ml of suspected blood or tissue; place 1 ml of *normal* blood or tissue in the other. Heat *very* gently at low heat. The normal blood will char to a brown-black color whereas, if carbon monoxide is present, it will remain brick red. The test is specific and sensitive to 40 percent carbon monoxide saturation.

2. Take 1 drop of blood and dilute with 10 to 15 ml of water. Compare with normal blood diluted in the same manner. Blood containing carbon monoxide is pink. (Sensitive to 50 percent carbon monoxide saturation.)

3. Dilute 1 to 2 drops of blood with about 15 ml of water so that it is a faint pink. This is performed parallel with blood positive for carbon monoxide and a negative blood blank.

    Positive CO blood can be made by bubbling CO gas through blood. Drop (dropwise) 12 ml of H_2SO_4 on 25 ml of formic acid and bubble the CO through a $CaCl_2$ drier and then through blood. Saturation (100%) usually takes about 20 minutes.

    To each of three solutions (unknown, positive known, and negative known), quickly add about 5 drops of 25% NaOH; quickly place thumb over top of each and quickly shake individually.

    The normal (negative) blank will *immediately* turn a straw yellow color, whereas the blood containing more than 20% carboxyhemoglobin will also turn a straw color *but* will delay 5 to 60 seconds or more before it is straw color. The intensity of the original (pink) cherry red plus the time of persistence may easily help to approximate small, moderate, or large amounts.

    This test is specific for carboxyhemoglobin and is positive for levels above 20 percent saturation. The simplicity of this test should lend itself to emergency and presumptive use: *only* fetal hemoglobin interferes (positive).

4. Microdiffusion technic (Feldstein). See Section I.

   Seal with 10% H_2SO_4.

   Outer compartment: 1 ml of blood spread plus 2 ml of 10% H_2SO_4 as expellant.*

   Inner compartment: 2 ml of palladium chloride (11 mg $PdCl_2$ in 25 ml of 0.01N hydrochloric acid; gently (H_2O bath) heat to dissolve.

   Diffusion time is 2 hours at room temperature (30°C). Reduction of $PdCl_2$ to gray or black is positive for carbon monoxide. H_2S (putrefaction) interferes.

   Serial standards of carbon monoxide (5, 10, 20, 30, 40, 50, and 60%) can be made by diluting 100 percent saturated carbon monoxide blood with normal blood.

   This test is sensitive to 5 percent CO saturation.

5. Dilute 1 ml of blood with 9 ml of water. Add 10 ml of a pyrotannic acid solution (1 gm of pyrogallic acid and 1 gm of tannic acid in 100 ml of water); stopper, shake, and allow to stand 15 minutes. Normal blood is gray-brown; blood containing carbon monoxide retains a pink color proportional to saturation. These should be compared with standards similarly treated. Standards are prepared by saturating blood with carbon monoxide (gas) for 1 hour and assuming this to be 100 percent saturated. These are serially diluted with blood to yield varying required standards and then treated with pyrotannic acid. If kept in the dark, these standards are stable for at least 6 months. This test is sensitive to about 20 percent carbon monoxide saturation (specific).

6. Measurement of carboxyhemoglobin by Co-Oximeter (Model 182, Instrument Laboratory Inc., Lexington, MA) (Freireich, Dubowski, and Luke):

   Collect *fresh* capillary, venous, or arterial blood in a tightly closed container, using dry sodium citrate or dry sodium edetate or sodium heparin as anticoagulant. Nonhemolyzed blood may be preserved at 4°C for at least 24 hours.

   For *unhemolyzed postmortem* blood, approximately 5 ml

---

*Substitution of 5% $AgNO_3$ as expellant will minimize interference of H_2S (Cohn).

are centrifuged; the supernatant plasma is removed and discarded. Dilute the cell volume (1:1) with zeroing solution. Add 10 mg of sodium hydrosulfite and shake the mixture. If clots are present, homogenize the entire mixture with a tissue grinder. Recentrifuge the resultant mixture (in a closed container); the supernatant solution is removed and saved for analysis.

For *hemolyzed* blood, mix well; take approximately 3 ml and dilute 1:1 with zeroing solution. Follow instructions as for unhemolyzed blood.

After the instrument has warmed up, inject sufficient zeroing solution (using a regular 2 or 5 ml disposable syringe) into the sample port to completely fill the spiral plastic tubing: it has to be free of air bubbles. Leave the syringe attached to the sample port. Turn on the pump to carry out the zeroing cycle. Turn on the digital display for each channel (Hb, HbO_2, HbCO) and set each to zero; repeat several times until each channel is self-settled to zero.

To the syringe attach a filter with a microfiber glass prefilter pad. Draw about 2 ml of blood or supernatant into the syringe. Remove the microfilter; inject the specimen into the sample port until the reservoir is filled.

Turn on the pump and read the concentrations of Hb, O, and CO on each channel; the number read will be the percentage in blood. Repeat two or three times and average.

Between samples, flush with zeroing solution and reset each channel to zero. When all samples have been measured, inject a cleaning solution (70 m mol sodium hypochlorite), leave at least 5 minutes, flush with zeroing solution, and turn off the instrument.

Reagent: Zeroing solution—10.6 gm octylpnenoxdecaethanol/liter.

Treatment

Immediately remove patient from exposure with minimal activity; carry in horizontal position; minimize energy used and oxygen demand. Any exertion may cause patient to collapse because of low oxygen reserve.

Oxygen (pure) is indicated; so is artificial respiration if breathing is labored or shallow. It is most urgent to prevent or abate anoxia.

Circulation may be improved by *gently* rubbing extremities. Keep patient warm and *quiet.* Avoid all strain. Complete bed rest. Be alert to a delayed relapse several hours later.

Small amounts of whole blood transfusions have sometimes been suggested but perhaps are not necessary since carboxyhemoglobin (although fixed) is not a lasting union. In 3 hours, about 50 percent of the combined carbon monoxide is removed by ordinary breathing. Oxygen therapy greatly facilitates this removal (about 50% in 30 minutes).

Giving respiratory stimulants or methylene blue is of no practical value and *is even dangerous.*

Supportive measures are usually necessary. Pulmonary edema and/or pneumonia would be possible complications.

In an acute episode of carbon monoxide poisoning where either the concentration (c) or time exposure (t) is sufficiently high (above $c \times t = 1500$) to produce a *coma* and *anoxia,* there is always a possibility of damage to the heart and brain. The more profound the coma (and anoxia) and the longer the time exposure, the more severe and the more certain is this damage to the brain and heart. During and following such an episode, be certain to minimize the oxygen demand of the patient. Complete bed rest is mandatory; monitor all vital functions.

Brain damage may be estimated by neurologic testing and is also confirmed by psychologic performance tests specially designed for the purpose.

In an exposure to carbon monoxide where the concentration and the time interval of exposure ($c \times t$) was not sufficient to produce unconsciousness or coma, the anoxia can in itself be a terrifying experience and a discomfort. There can also be a possibility of irritation to the nose, throat, and lungs due to impurities, residual brain damage is unlikely.

CARBON TETRACHLORIDE (CCl₄)

Synonym: Chlorinated hydrocarbon.

Uses: Formerly used as cleaning agent, degreasing agent, fire extinguisher, fumigant (Chlora Sol), vermicide, antihelmintic, dry cleaning agent.

Properties: Heavy, colorless, nonflammable liquid. Sweet penetrating odor. Bp 76°C. Soluble in ethanol, ether, or chloroform. Extremely toxic.

MLD: Approximately 4 ml/70 kg person.

LETHAL BLOOD LEVELS: Any traces.

Remarks: Carbon tetrachloride, when thrown on fires or when heated, produces phosgene, which is very toxic. Inhalation while cleaning clothes or window blinds has caused fatalities. Agent is absorbed rapidly through all surfaces, including skin; presence of oil or alcohol enhances rapid absorption, and a greater toxicity.

Symptoms

ACUTE: In acute poisoning due to *inhalation* of high concentrations, as in its use as a dry shampoo or rug or venetian blind cleaner, there is a direct toxic action on the myocardium as well as central depressor and peripheral vasodilator actions. Other reactions include a sense of fullness in the head, dizziness, headache, CNS depressant, ventricular fibrillation, stupor, unconsciousness. Death may occur within several minutes by cardiac arrest.

IMMEDIATE: After *oral ingestion* of a large amount of this compound, there is a feeling of warmth in the stomach region followed by inebriation, hiccoughs, convulsions, headache, abdominal pain, nausea, vomiting, and diarrhea. Death may occur as a result of cardiovascular collapse or respiratory failure.

Recovery from the immediate effect of the poison does not preclude possibility of a relapse, and careful observation of patient is necessary for at least 3 or 4 days. Carbon tetrachloride exerts a toxic effect that may be *latent* but is still acute on the liver and kidneys. Twelve to 36 hours after ingestion, there may be headache, muscular pain, general malaise, nausea, vomiting, diarrhea, abdominal tenderness (especially liver area), and jaundice.

DELAYED: There are some signs, symptoms, and pathology that may not manifest until from 2 to 8 days after exposure. The headache and malaise persist, as do the gastrointestinal symptoms and, at this point, it is not unusual for bloody stools to appear. Clinical signs of hepatitis may appear—with a large tender liver and increasing amount of jaundice, as well as an oliguria or anuria resulting from direct kidney damage. There is usually some back pain associated with this, along with an increase in nonprotein nitrogen, and potassium in blood as a result of renal failure. Other effects include acidosis and marked nervousness with convulsions, stupor, and possibly death. Death may be due to potassium intoxication or a generalized reaction due to retention of toxic waste products.

Hypertension may not appear immediately but usually a few days after the kidney damage becomes apparent. The acute liver damage is at a maximum in 48 hours, and there have been several cases reported where evidence of liver damage had cleared before the kidney effects became apparent. Death due to nephrosis may usually be averted because the lesion may repair itself in time and recovery may occur if patient can be carried through this period.

Identification

Separated by steam distillation.

1. Odor of carbon tetrachloride on breath or in vomitus. Positive Fehling's tests for sugar in urine.

2. Colorless heavy liquid. Bp 76°C.

3. *Isonitrile test:* Place a small amount of suspected liquid in 10 ml of water, or use 10 ml of distillate. Then add 1 ml of purified aniline and 2 ml of 20% sodium hydroxide and gently heat this mixture for several minutes. A positive result produces a foul odor of phenylisonitrile (skunk odor). Other chlorinated hydrocarbons, e.g. chloral and chloroform, also give positive test.

4. *Pyridine test:* To 1 ml of suspected fluid or 10 ml of distillate, add 5 ml of 30% sodium hydroxide and 5 ml of purified pyridine. (Solid KOH, 2 gm, is stored with pyridine to minimize false reaction). Gently heat for 5 to 10 minutes on a steam bath.

A pink-red color may indicate carbon tetrachloride. Chloral hydrate, chloroform, or other chlorinated hydrocarbons such as chlorobutanol, DDT, and trichloroethanol also give similar reactions. If distillate or test solution is very dilute, first concentrate it by extraction with *n*-heptane and then do test on this. Microdiffusion test may be employed directly on biologic specimen.

For details and quantitation, see under Chloral Hydrate.

5. *Rapid screening by Fujiwara modification* (Bonnichsen and Maehly) :

a. Twenty (20) ml of urine or tissue distillate plus 2 to 3 gm KOH and 2 ml of pyridine (best grade) are vigorously shaken in a test tube. Gently heat in water bath below boiling for several minutes. A pink to violet color is positive. A reagent *blank must* always be made to rule out reagent (especially pyridine) contamination.

b. Twenty (20) ml of urine or tissue distillate, 2 to 3 gm KOH plus 0.5 ml, and 0.4 ml of acetonitrile are mixed and treated as above in test a. A reagent blank must be performed.

For carbon tetrachloride, test b is more intense. For chloroform and other chlorinated hydrocarbons, test b is the same or less intense than test a. For trichloroethylene, test b fades rapidly.

6. NIR; GC: See Section I.

7. Reflux 2 hours with sodium hydroxide and titrate for organic-bound chlorides, which are now ionic chlorides.

8. *Beilstein test:* Burns with a green flame with copper oxide heated on a copper wire. All chlorinated hydrocarbons → green flame.

9. Liver and kidney function tests may be suggestive for delayed action.

10. Microdiffusion: See Section I.

Treatment

Gastric lavage with caution with saline solution, followed by saline cathartics. Avoid fats, oils, alcohol, epinephrine, ephedrine, or related stimulants. Remove contaminated clothing and wash body. Artificial respiration and oxygen therapy as needed.

Treatment is aimed at keeping patient alive until liver and kidney damage subsides. Supportive measures are essential! Regulate fluid intake and electrolyte balance! *Caution:* fluids only if renal function is adequate!

Guard against liver and kidney damage. Hemodialysis may be required to control blood electrolytes. Return to normal liver and kidney function may take several months.

Sulfhydryl compounds (methionine and cysteine) have been reported of some use.

Guard against possible secondary infection.

General symptoms and treatment similar for dichlorhydrin.

CHLORAL HYDRATE ($C_2H_3Cl_3O_2$)

Synonyms: Chloral; "Mickey Finn;" "Knock-out drops." Trichloroacetaldehyde monohydrate; Noctec.

Uses: To arrest convulsive seizures, powerful hypnotic.

Properties: White crystalline. Pungent aromatic pear odor. Bitter taste. Mp 52°C bp 98°C with dissociation. Soluble in water, ethanol, or ether; volatile and is isolated by distillation.

MLD: Approximately 5 gm/70 kg person. Therapeutic dose is 0.5 to 2 gms (oral).

BLOOD LEVEL THERAPEUTIC: 1 mg%; lethal, 10 mg%.

Remarks: Alcohol enhances absorption and hides bitter taste; synergistic with alcohol and should not be used if patient is still intoxicated.

Symptoms: Bitter taste and pungent odor; breath has a pear odor. Irritation of gastrointestinal tract, blanching of lips. Rapid response within 15 minutes; drowsy, sleep, deep coma that may last 10 hours with little aftereffect other than some nausea or vomiting. Depression of central nervous system including cardiovascular and respiratory depression; slow and feeble pulse, circulatory collapse and death. Prolonged (chronic) use may produce fatty changes in liver and kidney damage.

Identification

Isolated by direct distillation (catch distillate in dilute 5% hydrochloric acid); or can be separated by ether or heptane extraction.

1. Chloral hydrate is also eliminated in urine as urochloralic acid and as the glycuronate. False-positive Fehling's test for reducing sugars, but negative with Benedict's test for sugar.

2. Place a small amount of suspected liquid in 10 ml of water, or use 10 ml of distillate. Then add 2 ml of purified aniline and 4 ml of 20% sodium hydroxide and gently heat for several minutes. A positive result produces a foul odor of phenylisonitrile (skunk odor). Other chlorinated hydrocarbons such as chloroform and carbon tetrachloride also give positive results.

3. Blood determination of chloral hydrate or chloroform: To each of two glass-stoppered tubes or graduated cylinders, add 2 ml of blood or tissue distillate (equivalent to 2 gm of tissue). Cool both in an ice bath. In one of the solutions only, pipette 1 ml of 30% potassium hydroxide. Add 6 ml of heptane (CP) to both tubes, shake, and draw off a 5 ml aliquot of heptane after the solutions have separated. Put the heptane into two tubes, each containing 2 ml of 30% of potassium hydroxide and add 4 ml of purified pyridine (CP). Shake the tubes and immerse them in a water bath at about 80°C for 10 minutes. Cool; then centrifuge. A dark pink to red color in the test tube to which alkali had initially been added indicates the presence of chloral hydrate. A similar color in the other test tube indicates the presence of chloroform.

   This test is sensitive to 5 μg. The concentration may be determined by reading the red color in a spectrophotometer at 520 nm or by visual comparison with standards similarly prepared. (Pyridine must be pure and blank must be tested each time.)

   This test is positive for carbon tetrachloride and other chlorinated hydrocarbons, also trichloracetic acid.

4. Chloral hydrate (quantitative): Saturate 5 ml of urine (or

5 gm of blood or ground tissue with 5 ml of water added) with sodium chloride. This mixture is directly distilled (steam distilling is unsatisfactory). Collect 5 ml of distillate. This distillate, plus 5 ml of pyridine (best grade), plus 4 gm KOH are vigorously shaken and then placed in a water bath for 2 minutes, below boiling.

Transfer 3.0 ml of the pyridine layer and 1.0 ml of water to 1 cm cuvette. Read at 530 nm.

Seventy-nine (79) μgm of chloral hydrate has an absorbance of 1.00 (Bonnicksen).

5. Chloral hydrate → trichloroethanol + trichloroacetic acid. Trichloroethanol: prepare sodium tungstate-sulfuric acid, protein free filtrate, then distill to convert into formaldehyde; test with chromotropic acid. (See Formaldehyde—page 342).

Trichloroacetic acid: do Fujiwara test directly on serum, as described above in test 3. Use normal serum as blank. Read at 550 nm.

6. Microdiffusion: See Section I.

To differentiate, do tests 7, 8, 9, and 10.

7. Distill directly into CCl_4 (spectroscopic quality) and then scan in NIR: See Section I.

8. GLC: Stainless steel column 5 inch by $\frac{1}{8}$ inch o.d.; 15% FFAP (free fatty acid phase); 60–80 mesh acid-washed chromosorb W; electron capture detector; injection part 165°C, column 105°C (for separating chloral hydrate and trichloroethanol; 120°C for trichloroethanol alone; carrier gas, nitrogen; flow rate 8 ml/minute.
Reference: Jain et al.: *Am Acad Foren Sci, 12:*497, 1967.

9. Use 10 ml of distillate plus 10 drops of resorcinol (saturated) and 3 ml of sodium carbonate (saturated). Allow to stand for 1 hour. Pour contents into a beaker containing 10 ml of water: chloral will produce a pretty green fluorescence; chloroform or carbon tetrachloride will not.

10. Chloral hydrate + Nessler's reagent → brick red precipitate. Chloroform + Nessler's reagent → nothing.

11. Chloral hydrate distilled with sodium hydroxide → chloroform (typical odor).

12. TLC (Bonnischen and Maehly) :
Solvent: Methanol:NH_4OH (70:1) .
Spray: Resorcinol (10% in ethanol) ; then spray with alcoholic KOH (10%) → violet
Rf = 80

Treatment

Maintain all vital signs; maintain patent airway and remove secretions with suction; use oxygen as necessary.   Supportive. Maintain blood pressure, water, and electrolyte balance; guard against cardiovascular collapse.   Do not use stimulants.   See under Barbiturates.

CHLORATES ($KClO_3$)

Derivatives: Potassium or sodium chlorate.

Uses: Throat gargle, mouthwash, matches, fireworks, toothpastes, weed killer.

Properties: White crystalline.   Sold as powder and tablets; powerful corrosive, powerful oxidizing agent, H_2O soluble.

MLD: Approximately 10 gm/70 kg person.

Remarks: Rare poisoning; occasional accidental swallowing in children.   Produces a marked methemoglobinemia; acetanilide, aniline, bromates, nitrobenzene, nitroglycerine, amino and nitro compounds, and nitrites also produce methemoglobinemia.   Well water when contaminated with surface drainage may convert to nitrites in infants; pickled meat with $NaNO_2$ or nitrates.

Symptoms: Nausea, vomiting, abdominal pain, diarrhea, pain in throat, thirst, pallor, corrosion of throat and stomach; marked methemoglobinemia: *chocolate-colored blood* or cyanosis may be evident with blood levels at 20 percent.   Liver and kidney damage may develop with jaundice, nephrosis, and anuria after a delayed period; *hemolysis* and red-colored urine are noted.   At levels of 60 percent of methemoglobinemia and above, there is extreme weakness due to oxygen lack.   Other effects of methemoglobinemia include tachycardia, headache, dizziness, mild confusion, dyspnea, salivation, ataxia, drowsiness, flushing of skin, palpitations, visual disturbances, fall in blood pressure, weak pulse, collapse, cerebral anoxia, respiratory and/or cardiac failure, convulsions before death.

Identification

Chlorates are *rapidly* changed in the body, so tests should be made *promptly*. Identification is most satisfactory in stomach lavage or vomitus or from drinking-glass residue. Suspend stomach contents or vomitus in water and then filter and test directly.

1. To clear filtrate add several drops of indigo Carmin (0.01%) plus several drops of H_2SO_4 (10%) → blue. Then add several crystals of Na_2SO_3 and the blue color fades. Bromates and hypochlorites also give the same reactions.

2. To another clear aliquot, add 2 ml of silver nitrate (10%) → white precipitate of chlorides. This is filtered and the precipitate discarded. Chlorates give no silver precipitate. Filtrate is mixed with 2 ml of nitric acid (10%) and 2 ml of formaldehyde (38%), which converts chlorate to chlorides, which is precipitated as the silver chloride (white).

3. To another clear filtrate aliquot add starch solution + KI solution + HCl → I_2 is liberated, which reacts with starch → blue-black.

4. To 5 ml of vomitus, add 5 ml of trichloroacetic acid (20%). Filter.
   a. Filtrate plus 2 drops of aniline plus 1 ml of hydrochloric acid → blue-green.
   b. Filtrate plus 1 ml of diphenylamine (2% in sulfuric acid) blue. (Bromates and nitrates also react.)

5. Heparinized venous blood has brown hue (methemoglobin) that will not turn red when oxygenated by frequent shaking with air.

6. One (1) ml of blood methemoglobin (brown) plus 2 drops of 5% potassium cyanide → immediately turns red. (Sulfhemoglobin does not.)

7. Methemoglobin in blood. See Aniline.

Methemoglobin is converted to hemoglobin on standing at room temperature. If sample can not be analyzed immediately, freeze it.

Blood should be heparinized or EDTA treated; all reagents should be reagent quality and freshly prepared.

Treatment

Activated charcoal, or milk, or dilute sodium thiosulfate, then gastric lavage, if early, with great care. Avoid emetic. Give demulcents. Keep patient warm and quiet. Maintain water and electrolyte balance. Avoid acids, lemonade, or fruit drinks. Minimize oxygen demand by bed rest. Artificial respiration and oxygen therapy to support respiration as needed; and general supportive measures.

Little treatment required for methemoglobinemia if less than 30 percent and if exposure has been removed. Normal conversion back to hemoglobin is at a rate of more than 0.5 gm per hour.

Methylene blue is reported *not* effective in chlorate-induced methemoglobin. Whole blood or exchange transfusion may be helpful in severe cases. Ascorbic acid, or sodium ascorbate, or thionine have been reported to be of some help to hasten conversion. Dialysis may also help to hasten removal of chlorates.

Treat for possible liver and kidney damage; and corrosion.

General symptoms and treatment are similar for potassium bromate poisoning.

TEST FOR BROMATE IN URINE: 2 ml of urine plus 1 ml of 4N hydrochloric acid; centrifuge, add 1 ml of 0.01% Evans blue → color fades. Nitrites interfere but are removed by 0.3 gm of urea.

CHLORDANE ($C_{10}H_6Cl_8$)

Synonyms: Octachlor; Velsicol 1068; octachlorohexahydro-methanoindene.

Uses: Insecticide.

Properties: Dark brown, viscous, oily liquid. Insoluble in water; soluble in most organic solvents.

MLD: Approximately 8 gm/70 kg person.

Remarks: More toxic than DDT.

Symptoms: Absorbed through all portals including skin. Gastrointestinal irritant; nausea or vomiting may be delayed. Central nervous system stimulant, neurologic symptoms, anorexia, weight loss, possible liver and kidney damage, hyperexcitability, tremors, convulsions, depression; convulsions again followed by depression, respiratory failure.

Identification

Liver and kidney function tests may be of presumptive value.

1. *Beilstein test:* Thick copper wire dipped in copper oxide and heated to make a bead at end is dipped in any chlorinated hydrocarbon and heated; will burn with a *green* flame.
2. Extract with *n*-hexane: To 1 ml of extract, add 3 ml of Davidow's reagent. Heat in a test tube for 30 minutes in boiling water → red.

   Reagent: 1 volume of diethanolamine to 2 volume of IN alcoholic KOH.
3. TLC: See Section I.
4. GC: See Section I.

Treatment

Wash contaminated skin with soap and water. Use gloves while treating.

Emetics or gastric lavage and saline cathartics (NaSO₄) ; avoid oil demulcents or laxatives. Epinephrine should not be used (in any halogenated insecticide poisoning). Control irritability or convulsions with Valium or short-acting barbiturates, with caution. Quiet and rest are essential. Symptomatic treatment and supportive measures as required for respiratory, liver, or kidney involvement.

General symptoms and treatment for endrin are similar to chlordane; however, endrin is more toxic.

CHLORINATED HYDROCARBONS

Carbon tetrachloride: See under Carbon Tetrachloride.

Chloroform: See under Chloroform.

Dichloroethylene (acetylene dichloride): Colorless liquid. Mild odor. Used in perfumes, textiles, paints, varnishes, glues, soaps, rubber. Strong narcotic action; damages central nervous system with paralysis of sensory fibers of the trigeminal and optic nerves. Absorbed through all portals.

Ethyl chloride: Odorless colorless gas at room temperature. Used as local anesthetic, refrigerant, insecticide. Absorbed through all portals. Rapidly hydrolyzed to ethyl alcohol and hydrochloric acid. Symptoms typical to ethyl alcohol but effects are fleeting. In addition, it has a depressant effect on the heart and may produce ventricular fibrillation. The anesthetic effect disappears rapidly.

Ethylene dichloride (1,2-dichloroethane): Colorless oily liquid. Pleasant odor (sweet) ; sweet taste. Used as degreasing agent and solvent for oils, rubber, soaps, etc. Absorbed through all portals. Exerts a powerful narcotic action. Symptoms similar to chloroform and carbon tetrachloride.

Methyl bromide: Colorless gas, sweet ethereal odor. Soluble in water, alcohol, chloroform. Used as vermicide. Absorbed through all portals. Similar in action and symptoms to methyl chloride. Prognosis is poor. See under Methyl Bromide.

Methyl chloride: Colorless gas, sweet ethereal odor. Soluble in water, alcohol, and chloroform. Used as refrigerant. Absorbed through all portals. Rapidly hydrolyzed to methyl alcohol and hydrochloric acid. Typical symptoms of methyl alcohol; formates may be found in urine. Delayed symptoms (years later) : hallucinations, loss of memory, temporary blindness. Prognosis is poor.

Pentachloroethane: Similar to tetrachloroethane in properties and action.

Tetrachloroethane: Colorless liquid. Used as solvent for degreasing, and in paints, varnishes, resins. Strong narcotic effect; most toxic of the chlorinated hydrocarbons. Absorbed through all portals. Severe liver damage; MLD, 4 ml/70 kg person.

Tetrachloroethylene: Colorless liquid. Etherlike odor. Used in pharmaceuticals, soaps, solvents. Narcotic action but less potent than chloroform or carbon tetrachloride. It is the least toxic of the chlorinated hydrocarbons. Absorbed through all portals.

Trichloroethane (methyl chloroform): Colorless liquid used as cleaner and industrial solvent. Strong narcotic action similar to chloroform and carbon tetrachloride. Absorbed through all portals. "New carbona."

Trichloroethylene (Trilene): Colorless liquid. Mild odor. Used in perfumes, anesthetics, rug cleaning, textiles, paints, varnishes, glues, rubber. Strong narcotic action. Damages central nervous system with paralysis of fifth and optic nerves. Absorbed through all portals. Metabolized and eliminated in urine as trichloroethanol and trichloroacetic acid. Positive for Fujiwara test.

Tests and Treatment—supportive.

Generally similar to carbon tetrachloride.

NIR; GLC; distill into *n*-hexane and read in UV spectrophotometer: See Section I.

CHLORINE (Cl₂)

Synonyms: Chlorine gas; chlorine water; Javelle water; Clorox; Purex; Rox; NaOCl.

Uses: Bleaching agent (industrial) for cotton and paper; water purification and sewage treatment; mildew remover; distributed as liquified (compressed) chlorine; or HTH, chloramine T, or similar high test hypochlorite to liberate chlorine gas.

Properties: Green-yellow gas with pungent, irritating odor that can be detected in even low concentrations such as 3 ppm; heavier than air; unless a person is "trapped," he will not voluntarily stay in an atmosphere containing over 10 ppm because it is so painfully irritating; causes severe choking, coughing, and gasping for air.

MLD: Approximately 500 ppm; 1000 ppm rapidly fatal; 50 ppm is dangerous.

Symptoms

Sharp penetrating irritating odor, lacrimation, choking, gagging, salivation, nausea, vomiting; strong irritation to eyes, nose, and throat; difficult breathing (burning and painful), pulmonary edema, bronchial congestion, sneezing, bronchitis, asphyxia, cyanosis, pallor, cold clammy skin, collapse, death.

Inhalation of small amounts causes few or no symptoms. In

larger amounts, it is a powerful irritant to the mucous membranes of the eyes, nose, and throat. Inhalation of 30 ppm causes immediate choking, coughing, and burning pain in chest.

Temporary disability usually occurs and the vast majority of these patients make a complete recovery (even those that develop a patchy pneumonitis).

Permanent disability is rare and results only when extensive denuding of the fine bronchioles has occurred. Such a rare case may have symptoms of bronchiolar spasm or stenosis. There is no evidence that exposure to chlorine gas predisposes to the later development of tuberculosis or lung cancer. (Johnstone and Miller.)

Acute symptoms usually subside in 12 to 24 hours but may develop into pneumonia and/or bronchitis. (Von Oettingen.)

Sudden death is also possible from asphyxia (cyanosis), shock, reflex spasm in the larynx or massive pulmonary edema.

The rarity of permanent disability is supported by two massive accidental chlorine spills, one involving 418 entrapped persons in a subway train (Chasis et al.) and one involving about 1,000 inhabitants living near an overturned railroad tank (Joyner and Durel.)

Identification
1. Irritating, pungent, green-yellow gas; heavier than air and hugs the ground at lowest level.
2. Easily bleaches cloth.
3. Dissolves in water → hydrochloric acid (HCl) + hypochlorous acid (HOCl).
   a. blue litmus → red.
   b. Nascent odor of chlorine and hydrogen chloride.
   c. add silver nitrate (10%) → white precipitate, which does not dissolve when adding HNO_3
   d. Leak is easily detected by the white heavy clouds produced (NH_4Cl) when in contact with open bottle of (concentrated) ammonium hydroxide.
4. Distill onto KI: starch (paper) → black.
5. Distill into *o*-tolidine solution → orange.

Treatment

Remove from exposure; wash all exposed body area with sodium bicarbonate solution. Keep warm and quiet. Oxygen or artificial respiration as necessary. Maintain all vital signs. Guard against respiratory difficulties due to pulmonary edema. Maintain body fluids and electrolyte balance. Codeine to depress cough reflex. Guard against (or treat) secondary infection.

Do not attempt to neutralize chlorine with chemicals or drugs. No salves or ointments should be applied for 12 hours. Chlorine is very reactive with many chemicals. Supportive!

References

Chasis, H., Zapp, J.A., Bannon, J.H., Whittenberger, J.L., Helm, J., Doheny, J.J., and MacLead, C.M.: *Occup Med, 4:*152-176, 1947.

Johnstone, R.T. and Miller, S.E.: *Occupational Diseases and Industrial Medicine.* Philadelphia, Saunders, 1960.

Joyner, R.E. and Durel, E.G.: Accidental liquid chlorine spill in a rural community. *J Occ Med, 4:*152-154, 1962.

Von Oettingen, W.F.: *Poisoning.* New York, Paul B. Hoeber Inc., 1952.

CHLOROFORM (CHCl₃)

Synonyms: Trichloromethane.

Uses: Anesthetic, medicinals, sedative, antiseptic, solvent in industry.

Properties: Heavy colorless liquid. Volatile, strong odor, burning sweet taste. Bp 61°C. Insoluble in water; soluble in fats and oils.

MLD: Approximately 15 ml/70kg person.

Remarks: Should not be commonly used for anesthesia (too dangerous). Not metabolized in the body. Light anesthesia, 7 mg%; deep anesthesia, 15–25 mg% (Curry); lethal, 40 mg% in blood (liver is higher).

Symptoms: Odor of chloroform (sweet), dilated pupils, acidosis, apnea, irregular respiration, cold clammy skin, cyanosis, slow weak irregular pulse, coma; respiratory but especially circulatory depressant; acute cardiac failure, early fall in blood pressure, myocardial damage, oliguria or anuria, ventricular fibrillation, fatty infiltration and degeneration of liver, slight renal damage, deep narcosis, death terminally from cardiac arrest and/or respiratory failure.

Identification

Volatile steam distillation separation.

1. Place a small amount of suspected liquid in 10 ml of water, or use 10 ml of distillate. Then add 3 ml of purified aniline and 5 ml of 20% sodium hydroxide and gently heat for several minutes. A positive result produces a foul odor of phenylisonitrile (skunk odor). Other chlorinated hydrocarbons such as chloral hydrate also give a positive test.

2. Clear, colorless, nonflammable liquid, but vapors burn with a green flame. Sweet characteristic odor. Bp 61°C.

3. To 1 ml of suspected liquid plus 10 ml of water or 10 ml of distillate, add 5 ml of purified pyridine plus 5 ml of 30% sodium hydroxide; gently heat for 5 to 10 minutes on steam bath. A pink-red color indicates chloroform. This color is proportional to concentration and can be compared with standards similarly prepared. Carbon tetrachloride and chloral also give positive results.

4. Urine gives false Fehling's test for sugar.

5. Chloroform + resorcin + sodium hydroxide → red color with heat (blank gives purple color, which fades).

6. Ragsky reflux → titrate chlorides, after liberating chlorides by refluxing (reflux with strong sodium hydroxide for several hours).

7. Liver and kidney function tests may be of presumptive value.

8. Copper wire burns with green flame (Beilstein test). This is a test for chlorinated hydrocarbons.

9. Microdiffusion; NIR; GC: See Section I. Also see under Chloral Hydrate.

Treatment

Induce vomiting or gastric lavage with warm water or milk if ingested. Demulcents. Artificial respiration and oxygen therapy. Low-fat, and high-carbohydrate diet and B complex vitamins for possible liver damage.

Maintain body heat, electrolyte and fluid balance; maintain

adequate airway, respiration, and normal blood pressure. Prevent hypoxia. Symptomatic and supportive measures for prolonged coma; guard against secondary infection and depression.

CHLORONAPHTHALENE ($C_{10}H_7Cl$)

Synonym: Halowax.

Use: Insulation.

Symptoms: Gastrointestinal upset, dark urine, jaundice, liver damage, convulsions, coma.

Identification

See test for naphthalene in urine (under Mothballs).

Treatment

Valium or ether or short-acting barbiturates to control convulsions (with caution); then gastric lavage. Avoid fat or oil demulcents. Support against possible liver damage, oxygen and artificial respiration if needed.

CHLOROPICRIN (CCl_3NO_2)

Synonyms: Trichloronitromethane; nitrochloroform.

Uses: Disinfectant for cereals and grains, insecticide, parasiticide. Commercially available. War gas (sternutator); Tear gas.

Properties: Liquid. Intense odor. Soluble in petroleum ether, ether, and alcohol; insoluble in water. Bp 120°C. Solidification, 69°C. Toxicity resembles chlorine gas.

MLD: Concentration of 2 mg per liter, inhaled for 10 minutes, is lethal.

Symptoms: Sharp penetrating odor. Produces severe irritation in upper respiratory passages. Strong lacrimatory properties, peculiar form of frontal headache, conjunctivitis, apprehension, pulmonary edema. *Oral:* Severe nausea, vomiting, colic, diarrhea, flow of tears.

Identification

Separated by steam distillation.

1. UV in ethanol: maximum density, 275 nm; minimum density, 255 nm.

2. TLC (hexane:acetone) : See Section I.
3. NIR: See Section I.

CHLOROTHIAZIDE (DIURIL)

Properties: Carbonic anhydrase inhibitor, diuretic. Chemically related to sulfanilamide group. White crystalline. Low solubility in water; soluble in sodium hydroxide but decomposes on standing. Potentiates hypotensive drugs such as ganglionic blockers or hydralazine.

Symptoms: Dehydration and sodium and potassium loss. Fluid and electrolyte imbalance; may produce dry mouth, thirst, drowsiness or restlessness, muscular fatigue and pain, hypotension, nausea, vomiting, tachycardia, mental confusion, delirium, convulsions, shock, coma.

Identification

1. UV spectrophotometry: Maximum density, 291 nm; $E_{1cm}^{1\%}$, 450.
2. Merck Sharp & Dohme method: Prepare a protein-free filtrate (1:20) by adding 1 ml of plasma and 4 ml of 20% PTS solution to 15 ml of water. Dilute urine samples or aqueous standards may be prepared similarly so that the final concentration of PTS is 4 percent.

    Transfer 5 ml of protein-free filtrate (which should contain 5–40 μg of chlorothiazide) to a test tube with 1 ml of 3.75N sodium hydroxide. Heat tube in water bath for 30 minutes. Allow solution to cool; then 5 ml is transferred to a colorimeter tube. Acidify with 1 ml of 6N hydrochloric acid and add 0.5 ml of sodium nitrite. Mix contents gently. After 3 minutes, add 0.5 ml of ammonium sulfamate to destroy excess nitrite. The contents are again gently mixed.

    In about 5 minutes, add 0.5 ml of the EDH reagent and again gently mix. Allow the color to develop fully (which takes about 10 minutes). Read in colorimeter at 515 nm.

    Standardization: The color produced by chlorothiazide in amounts of 5 to 40 μg, when carried through the procedure, is reproducible and follows Beer's law. It is convenient to prepare standards that contain from 1 to 6 μg per milliliter of chlorothiazide in 4% PTS, so that 5 ml portions may be measured directly at 515 nm.

Reagents:

- 20% *p*-toluenesulfonic acid (PTS)
- 3.75N sodium hydroxide
- 6N hydrochloric acid
- 0.1% sodium nitrite (fresh)
- 0.5% ammonium sulfamate (fresh)
- 0.1% *N*-(1-naphthyl)-ethylene diamine hydrochloride (EDH) (fresh)

Treatment

Withdraw drug; correct fluid and electrolyte imbalance. Supportive.

CINCHOPHEN ($C_{16}H_{11}NO_2$)

Synonyms or derivatives: Atophan; neocinochophen (Tolysin); phenylquinoline; phenylcinchoninicum.

Uses: For gout. Analgesic, antipyretic.

Properties: Small, colorless, needlelike crystals or a white or yellowish white powder. Mp 213–216°C.

MLD: Approximately 5 gm/70 kg person.

Remarks: Mp 215°C with partial decomposition. Usually encountered as chronic poisoning.

Symptoms: Nausea, vomiting, diarrhea, malaise, tinnitus, liver tenderness and pain, yellow atrophy, jaundice, renal damage, acidosis, severe gastric corrosion, albuminuria, skin rash, anorexia, increased bile production, vasomotor disturbances, lowered body temperature, analgesia, increased uric acid excretion in urine, itching, stupor followed by death in coma, which may be delayed as long as a week.

Identification

1. Extracted by acid-ether solution.
2. No simple tests for cinchophen; however, a saturated solution in hot dilute hydrochloric acid will precipitate reddish brown crystals if platinic chloride is added.

3. UV spectrophotometry: See Section I.
4. Increased uric acid, chloride, and urea in urine may be presumptive tests.

Treatment

Gastric lavage and emetics if acute. Saline cathartics (25 gm of sodium sulfate) . Treat as for Salicylates.

Prognosis poor after severe symptoms have developed. Supportive therapy for kidney and liver damage.

Maintain body heat and fluid balance.

Symptomatic and supportive measures. Guard against gastric perforation, acidosis, electrolyte and fluid imbalance, and secondary infections.

COCAINE ($C_{17}H_{21}NO_4$)

Synonyms: "Snow;" neurocaine; benzoyl methyl ecgonine.

Uses: Local anesthetic on mucous membranes; not to be injected.

Properties: White shiny crystals; mp 98°C; basic; bitter and numbing to taste; soluble in chloroform or ethanol or ether (in small amounts) .

MLD: Approximately 500 mg (oral) for a 70 kg person; much less by mucous contact.

Remarks: Alkaloid, sympathomimetic, CNS stimulant; death may be immediate by respiratory and circulatory failure, usually within 30 minutes; if patient survives several hours, prognosis is good. Metabolizes in man to ecgonine.

Symptoms

ACUTE: Restlessness, excitability, euphoria, confusion, increased blood pressure and pulse rate, numbness, dry skin and dry mouth, chills, fever, sweating, pallor, muscle spasms, tachycardia, abdominal pain, nausea, vomiting, dilated pupils, delirium, increased reflexes, convulsions, hypotension, irregular respiration, circulatory and respiratory difficulties, coma, death (can block heart conduction system) .

CHRONIC: Some of the above plus loss of the sensation of cold, hunger, tiredness, or pain; loss of weight; perforation of nasal septum (constricts blood vessels) if sniffed; pitting of cornea if locally applied; paranoia, hallucinations, mental deterioration. Possible fatty changes in kidney and liver and congestion in the gastrointestinal tract and in the brain.

Identification

Urine or bile: Cocaine + metabolite ecgonine.

Neutral or barely alkaline with NH_4OH is extracted with ether or chloroform; separate and evaporate solvent with a stream of air (high heat or strong alkali decomposes cocaine).

1. UV spectrophotometry: See Section I.
   In 0.5N H_2SO_4: Maximum density, 232, 274 nm; $E_{1cm}^{1\%}$, 520, minimum density, 260 nm.
   In ethanol: Maximum density, 233 nm.

2. TLC: See Section I.

	$CHCl_3$:meOH (9:1)	meOH:NH_4OH (200:3)	isopropyl ether:ethanol (80:20)
cocaine	95 Rf	73	71
Lidocaine	80	74	14

3. GLC: See Section I.
   2 ft; 2.5% SE-30 column at 210°C (Finkle).
   FID; N_2 carrier gas
   Cocaine Rt 0.29 relative to pentobarbital 3.5 minutes.
   Metabolite Rt 0.45 relative to pentobarbital 2.5 minutes.

4. Crystal tests: See alkaloids.
   a. Wagner's → brown precipitate
   b. Mayers → white precipitate
   c. platinic chloride → pale yellow precipitate
   d. picric acid → yellow precipitate
   e. gold chloride →yellow precipitate (mp 198°C)

5. Color tests: See Alkaloids.
   a. Mandelin → orange
   b. Meckés → colorless → light red → yellow (by heat)
   c. Marquis → wine red (by heat)
   d. sulfuric acid → water bath for 5 minutes; add 2 drops of water → methyl benzoate (peppermint odor)

6. Physiologic tests:
   a. Numbness sensation when "trace" is placed on tip of tongue.
   b. 1 drop (neutralized) placed in cat's eye → dilated pupil.
7. Other special color or precipitate tests:
   a. cobalt thiocyanate (2% in H_2O)

   cocaine → blue "flaky" precipitate is formed, which is not dissolved by 3 drops of freshly prepared solutions of stannous chloride.

   procaine hydrochloride (Novocaine) → blue precipitate, which is soluble in $SnCl_2$

   lidocaine (Xylocaine) → blue color

   dilucaine (Nupercaine) hydrochloride → intensely blue precipitate soluble in $SnCl_2$

   tetracaine (Pontocaine) hydrochloride → intensely blue flaky precipitate is formed, is soluble in $SnCl_2$.

   Heroin, morphine, codeine, methadone, and quinine interfere by giving a similar reaction; Demerol does not interfere.

   Reference: Methods of Analysis for Alkaloids, Opiates, Marihuana, Barbiturates and Miscellaneous Drugs. Publication No. 341 (Rev 12-66). Internal Revenue Service.

   b. cocaine (30 mg) in 2 ml H_2O + 2 drops NH_4OH → heavy precipitate

   procaine → negative

   c. cocaine + 5 drops chromic acid (5%) → orange-yellow precipitate on adding 1 ml HCl → precipitate darkens

   procaine → negative
8. Enzyme multiplied immunoassay technic (EMIT). Kit is available by Syva.

Treatment

Control convulsions with ether, diazepam, or short-acting barbiturates. Wash away from skin or mucous membrane. Delay gastric absorption with activated charcoal and/or milk, then remove by gastric lavage or emesis followed by catharsis. Maintain patent airway and adequate respiratory exchange; supportive and monitor with EKG.

TREATMENT FOR CHRONIC EXPOSURE: Withdrawal of drug; this

does not produce withdrawal symptoms. Supportive for possible kidney or liver involvement and other related symptoms. Chronic users can tolerate very large doses.

CODEINE $(C_{18}H_{21}NO_3)$

Derivative: morphine (methyl morphine).

Uses: Analgesic, for coughs.

Properties: Basic, alkaloidal, white crystalline. Mp 155°C.

MLD: Approximately 800 mg/70 kg person.

APPROXIMATE BLOOD LEVELS: Therapeutic 0.003 mg/dl; lethal, 0.5 mg/dl; half-life 5 hours.

Remarks: Less toxic than morphine. Parasympathomimetic. Metabolizes in man to morphine.

Symptoms: Muscular weakness, disturbed vision and hearing, nausea, dizziness, delirium, constriction of pupils (occasionally dilatation), dyspnea, depression of cough reflex, constipation, respiratory depression, collapse, coma.

Identification

Isolated with alkaline-chloroform extraction. See Alkaloids.

1. Residue is dissolved with 1 ml of acetic acid (1%).

    Use 1-drop aliquot portions for spot-precipitant tests and examine for typical crystals.
    a. Wagner's reagent → brown precipitate
    b. Mayer's reagent → white precipitate
    c. picric acid → yellow precipitate
    d. potassium iodide → long needles
    e. Marme's →dark rosette

2. Small aliquot portions of residue are transferred to spot plate and color reagents applied.
    a. sulfuric acid + sugar → red (with heat)
    b. sulfuric acid + potassium chromate → olive green
    c. sulfuric acid → colorless → blue → red (by heat)
    d. nitric acid → orange → yellow
    e. nitric acid + sulfuric acid → colorless → blue (by heat)
    f. Fröhde's reagent → green → red-brown

g. sulfuric acid + ferric chloride, 1 drop (10%) + heat → blue color after brief foaming

h. Mandelin's reagent → green → blue

i. Marquis' reagent → reddish violet → blue-violet

j. Oliver's reagent → no color

Refer to section on alkaloids for reagents and technics. To differentiate between morphine and codeine, refer to Alkaloids and morphine.

3. UV spectrophotometry; TLC; GC: See Section I.

Treatment

Activated charcoal or proteins. Gastric lavage with dilute potassium permanganate (1:10,000). Sodium sulfate (25 gm) with half a glass of warm water.

Artificial respiration and oxygen therapy as needed. Maintain body heat, fluid balance, and respiration. Supportive measures.

Naloxone is specific and especially good. Treatment generally similar to morphine.

COLCHICINE ($C_{22}H_{25}NO_6$)

Synonyms: *Colchicum* (autumn crocus) ; colchicein.

Uses: Gout, diuretic, purgative.

Properties: Pale yellow amorphous scales or powder. Soluble in ether, chloroform, or alcohol; insoluble in petroleum ether, which is a good way to eliminate impurities of fats or oils. Turns dark on exposure to light.

MLD: Approximately 30 mg/70 kg person.

Remarks: Mp 142–146°C. This drug is *slow* in action, producing symptoms several hours after administration in large as well as small doses. Death may be delayed 24 hours or more. May be detected *even* 8 days later in organs, urine, and stomach lining.

Symptoms: Burning in mouth and throat with difficulty of swallowing, violent gastrointestinal irritation, nausea, vomiting, profuse watery and bloody diarrhea, abdominal pain, profuse salivation, dilated pupils, kidney damage, hematuria, oliguria, irregular pulse and respiration, great prostration, cold sweaty skin, muscular pain, convulsions, paralysis of limbs, respiratory paralysis, collapse, asphyxia, death.

Identification

Classified as an alkaloid. Isolated by alkaline-chloroform extraction.

1. Aqueous solution is neutral to litmus.
2. Dilute acid solution of colchicine is precipitated by most of the alkaloidal precipitants except platinic chloride and picric acid.
3. Small traces of tablets or alkaloidal residue from evaporated alkaline-ether extract is placed in an indented spot porcelain plate or glass plate and is acidified with 1 drop of (2%) acetic acid. The following alkaloidal precipitants are added in micro-amounts, and crystal appearance and structures are studied and compared with known samples.
   a. gold chloride → yellow amorphous precipitate → crystalline form on standing
   b. Wagner's reagent → brown precipitate (if present in fair amounts)
   c. Mayer's reagent → white precipitate (if present in fair amounts)
   Refer to Alkaloids.
4. Small traces of alkaloidal residue or tablets are placed in an indented porcelain plate or glass plate and the following color tests are performed by the addition of 1 drop of each respective reagent to a new sample. Record all colors, absence of colors, or color changes; compare with actions on known. See Alkaloids.
   a. alcoholic solution of colchicine + ferric chloride → garnet red color
   b. Mandelin's reagent → blue-green → greenish brown (Dissolve 1 gm of ammonium vanadate in 100 ml of concentrated sulfuric acid.)
   c. Fröhde's reagent → brownish orange to yellowish green (0.2 gm of molybdic acid in 10 ml of concentrated sulfuric acid.)
   d. Mecke's reagent → citron yellow to yellow-brown (by heat)

(0.5 gm of selenious acid dissolved in 100 ml of concentrated sulfuric acid.)

    e. concentrated nitric acid → violet-red to green to yellow; add potassium hydroxide → red-orange

    f. Erdmann's reagent → blue; add potassium hydroxide → red (Sulfuric acid plus nitric acid.)

    g. Marquis' reagent → yellow (Sulfuric acid plus formaldehyde [25:1].)

    h. sulfuric acid → colorless → blue (by heat) → red (by nitric acid)

5. UV spectrophotometry. (In ethanol or chloroform; does not form salts.) See Section 1 — page 106.

6. Thin Layer Chromatography (TLC) —Kovatsis and Heyndrickx: Solvent developer: Chloroform:acetone:methanol (40:45:15) , Rf 50.

Spray: Vanadate reagent (0.05 gm% in 20% H_2SO_4) → yellow followed by iodoplatinate (3.8 gm KI + 0.38% $PtCl_4$ in H_2O) green brown spots. (sensitivity, 15 μg) .

Treatment

Charcoal or milk and gastric lavage if not in convulsions. Control convulsions with Valium or carefully with short-acting barbiturates. Morphine for pain; calcium gluconate if colic is severe; Atropine as an antispasmodic. Symptomatic and supportive measures. Support against cardiovascular or respiratory difficulties. Maintain respiratory exchange, blood pressure, water, electrolyte and heat balance.

Symptoms and treatment generally similar for colocynth.

COPPER (Cu)

Derivatives: Copper sulfate; copper acetate; copper arsenite.
Blue vitriol: copper sulfate.
Paris green: copper acetoarsenite.
Scheele's green: copper arsenite (ortho) .
Brunswick green: copper carbonate plus chalk.
Mountain green: native copper carbonate.

Uses: Insecticides, fungicides, alloys.

Properties: Blue or green, crystalline.

MLD: Approximately 15 gm of copper sulfate for a 70 kg person. Copper arsenic compounds are far more toxic; oxide is less toxic.

APPROXIMATE BLOOD LEVELS: Therapeutic (normal), 0.15 mg/dl; lethal, 0.6 mg/dl.

Remarks: Copper is relatively nontoxic; it is usually the associated negative radical that is far more toxic and is therefore the agent requiring treatment. Cumulative. Copper is a normal human constituent; urine may contain up to 0.1 mg per diem output (increased in Wilson's disease).

Symptoms: Metallic taste, nausea, vomiting, diarrhea (stool has dark green color), abdominal pain, gastric lavage has bluish tint, salivation, kidney irritation, thirst, irregular pulse and respiration, headache, giddiness, cold sweat, clammy skin, kidney and liver damage, delirium, convulsions, paralysis, exhaustion, pain in chest, coma, collapse.

Identification

Digest with nitric acid, sulfuric acid, perchloric acid.

1. unknown + 1 ml of concentrated ammonia → intense blue color
2. Dithizone: Titration extraction at pH 4; 1 ml of dithizone ≅ 3.5 µg of copper. Digest urine as described under Acid Digestion in Section I. Then titrate as described under Mercury Compounds.
3. unknown + potassium ferrocyanide solution (10%) → red-brown precipitate
4. unknown + sodium hydroxide solution (10%) → blue precipitate
5. unknown + hydrogen sulfide (hydrogen sulfide gas) → black precipitate
6. unknown + ammonium carbonate solution → light blue precipitate
7. unknown + potassium iodide solution → brown precipitate
8. Natelson: To 1 ml of cell-free serum, add 1 ml of 1.2N hydrochloric acid. Allow to stand 5 minutes. Add 1 ml of 20%

trichloroacetic acid; mix and allow to stand 5 minutes. Centrifuge 15 minutes at 2500 rpm; to a 2 ml aliquot add 1.5 ml of trisodium phosphate (saturated solution 100 ml + 5 ml of 10% NaOH) until pH 7.5–9.0. Test with pH paper. Add 0.2 ml of biscyclohexanone-oxalyl-dihydrazone reagent. Let stand 15 minutes. Read before 1 hour at 600 nm. Normal: 80–160 μg of copper per 100 ml.

Reagent: Biscyclohexanone-oxalyl-dihydrazone (saturated): Dissolve 500 mg in 100 ml of 50% ethyl alcohol available from G. Frederick Smith Chemical Co.

9. Atomic absorption.

Treatment

Gastric lavage with charcoal or proteins (milk or albumin). Demulcents. Morphine for pain. Keep patient warm and quiet. Maintain fluid and electrolyte balance, support against liver and kidney damage and dehydration.

Oxygen and artificial respiration as needed.

Keep bowels open with cathartics (sodium sulfate, 25 gm). Supportive and symptomatic treatment.

Versenate (CaNa$_2$ EDTA) is effective to hasten elimination. Penicillamine (Cuprimine) has also been useful in copper elimination.

CORTICOSTEROIDS

Synonyms: Cortisone; Dacortin; Delta Genacart; fludrocortisone; Marsolone; methylprednisolone; Phenolone; prednisolone (Codelcortone; Delta-Cortef; Deltacortril; Delta-Stab; Di-Andreson-F; Hostacortin-H; Hydeltra; Hydrocortisone; PreCortisyl; Sterane; Sterolone) ; prednisone; triamcinolone.

Symptoms

IMMEDIATE: Anaphylaxis, prostration, coma, rigor, death (rare).

LATER: Hypertension and edema, disturbance of water and electrolyte balance.

Identification

1. UV spectrophotometer. See Section I.

H$_2$SO$_4$ (0.5N) : Maximum density, 241 nm.

NaOH (0.5N) : Maximum density, 247 nm.
Ethanol: Maximum density, 240 nm.

2. a. 0.2 mg prednisone + 1 ml H_2SO_4 → yellow
   b. 0.2 mg prednisolone + 1 ml H_2SO_4 → wine-red after 1 minute

3. TLC. See Section I.
   Developing solvents:
   • Chloroform:acetic acid (9:1) Rf 0.17 (prednisolone)
   • Methylene chloride:acetone (8:2) Rf 0.18
   • Chloroform:acetone (9:1)
   Spray
   • Phosphoric acid 30–40%
   • Vanillin (3 gm) + 0.5 ml H_2SO_4 + 100 ml ethanol → blue color
   • Phosphomolybdic acid (1.5 gm) in 100 ml ethanol heat plate to 110°C for 5–10 minutes; examine under UV light

Treatment

Supportive measures; maintain vital functions.

CURARE ($C_{38}H_{44}Cl_2N_2O_6$)

Derivatives: Tubocurarine chloride; Intocostrin; curarine. Flaxedil is curarelike.

Uses: Preoperative agent. Antispasmodic, muscle relaxant.

Properties: Basic white crystalline. Mp 161°C.

MLD: Approximately 50 mg/70 kg person.

APPROXIMATE BLOOD LEVELS: Therapeutic, 0.07 mg/dl; half-life, 1 hour.

Remarks: Alkaloidal. Blocks motor end plate. Far more toxic by injection; relatively nontoxic orally. Parasympatholytic, acts within 2 minutes.

Symptoms: Partial paralysis, head drop, dilatation of pupils, blurred vision (double vision), frontal headache, dizziness, euphoria, advanced paralysis. Consciousness not affected. Glycosuria frequently observed. Respiratory failure, death.

Identification

Isolated by alkaline chloroform or ethylene-dichloride extraction.

1. Residue is dissolved with 1 ml of 1% acetic acid. Use 1 drop aliquot portions for spot-test typical crystals.
   a. Wagner's reagent → brown precipitate
   b. Mayer's reagent → white precipitate
   c. picric acid → yellow precipitate
   Refer to Alkaloids.

2. Small aliquot portions of residue are transferred to spot plate and color reagents applied. See Alkaloids.
   a. sulfuric acid → blue → red
   b. nitric acid → purple
   c. sulfuric acid + nitric acid → violet-purple
   d. Fröhde's reagent → violet
   e. Mandelin's reagent → violet
   f. Mecke's reagent → light violet → red
   g. sulfuric acid (2%) → heat at 40°C → dryness → red color persists for 2 hours
   h. sulfuric acid + crystal of potassium dichromate → blue → red (persists). If strychnine → blue → red → colorless (fading purple) fades more rapidly.
   i. Biologic: inject into rabbit → head drop.

3. UV spectrophotometry: Extract with ethylene dichloride and read in 0.5N H_2SO_4.

4. RIA and by mass spectrometry.

Treatment

Cautiously, physostigmine. Artificial respiration and oxygen therapy. Catheterize frequently. Maintain fluid balance. Tensilon to reduce intensity of peripheral paralysis. Keep patient warm and quiet, and maintain respiration.

Muscular power usually returns in approximately 30 minutes, but diplopia may persist for 3 to 4 hours. After 6 hours, all symptoms usually disappear except for a feeling of tightness in the chest, which may last several days.

Note: Succinylcholine (Anectine) chloride, brucine, magnesium salts, and tetraethyl ammonium compounds also produce a curarelike paralysis with respiratory failure. Therefore, fundamental treatment is to maintain respiration and blood pressure.

CYANIDES (NaCN, KCN, HCN)

Derivatives: Sodium or potassium cyanide, prussic acid, hydrocyanic acid. Amygdalin glucosides in plants hydrolyze to cyanide and glucose. Nitriles, cyanamide, nitroprussides.

Uses: Metal polish, insect extermination, metallurgy, industry.

Properties: White crystalline salt; alkaline reaction.

MLD: Sodium cyanide, approximately 150 mg; potassium cyanide, 200 mg; hydrogen cyanide, 100 mg for a 70 kg person.

APPROXIMATE BLOOD LEVELS: Normal, 0.01 mg/dl; lethal, 0.5 mg/dl.

Remarks: Gas has an almond odor. Very toxic; immediate treatment is essential. May be absorbed through all portals. Death may occur within 5 minutes, or may be delayed several hours.

Symptoms: Following oral ingestion, the stomach is strongly alkaline; local irritation of mucous membranes, burning tongue, perspiration, flushing, throat irritation, salivation, headache, vertigo, tinnitus, fainting, vomiting, photophobia, almond odor vomitus, irregularities of pulse, irregular rapid respiration, convulsions, histotoxic anoxia, excitement, cherry red blood, coma, convulsions, partial paralysis, death usually within a few minutes due to respiratory arrest (sometimes may be delayed.)

Amygdalin glucosides (apple, almond, apricot, peach pits), in addition to above cyanide symptoms, produce high fever, elevated blood glucose, and positive glucose test in urine.

Identification

Direct on tissue or fluids.

1. Five (5) ml of tissue slurry or fluids is slightly acidified with tartaric acid in Erlenmeyer flask fitted with a "loose" cork.

    Schonbein test reagent: dip strip of filter paper into a 10% alcoholic solution of guaiac resin; air dry; then moisten with 0.1% $CuSO_4$. This strip is held with loose cork and is suspended in head space in an Erlenmeyer containing the specimen. Gently warm Erlenmeyer on low H_2O bath at 37°C → reaction may be immediate or may take 15 minutes (depending upon concentration). Blue color may suggest the presence of cyanide, H_2O_2, ozone, chlorine, nitrogen oxide, or sulfides (H_2S). Confirm cyanide by following test.

2. One (1) ml of 10% sodium hydroxide is placed in center, then 1 ml of blood, or gastric contents in outer chamber of a microdiffusion "Conway cell." See Section I.

Several drops of 10% sulfuric acid is placed in rim as a liquid seal; then overlay the specimen with 1 ml of H_2SO_4 (10%). *Immediately* cover and gently twist lid to make a liquid seal in rim.

Allow to liberate volatile (HCN) cyanide from specimen to absorb into the sodium hydroxide (about 1 hour at room temperature).

Remove the lid and add 5 drops of (10%) fresh $FeSO_4$. Add dropwise HCl to (just) dissolve the brown precipitate of $Fe(OH)_3$.

When the brown is completely dissolved a blue color indicates presence of cyanide as Prussian blue fine precipitate. This color is proportional to concentration and is sensitive to 0.1 mcg/dl and is specific using the above procedure.

0.1 mcg/ml (+ −)		0.5	++
0.3	+	1.0 mcg/ml	+++
		3.0	++++

Steam-distillation separation (collect distillate in 10% sodium hydroxide to prevent loss). See Section I.

3. To 20 ml of distillate, add several drops of sodium hydroxide (10%); plus several drops of fresh ferrous sulfate (10%) → brown precipitate of ferric hydroxide. Dropwise add hydrochloric acid until precipitate just disappears; a new precipitate of Prussian blue (deep blue) will appear if cyanide is present (specific).

4. To 20 ml of distillate, add 10 ml of ammonium polysulfide. Evaporate on water bath to dryness → ammonium thiocyanate. Dissolve with approximately 5 ml of water; then acidify with

hydrochloric acid. Filter and add a few drops of ferric chloride → a deep red color (ferric thiocyanate).

5. To 20 ml of distillate, add 5 ml of silver nitrate (10%) → white precipitate. (Hydrochloric acid interferes.)
6. Make 20 ml of distillate alkaline with sodium hydroxide (10%). Add 3 ml of picric acid and gently heat → red color. (Creatinine and blood sugar interfere.) Blood is unsatisfactory.

Note: *Cyanide* (HCN) in traces may sometimes be generated in fires in conjunction with carbon monoxide and can later be found in the blood of the victim in addition to the finding of carbon monoxide. Levels of CN may range 50 to 200 μg% in blood; also found with heavy smokers.

Treatment

Immediate action is essential. Death is rapid.

Sodium nitrite, 3%, in 10 ml of normal saline given slowly intravenously. Then follow with sodium thiosulfate: 25% (50 ml) intravenously. Repeat if necessary. Kit (Lilly) available.

If above is not available, inhalation of several pearls of amyl nitrite every 3 minutes.

Administer vasopressor drugs to prevent fall in blood pressure; oxygen as needed.

If taken orally, induce vomiting or gastric lavage, after given above treatment.

Artificial respiration or oxygen therapy to maintain breathing. (Heart sometimes continues when respiration stops.)

Recumbent position, keep patient quiet and warm; supportive.

DDT ($C_{14}H_9Cl_5$)

Synonyms: Dichlorodiphenyltrichloroethane; 1,1,1,-trichloro-2,2-bis (*p*-chlorophenyl) ethane.

Uses: Insecticide, was common. Available as 10% in talcum, 5% in kerosene; 50% wettable. Uses are now restricted in United States.

Properties: White crystalline. Not very soluble in water. Neutral. Mp 109°C.

MLD: Approximately 15 gm/70 kg person. DDD is less toxic.

APPROXIMATE BLOOD LEVELS: Normal, 0.001 mg/dl; lethal, 0.5 mg/dl; half-life, 1 year.

Remarks: Its greater toxicity may be due to its vehicle—kerosene. Death may be delayed 24 hours or more, but usually occurs in 5 to 24 hours. Fat soluble; is stored in tissue fat.

Symptoms: Acts on central nervous system; symptoms may appear within 1 hour. Nausea, vomiting, diarrhea, anorexia, mental anxiety, giddiness, stiffness and pain in jaw, sore throat, tremors, numbness and partial paralysis of extremities, hyperactive knee jerk, loss of proprioceptive and vibratory sensation of the extremities, delirium, convulsions, respiratory arrest. Pulmonary edema probably due to paralysis of respiratory center. Injury to liver and kidney, collapse, death. Symptoms may be delayed several months.

Identification: Vomitus or gastric lavage or residues

1. Extract with 4 times its volume with petroleum ether. Separate, and gently evaporate. Pick up residue with 5 ml of n-hexane (spectral grade). Micro filter and read in UV spectrophotometer. Maximum density is 235 nm. See Section I.

2. To 5 ml (dissolved in n-hexane in Test 1 above), add alcoholic NaOH → evaporate to dryness. Cool. Add 5 drops mixture (CCl_4 + H_2SO_4 + HNO_3). Shake vigorously → green color (fades in about a minute).

3. Wipe some DDT onto a cotton swab; dissolve in ethanol and then transfer a small aliquot into 5 ml of anhydrous hot pyridine containing a pinch of xanthydrol and one pellet of solid KOH → red color. Sensitive to 10 μg. Use hood.

4. Residue is re-extracted with acetone and then evaporated (carefully) to dryness. After nitrating, DDT and related compounds give a rose-blue color with KOH; and a bright blue-purple with acetone and alcoholic KOH. Sensitive to 1 μg.

5. Beilstein test: Copper wire heated with CuO; burns green with chlorinated hydrocarbons.

6. Thin layer chromatography (TLC), See Section I.

7. Gas chromatography with electron capture detector.

8. For chronic exposure kidney and liver function tests may be of some presumptive value, but nonspecific.
Note: DDT is stored in fat depots.

9. Tentative AOAC:

Use a 5 ml sample; extract with 15 ml of acetone; filter and evaporate acetone. Dissolve extract with alcohol and add several pellets of potassium hydroxide. Reflux for 1 hour. Add 50 ml of water and cool; then add sufficient nitric acid to neutralize plus 1 ml in excess. Add exactly 40 ml $N/10$ standard silver nitrate; add until no more precipitate is produced, plus small excess. Add 0.5 gm of ferric sulfate and 5 ml of nitrobenzene. Back titrate the excess $AgNO_3$ with standard $N/10$ NH_4SCN until a faint pink end point.

Calculate percent of DDT on the basis that 1.00 mg of chlorine = 10 mg of DDT: $0.00355 \times 20 \times 10 = \%$ DDT.

Treatment

Emetics or gastric lavage, and saline laxatives. Avoid oil laxatives (or oils in general). Epinephrinelike drugs should be avoided.

Control convulsions with Valium or short-acting barbiturates. Guard against fatal ventricular arrhythmias.

Quiet and rest are especially necessary; Low-fat, high-glucose diet, and other supportive measures for liver damage.

Calcium gluconate (4–10 cc of 10% solution IV). Maintain body heat and fluid balance.

DDD or Dilan is less toxic; aldrin or dieldrin is more toxic than DDT. General symptoms and treatments are similar.

DEMEROL ($C_{15}H_{21}NO_2$)

Synonyms: Meperidine; pethidine; isonipecaine.

Uses: Substitute for morphine. Antispasmodic, narcotic, analgesic.

Properties: Basic. Bitter taste. Mp 186–189°C. Soluble in ethanol, $CHCl_3$, or ether.

MLD: Approximately 1 gm/70 kg person.

APPROXIMATE BLOOD LEVELS: Therapeutic, 0.05 mg/dl; lethal, 1 mg/dl; half-life, 3 hours.

Remarks: Similar to morphine in action but less toxic; less habituation and addiction. Not to be used intravenously.

Symptoms: General symptoms similar to morphine, but effects are not as lasting. Relaxation of smooth muscles, euphoria, dizziness, perspiration, dry mouth, nausea and vomiting, short-lasting drowsiness, some mental confusion.

Pupils are unaltered (possible dilatation) ; overdose may cause excitement, tremors, or even convulsions; blurred vision, disorientation, hallucinations, tachycardia.

Side reactions may be similar to symptoms for atropine overdosage; thus, the two may be confusing.

Identification

Alkaline-chloroform extraction, also by alkaline distillation. Five minute HCl-hydrolysis is suggested.

1. A small portion of residue is dissolved with 1 ml of acetic acid (2%). Use 1-drop portions in a spot plate and, with microtechnic, do alkaloidal precipitate tests. Technic and reagents described under Alkaloids. Examine for typical crystals.
   a. picric acid (sat.) → amorphous → large rosette crystals.
   b. sodium nitroprusside (5%) → amorphous → bladelike plate or small hexagonal crystals
   c. potassium dichromate (5%) → long yellow needles (in 6N hydrochloric acid)
   d. potassium iodide (20%) → long or short blunt needles

2. Make 100 ml of urine alkaline with sodium hydroxide. This is then distilled into 5 ml of 1% hydrochloric acid; collect 50 ml of distillate.

   Transfer distillate to a separatory funnel and make alkaline with NH_4OH. Extract with 50 ml of chloroform and again with 25 ml of chloroform. Combine the chloroform extracts, add 2 drops of hydrochloric acid, and evaporate. Pick up with 3 ml of water and read in UV spectrophotometer. See Section I. Maximum density, 263, 257, 251 nm; $E_{1cm}^{1\%}$, 9; minimum density, 261, 254, 248 nm.

3. TLC: See Section I.
   Developing Solvents:
   • Benzene:Acetone:NH_4OH (100:20:6)
   Shake and discard excess NH_4OH

Demerol	34 Rf
Phenergan	51
Benadryl	42
Cocaine	84
Elavil	56
Serax	12
Codeine	07

4. GLC: (Rouseau) See Section I.
   Column, SE 30, 4%, Ch. WAW, DMCS S steel, 5 foot by $\frac{1}{8}$ inch; injector 210°C; column 170°C; detector 210°C; Carrier: N; 35 ml/minute; retention time, 2.15 minute.

Treatment

Charcoal and then gastric lavage if taken orally and if patient is not yet depressed. Symptomatic and supportive measures similar as for Morphine. Naloxone (Narcan) is an excellent specific antidote. See under Morphine.

DETERGENTS (phosphate types)

Uses: Dishwashing, general household, industrial cleaning agent.

Properties: May contain sodium tripolyphosphates, sodium silicates or metasilicate, sodium sulfate, trisodium phosphate, nonionic sufactant, chlorinated isocyanuric acid, sodium carbonate. If ammoniated, see under Ammonia.

Symptoms: Corrosive burning of mouth, throat and esophagus; pain in the digestive tract, intense thirst, dysphasia, nausea, vomiting, diarrhea, collapse with rapid feeble pulse, clammy skin, shallow and difficult breathing. Delayed action may include intense swelling and ulceration of mouth, throat, and esophagus. Esophageal stricture and gastrointestinal complications may be possible with high alkalinity. Hypotension, shock, low blood calcium, tetany.

Identification

Very alkaline to pH test paper. Test for Phosphates.

Treatment

Immediately irrigate eyes (gentle stream) with water, if contacted; assure complete flushing.

Mouth contact: flush copiously with water; avoid gagging or swallowing the rinse water. Melted butter, vegetable oil, or margarine may serve as demulcent.

If ingested: Give water or milk immediately for diluent effect, and give citrus fruit juice or vinegar mixed with equal parts of water for neutralization, then give demulcents. Do not induce vomiting. *Carefully evaluate* before doing a gastric lavage.

Corticosteroids and supportive measures to minimize stricture of the esophagus. Maintain water, electrolyte, body temperature, and blood pressure. Calcium gluconate for hypocalcemia and Valium for convulsions.

Also see under Alkalies.

2,4-DICHLOROPHENOXYACETIC ACID
2,4,5-TRICHLOROPHENOXYACETIC ACID

Synonyms: 2,4-D; or 2,4,5-T esters or salts.

Uses: Weed or shrub killer, herbicide; Weed B-gon.

Symptoms: Throat and gastric pain, skin flushing, high fever, weakness, lethargy, visceral congestion, myotonia, hypotension; possible sudden death by ventricular fibrillation. Delayed action may produce weight loss, anorexia, bronchopneumonia (however, chest signs may be few or even absent), acute pulmonary edema, muscle weakness, liver and kidney damage, hepatomegaly, albuminuria.

Identification

Acid-chloroform extraction.

1. Heat gently with sulfuric acid and a pinch of chromotropic acid → purple (sensitive to 0.05 μg 1 ml).
2. Reflux with sodium hydroxide and then titrate for total organic chlorides. See under DDT.

3. Read in UV: 0.5N NaOH.

Maximum density, 230, 284, 290 nm; minimum density, 258, 289 nm; $E^{1\%}_{1cm}$, 97.

4. Extract stomach contents with alcohol and reflux; filter and concentrate by distillation with reduced pressure (Repetto and Menendez).

   a. Aliquot for TLC and GC

     Solvents:

      • Benzene:ethanol (1:1)

      • Acetone:ethanol (1:1)

     Sprays:

      • Ammoniacal $AgNO_3$ in acetone → expose → UV → dark spots.

      • Chromotropic acid in H_2SO_4 (50%) + heat → dark purple.

   b. Decolorize with decolorizing charcoal if necessary. Residue + 2 ml H_2SO_4 + 5 mg chromotropic acid. Heat to charring point → cool → stand → violet color.

5. Extarct with *n*-heptane; read in UV spectrophotometer with hexane reference blank.

Maximum density 283, 292 nm; minimum density 250, 289 nm.

Treatment

Generally similar to kerosene. Give quinidine sulfate orally to relieve myotonia if present and to suppress ventricular arrhythmias. Activated charcoal or milk, then gastric lavage with care. Saline cathartics (Na_2SO_4—30 gm). Symptomatic and supportive for fever or convulsions or cardiac arrhythmias. Maintain water and electrolyte balance. Maintain an alkaline urine with $NaHCO_3$ during myoglobinuria.

DIELDRIN ($C_{12}H_8Cl_6O$)

Similar compounds: Aldrin; endrin (most toxic).

Uses: Insecticides.

Properties: Chlorinated hydrocarbon. Soluble in petroleum ether, fats, or oils; insoluble in water. Can be absorbed through all portals including skin.

Remarks: Serum has highest concentrations during the first day; thereafter, serum has the least and brain and muscle tissues have a higher concentration. After several months the fat layers contain residual amounts.

Symptoms: Nausea, vomiting (sometimes absent when *very* large amounts are ingested in a short interval) ; acts as a central nervous system stimulant producing hyperirritability and violent convulsions and/or coma, cyanosis, dyspnea, abdominal pain, salivation. Vomiting unless treated will reoccur at short intervals ($\frac{1}{2}$ hour) but will stop usually when the central nervous system symptoms start to appear. E.E.G. may be abnormal for several months after exposure.

Identification

One hundred (100) ml of urine or stomach contents is vigorously (mechanically) extracted with 3×50 ml of *n*-hexane serially in a glass-stoppered bottle. Collect and wash hexane with water and then with 2% NaOH and once again with water. Remove unwanted lower layer each time by suction with a capillary tube. Finally the hexane is dried with anhydrous NaSO$_4$. Transfer extract to a test tube and evaporate to dryness on a water bath at about 40°C with a gentle stream of clean air (Cueto and Hayes).
1. GLC: Pick up above with hexane and inject. See Section I.
2. TLC: See Section I.
3. Extract stomach contents with petroleum ether, then evaporate; pick up residue with carbon tetrachloride. Read in NIR. Compare with standards.

Treatment

Control convulsions with Valium or short-acting barbiturates; dose just sufficient to control convulsions. Continue as needed until hyperirritability subsides.

Decontaminate body (skin) with soap and water. Use gloves. Gastric lavage or emetics; caution against aspiration. Saline cathartics (sodium sulfate, 30 gm in half a glass of water) .

Avoid fats or oils; do not use epinephrine, or related agents.

Calcium gluconate may be used in addition to short-acting barbiturates or Valium.

Supportive measures as necessary.

DIGITALIS GLYCOSIDES

Synonyms or group members: Digitalis, digitoxin, digoxin, gitoxin, Difoline, gitalin, Digalen, Digitalon, digitonin, digitin; foxglove, fairy gloves, purple foxglove. Neoside is digitalislike.

Uses: Medicinal (cardiac).

Properties: Extracted from leaves *(Digitalis purpurea)*. Insoluble in water or ether; soluble in chloroform or ethanol (neutral).

MLD: Approximate quantities for a 70 kg person:

digitalis:	2 gm
digitoxin:	3 mg
digoxin:	10 mg
gitalin:	15 mg
Digilanid-C	15 mg

APPROXIMATE BLOOD LEVELS: For digitoxin, therapeutic, 0.002 mg/dl; lethal, 0.005 mg/dl; half-life, 6 days. For digoxin, therapeutic, 0.0001 mg/dl; lethal, 0.001 mg/dl; half-life, 36 hours.

Remarks: Are grouped as glycosides. Overdose parenterally may produce death in less than 5 minutes.

Toxic symptoms may start to appear several hours after oral overdose. Even two or three times a therapeutic dose may sometimes bring on toxic symptoms. This may vary with the sex and age of the patient. Children appear to tolerate larger amounts than adults.

Symptoms: Oral symptoms may be slow in onset, i.e. delayed several hours. Nausea, abdominal pain, vomiting, drowsiness, slow irregular pulse; loss of appetite, salivation, cold extremities, giddiness, persistent vomiting, diarrhea, headache, generalized weakness. Delirium and hallucinations, visual disturbances of multiple nature, blurred vision, diplopia, disturbed color vision including mostly green and yellow and possibly red. Bradycardia, heart block, and cardiac arrhythmias of all types are possible; tremors, and occasionally convulsions. Death usually due to ventricular fibrillation or cardiac standstill.

Identification: Acid-Chloroform

Separate from stomach contents by dialysis for 24 hours; extract with 50 ml of chloroform by mechanical shaker. Filter and evaporate to near dryness. Transfer to a TLC plate.

1. TLC: See Section I
   Developing solvent:
   • Methylene chloride:methanol:formamide (85:14:1)
   • Methylene chloride:methanol:formamide (90:9:1).
   Spray: water (sensitivity 20 μg).

   Scrape off digitoxin spot and put it into a centrifuge tube containing 5 ml of xyanthydrol reagent. Stopper and agitate vigorously for 2 minutes. Loosen stopper and place in a water bath for 3 minutes, followed by an ice bath, and then centrifuge for 10 minutes at 2000 rpm.

   Digitoxin (5, 10, 20, and 30 μg) is quantitated by intensity of the rose-wine color. (Jelliffe: *Am J Clin Path, 47:*180, 1967.)

   Plate: 30 gm of silica gel G mixed with 60 ml of 0.05N sodium hydroxide (pH 7.0). Slurry spread in usual fashion at 250 μ.

   Reagent: Xyanthydrol was freshly prepared for each test: 30 mg dissolved in 100 ml of glacial acetic acid to which 1 ml of hydrochloric acid was added later.

2. (Johnston and Jacobs).
   Developing solvent: Benzene:ethanol 95% (7:3).
   Spray: 70% $HClO_4$:H_2O (15:100).

   Plate heated at 100°C for a few minutes. Approximately 1 μg of digitoxin, digoxin, ouabain, or lanatosides can be detected.

3. TLC: Extract with chloroform:methanol (1:1).
   a. *Solvent system #1:* Methylene chloride:methanol:formamide (80:19:1) (Stahl in Waldi)

      Detection: Freshly prepared aqueous 3% solution of chloramine (10 ml) is mixed, before use, with 40 ml of a 25% solution of trichloroacetic acid in 96% ethanol. After spraying, heat for 7 minutes at 110°C. Under UV, light blue spots appear; digitoxin gives a yellow spot.

b. *Solvent system #2:* Cyclohexane:acetone:acetic acid (49:49: 2).

Detection: Mix cautiously, while cooling, 5 ml of acetic anhydride with 5 ml of sulfuric acid. The mixture is added slowly, while cooling, to 50 ml of absolute ethanol. Prepare freshly before use. Spray plates; dry for 10 minutes at 110°C. Cool and spray again with fluorescein, 0.2% in ethanol. View under UV light.

4. Identification of digitoxin (0.1-mg) tablets: Pulverize and dissolve one tablet in a 10 ml Erlenmeyer flask with 5 ml of 80% ethanol. Heat for 10 minutes at 70°C with constant stirring to dissolve completely. Transfer quantitatively into a 60 ml separatory funnel using about 20 ml of water and then extract with five 4 ml portions of chloroform. After each extraction, carefully allow layers to separate and filter chloroform through dry filter paper to absorb droplets of water. Combine chloroform extracts into a 25 ml volumetric flask and bring volume up to 25 ml mark adding chloroform through the same filter paper.

A 10 ml aliquot is transferred and is evaporated to dryness with a stream of air. Dissolve residue in 2 ml of solution (0.3 ml $FeCl_3$ 10% and 50 ml glacial acetic acid). Then carefully underlay with 2 ml H_2SO_4 → brown ring at interface → light-green → blue which then diffuses into solution.

5. a. Another 10 ml aliquot is evaporated to dryness + Sanchez reagent (0.3 gm vanillin in 100 ml hydrochloric acid) → olive green → blue margin on gentle heat.

b. One (1) mg glycoside + 1 ml 1% alcoholic picric acid (fresh) + 1 ml of NaOH (carbonate free) → red-orange.

6. Digoxin (USP): Evaporate extract to dryness on steam bath and stream of air. To residue add 2 ml acid-$FeCl_3$ (60 ml acetic acid + 5 ml sulfuric acid + 1 ml $FeCl_3$ − 10%) → mix → green-green-blue.

7. Digitalis tablet is tan.

  a. Extract with alcohol; evaporate. Pick up with $CHCl_3$. Read in NIR with $CHCl_3$ reference blank; typical curve, identical with standard digitalis tablets. See Section I.

  b. Evaporate $CHCl_3$ → typical crystals; compare with standard digitalis.

8. RIA (kits available) .

Treatment

Prompt removal by gastric lavage and/or emesis and saline cathartic (30 gm of sodium sulfate in half a glass of lukewarm water) . Discontinue drug. Onset of symptoms may be delayed 6 hours; maximum effects may be delayed 15 hours; and duration of action may be even up to 1 month. Digitoxin is more toxic than digitalis; onset and duration of action are shorter. Antiemetics should be used to minimize the vomiting. Keep patient warm, quiet, and recumbent for several days; slight exertion may be fatal. Sedation for restlessness and excitement. Artificial respiration and oxygen therapy as needed. Supportive measures.

Dialysis is reportedly of little value and perhaps is even contraindicated.

Continued E.K.G. will indicate progress of treatment and condition of patient. Guard against arrhythmia.

General symptoms and treatment are similar for red squill, strophanthin, and ouabain.

DILANTIN ($C_{15}H_{11}N_2O_2$)

Synonyms: Diphenylhydantoin, phenytoin, Epamine.

Uses: Anticonvulsant, especially against grand mal epileptic convulsions.

Properties: Basic, white odorless powder. Soluble in water. Hygroscopic.

MLD: Approximately 2 gm/70 kg person.

APPROXIMATE BLOOD LEVELS: Dilantin—therapeutic, 1.0–2.0 mg/dl; lethal, 8 mg/dl; half-life, 24 hours. Phenobarbital—therapeutic, 0.5–1.5 mg/dl.

Remarks: Protects against hypersensitivity of nerve cells and anoxia.

Symptoms: Giddiness, ataxia, confusion, nervousness, tremors, dilated pupils, blurred vision, nystagmus, slurred speech, gastrointestinal upset, hyperglycemia, dysphagia. Hypertrophy of gums, increased capillary permeability, dry skin, itching, rash and purpura; agranulocytosis may result from prolonged use.

Identification

Acid-chloroform extraction:

1. Gives positive Koppanyi test as for barbiturates, but color is blue not lilac. Dissolve residue in 1 ml of chloroform and transfer to a micro test tube. Add 2 drops of cobalt acetate, mix, then overlay with isopropyl amine → purple interface.

2. Determination of Dilantin in presence of phenobarbital: (Goldbaum and Wallace: *Anal Chem 40*:978, 1968; and Ft. Gordon Pathology Hospital Staff.)

   Add 50 ml of chloroform (spectral grade) to each of three separatory funnels. Then add 5.0 ml serum to one; 5.0 ml of Dilantin standard (20 μg/ml) to another; and 5.0 ml of normal serum for Dilantin control blank. Shake well, separate, filter the chloroform layer, and collect 40.0 ml. Add 5 ml of 0.45N NaOH to each and shake well. Separate and transfer the NaOH layer to a test tube. Centrifuge for 5 minutes. If for Dilantin alone, skip step a for barbiturates and proceed for Dilantin with step b.

   a. For barbiturates: Transfer 2.0 ml of above NaOH extract into each of two test tubes. To first add 1.0 ml of 0.45N NaOH; to second add 1.0 ml of borate buffer and mix. Separate, and read in (Cary) UV spectrophotometer and obtain the differential UV curve by using the buffered extract in the reference compartment and the diluted NaOH extract in the sample compartment. Begin the spectrum at 305 nm with pen adjusted to the 0.300 absorbance line. The spectrum is ended at 230 nm.

   Verify the barbiturates by the shape of the differential curve. Barbiturates have a maximum absorbance at 260 nm with a minimum at 238 nm and isobestic points near 249 and 230 nm. Subtract baseline (0.300 absorbance) from absorbance at 260 nm. Corrected absorbance $\times$ 10.4 = mg/ dl of barbiturate.

b. For Dilantin after above barbiturate analysis: Combine both above extracts and evaporate in water bath at 50–60°C with vacuum to about 1 ml. Or if barbiturate analysis was not performed: Add 4.0 ml of the NaOH buffered extract into a centrifuge tube and then evaporate in water bath at 50–60°C with vacuum to about 1 ml.

Add 20 ml of 1% $KMnO_4$ (made in 7N NaOH). Stopper (with glass stopper only) and place in 80°C water bath for 8 minutes. Remove and cool. Add 4.0 ml *n*-heptane (spectral grade) and shake for 10 minutes. Transfer heptane and scan at 300–235 nm with *n*-heptane reference. Absorbance maximum at 247 nm is used for calculations when compared with standard curve.

Reagents:
- NaOH (0.45N)/3 ml NaOH (staturated) is diluted with $H_2O \rightarrow$ 110 ml.
- Borate buffer: Dissolve 61.8 gm boric acid and 74.6 gm potassium chloride in water and dilute to 1000 ml; allow to stand overnight. Filter any precipitate. Add 2 parts of NaOH (0.45N) to 1 part of above borate buffer using a pH meter to adjust to pH 10.5.

3. GC (Wallace). Barber-Coleman, 6 foot column packed with 2% Carbowax 20 M on gas chromatography Q, 100–120 mesh. Column at 200°C; carrier gas, nitrogen; flow rate, 50 ml per minute.

4. TLC: $CHCl_3$:ether (85:15), Rf 15. See Section I.

Treatment

Discontinue drug; gastric lavage with charcoal. Effects disappear within a few days after its administration is discontinued. Symptomatic and supportive treatment, and correct hyperglycemia if present.

3,5-DINITRO-ORTHO-CRESOL ($C_7H_6N_2O_5$)
(and related dinitrophenols)

Synonyms: DNOC, DN, DNP, Detel, Dinitrol, Sinox, Effusan, Elgetol, ND, nitrocapsine.

Uses: Insecticide (especially locusts) , fungicide, niticide.

Properties: Yellow crystalline. Bitter taste. Stains yellow. Mp 86°C. Soluble in acetone, chloroform, or benzene.

MLD: Approximately 0.5 gm/70 kg person; concentrations of 0.2 mg per cubic meter may be fatal.

Remarks: Symptoms and treatment generally are similar for other dinitrophenols.

Symptoms: Nausea, vomiting, gastrointestinal irritation, restlessness, hot and flushed, fever, sweating, dyspnea, thirst, fatigue, anxiety, excitement, increased respiratory rate, tachycardia, increased urine output, greenish-yellow urine, insomnia, chest pain, cyanosis, respiratory and cardiac difficulty, coma.

CHRONIC: Sweating, thirst, dyspnea, coughing, increased basal metabolic rate, loss of weight, general fatigue. Skin may be stained yellow. Neuritis, liver and kidney involvement.

Identification

1. Yellow color is discharged by hydrochloric acid
2. alcoholic solution + 1 ml of ferric chloride → yellow to deep red
3. warmed with a solution of sodium hypochlorite → chloropicrin (acrid odor)
4. Digested with 1% sodium hydroxide; filter. Filtrate is neutralized with sulfuric acid and then treated with a fresh solution of potassium cyanide → Purpurate (deeply colored; can be quantitated)
5. UV spectrophotometry: See Section I.
6. TLC: See Section I.

Treatment

Gastric lavage with sodium bicarbonate. Saline cathartics (25 gm of sodium sulfate) ; avoid oil laxatives or demulcents; Valium or short-acting barbiturates for excitement. Artificial respiration and oxygen therapy as required. Sponge and alcohol rubs to lower body temperature. Avoid antipyretic drugs! Fluids to guard against dehydration; sodium bicarbonate to correct acidosis; maintenance of electrolyte balance. Quiet and rest; symptomatic and supportive measures.

DITHIOCARBAMATES

Compounds: Ferbam, ziram, maneb, zineb, nabam.

Remarks: Local irritants, relatively low toxicity to man. Cause gastrointestinal upset, dermatitis, anorexia, weight loss after long exposure. Chemically similar to Antabuse and may therefore produce serious side reactions in the presence of alcohol.

Treatment

Gastric lavage, saline cathartics (25 gm of sodium sulfate).

DIOXANE

Remarks: Weak narcotic action, gastrointestinal irritant. Blood changes, anemia, dyspnea, liver and kidney damage possible.

Treatment

Symptomatic and supportive measures.

DORIDEN ($C_{13}H_{15}NO_2$)

Synonym: Glutethimide.

Properties: Insoluble in water; highly soluble in fats or oils; stored in fat depots. Rapidly hydrolyzed in alkali.

MLD: Approximately 10 gm/70 kg person.

Approximate Blood Levels: Therapeutic, 0.05 mg/dl; lethal, 4 mg/dl; half-life, 10 hours. Mild intoxication: about 1 mg% in blood; moderate intoxication: less than 2.5 mg; severe intoxication: above 3 mg% (about 10 gm intake) (coma).

Remarks: Long-lasting depressant, prolonged coma. Body fat, liver, or blood may be used for identification. Urine and bile contain the inactive metabolite. Synergism with alcohol or barbiturates.

Symptoms

ACUTE: Central nervous system depression; may have slow onset. Hypothermia followed by fever, diminished reflexes and lowered pain sensation, fixed and dilated pupils, Hypertension, pulmonary and cerebral edema, tachycardia, cyanosis, respiratory depression, deep coma, shock. *In children:* Fever, dry mucous membranes, laryngospasm, flushing closely resembling atropine poisoning.

Is slowly metabolized and eliminated. Depression lingers. Patient may regain consciousness and relapse into deep coma.

CHRONIC: Ataxia, tremors, hyporeflexia, slurring of speech, memory loss, delirium, irritability, fever, weight loss. Withdrawal symptoms include anxiety, convulsions, abdominal cramps, chills, numbness of extremities and difficult swallowing. Any or all of these may result from abrupt discontinuance.

Identification

Separated by ethyl acetate, petroleum ether, or chloroform.
1. Koppanyi test → blue-green → green.
2. TLC: See Section I.
   a. *Developer:* $CHCl_3$:ether (85:15). View under UV light and then spray.
      Spray: $Hg (NO_3)_2$ (1%) → black.
   b. *Developer:* $CHCl_3$:acetone (9:1). View under UV light and then spray.
      Spray: $HgSO_4$ and diphenylcarbazone (see under Barbiturates and TLC).

Compound	(a) Rf	(b) Rf	Color
Doriden	84	0.92	dark violet
meprobamate	20	0.24	white
phenobarbital	37	0.42	lilac
amobarbital	60	0.61	lilac
pentobarbital	56	0.64	lilac
secobarbital	60	0.72	blue

   c. *Developer:* Change the ratio to $CHCl_3$:acetone (75:25). *Doriden* now goes over the top.

3. Extract 50 ml of urine with 150 ml of ether. Filter the ether and evaporate gently in a white porcelain dish. Add to residue 2 drops of saturated hydroxylamine hydrochloride in ethanol and then add 2 drops of saturated potassium hydroxide in ethanol. Allow to stand about 30 minutes and carefully neutralize with hydrochloric acid to *barely* acidic; add 2 drops of ferric chloride (1.5% in 0.1N hydrochloric acid) → gives a violet color for Doriden (Hensel).

4. Extract 2 ml of plasma with 25 ml of chloroform. Also do a standard parallel at same time. Shake for 3 minutes and separate and filter $CHCl_3$ through Whitman #541 paper into a second separatory funnel. Add 5 ml of 0.45 N NaOH to the $CHCl_3$ filtered extract. Shake for 3 minutes. Separate and filter the $CHCl_3$ layer. Add 5 ml of 0.6N hydrochloric to the filtered extract; shake for 3 minutes.

   Transfer a 15 ml aliquot of the $CHCl_3$ layer to an evaporating dish. Carefully evaporate to dryness in an 80°C water bath using a stream of air. Remove from water bath as soon as evaporated to avoid destroying glutethimide.

   Pick up sample with a mixture of 2.0 ml of ethyl alcohol + 5.0 ml of *n*-hexane + 0.5 ml of distilled water.

   Mix for about 5 seconds to insure thorough mixing. Allow layers to separate. Remove hexane layer (top layer) by suction or dropper and discard. With remaining alcohol–water extract of standard and unknown transferred to silica cuvettes, set up blank and do standard and unknown as follows:

Blank	*Standard or Unknown*
1.0 ml alcohol-water (2.0/0.5)	1.0 ml of alcohol-water extract
2.0 ml ethyl alcohol	2.0 ml ethyl alcohol
1.0 ml distilled water	1.0 ml distilled water

   When all is set up, add 0.1 ml of 10N KOH to blank and quickly mix; with stopwatch ready, add 0.1 ml of 10N KOH to unknown or standard. Read and take absorbances at 1, 2, 3, 4, and 5 minutes against blank. *Read at 235 nm.*

   First do standard; then read unknown using the same blank.

Reference: Dauphinais and McComb: *Am J Clin Path, 44:*440, 1965.

5. GLC: See Section I.

6. Extract 5 gm of blood or homogenized tissue with 75 ml of chloroform. The chloroform layer is filtered through Whatman #41 filter paper.

The clear filtrate is shaken with 5 ml of 0.5N NaOH to remove barbiturates or other acidic compounds. Then it is again shaken with 5 ml of 0.5N H_2SO_4 to remove any basic compounds.

The chloroform layer is filtered through Whatman #41 paper to make it water-free and clear (approximately 50 ml). Evaporate gently to dryness with an air current. The residue (Doriden) is extracted with 2 ml of absolute alcohol and 5 ml of *n*-hexane (spectral grade). Add 0.5 ml of water and the two solvents separate into two layers. Mix, allow to settle, and then separate. Discard the *n*-hexane layer.

a. Add 1 ml of the clear alcohol extract to 2 ml of absolute alcohol.

b. Two (2) ml of a Doriden standard (50 μg/ml in alcohol) with hexane is run parallel to unknown.

c. Reagent blank of absolute alcohol and *n*-hexane. Discard hexane. Alcohol acts as a reference blank when KOH is added.

To each is added 1 ml of 0.2N KOH. Mixing time is recorded. Optical density is determined in a UV spectrophotometer against a reference blank.

Doriden in alcoholic KOH has a characteristic absorbance maximum at 235 nm and a minimum absorbance at 225 nm. Optical density is recorded at 235 nm at 8 minute intervals. Rate of hydrolysis (decay) of a Doriden standard is determined under identical conditions.

The half-life for Doriden under above conditions is about 17 minutes. The optical density at 235 nm after ten half-lives represents absorbing substances other than Doriden. This optical density is subtracted from each of the initial readings. On semilog paper, the correct optical densities are plotted against time. Optical density at zero time is determined by extrapolation. Using the above procedure, 50 μg of Doriden in 2 ml of plasma will have an optical density at zero time of aproximately 0.60 at 235 nm. Recoveries of all Doriden showed an error of 5 percent.

Reference: Goldbaum and Williams; Algeri.

Treatment

Carefully evaluate all reflexes (especially corneal and patellar). This is a guide as to depth of depression. At all times, maintain adequate respiratory exchange. Keep air passages open; prevent aspiration. Tracheotomy should be considered if indicated by excessive secretions and by difficulty in maintaining a clear airway; endotracheal intubation is a valuable aid for the first 48 hours. Give artificial respiration as needed.

Remove as much of the drug as possible by gastric lavage, taking every precaution to avoid aspiration. Avoid emetics if patient is depressed. Saline cathartic (30 gm of sodium sulfate) should further minimize absorption of drug.

Maintain adequate circulation with 5% glucose in water and/ or plasma expanders in dosage just adequate to maintain near normal blood pressure, as needed.

Place patient on side so as to minimize dangers of aspiration. Turn him at regular intervals to prevent hypostatic pneumonitis. Guard against secondary infection. Inflate lungs fully with room air at least once every 3 hours to diminish atelectasis. Careful observation for at least 24 hours after apparent recovery. Patient may awake and then later relapse into deep coma.

Maintain fluids, electrolyte balance, and body heat. Catheterize urinary bladder as necessary. Great caution is advised on administering parenteral fluids; cerebral and pulmonary edema may develop.

Mild analeptics such as Megimide (bemegride), Emivan, or Ritalin to just maintain reflexes and keep the E.E.G. active. These should not be used in an attempt to awaken the patient; in general, it is better to provide physiologic support of vital functions. *Intensive care is vital,* especially during the acute phase.

Coma may persist for days. Prognosis is good if anoxia and

pneumonia can be prevented. Supportive.

Hemodialysis in severe poisoning has been recommended, but it is reported that peritoneal dialysis is of doubtful value.

EMETINE ($C_{29}H_{40}N_2O_4$)

Synonyms: Ipecac, Dover's powders.

Uses: Expectorant, emetic, amebicide.

Properties: Basic, white amorphous powder. Soluble in alcohol, chloroform, and ether. Mp 74°C.

MLD: Approximately 200 mg/70 kg person.

Remarks: Alkaloid. Death may occur in 1 hour but usually is delayed several days. Systemic action is absent when drug is given orally.

Syrup of Ipecac is of low toxicity; Extract or tincture of ipecac is much more toxic.

Symptoms: Severe gastrointestinal irritation, nausea, vomiting, diarrhea, muscular pains, wrist drop, vertigo, dyspnea, convulsions, nephritis, cardiac depression, weakness and irregularity of heart rate, fall in blood pressure, myocardial necrosis, heart stopped in diastole.

Identification

Separated by alkaline-chloroform extractions.

1. Residue is dissolved with 1 ml of acetic acid (2%). Use 1-drop portions for spot-precipitant tests and examine for typical crystals. See Alkaloids.
   a. Wagner's reagent → brown precipitate
   b. Mayer's reagent → white precipitate
   c. picric acid → yellow precipitate
2. Small trace aliquot portions of residue are transferred to a spot plate and color reagents applied. See Alkaloids.
   a. nitric acid → orange-yellow
   b. nitric acid + sulfuric acid → green → yellow
   c. Mandelin's reagent → brown
   d. Marquis' reagent → brown
   e. Fröhde's reagent → red → brown-green

f. sulfuric acid → brown-green
g. calcium hypochlorite + drop of acetic acid → yellow-orange color

3. UV Spectrophotometry: See Section I.
4. TLC: $CHCl_3$:MeOH (85:15). See Section I.

Treatment

Gastric lavage with activated charcoal. Demulcents. Cardiac stimulants if needed. Valium or short-acting barbiturates with caution for convulsions.

Keep patient warm and quiet in recumbent position. Maintain fluid balance. Treat with supportive and symptomatic measures. Guard against kidney involvement.

EPHEDRINE ($C_{10}H_{15}NO$)

Synonyms: Ma huang, ephedrine sulfate or chloride.

Uses: Central nervous system stimulant, for asthma, respiratory stimulant, hypertensive agent, vasoconstrictor, cough syrups.

Properties: Sympathomimetic. Ephedrine HCl, Mp 218°C. Hygroscopic, Mp 40°, basic.

MLD: Approximately 600 mg/70 kg person.

Remarks: Is active when given orally. Effects superficially similar to those of epinephrine. Apparently no cumulative effects.

Symptoms: Hypertension, tachycardia, mydriasis, dry nasal mucosa, analepsis, motor restlessness, nervousness, insomnia, anxiety, delirium, inhibition of gastric and intestinal motility, cardiovascular collapse, death. Similar to epinephrine.

Identification

Separated by alkaline-chloroform extraction.

1. Typical crystals with alkaloidal precipitants. Refer to Alkaloids.
2. Test solution plus:
    a. salicylaldehyde + sulfuric acid → red
    b. sulfanilic acid + hydrochloric acid + sodium nitrite (10%) → colorless → much later → rose-red

c. potassium hydroxide (10%) → no color → evaporation → orange-red

3. Dissolve 10 mg in 1 ml of water plus 2 drops of hydrochloric acid (10%) and 0.1 ml copper sulfate (10%) followed by 1 ml of sodium hydroxide (20%) → reddish purple color.

    To this mixture, add 1 ml of ether and shake well → ether layer is purple and water layer is blue.

4. Dissolve 50 mg in 10 ml of chloroform → allow to stand → and on spontaneous evaporation → typical crystals (Mp 218°C).

5. UV Spectrophotometry; TLC: See Section I.

Treatment

Symptomatic, general supportive treatment. Gastric lavage with potassium permanganate (1:10,000). Sedation with Valium or short-acting barbiturates. Generally similar to amphetamine and epinephrine.

EPINEPHRINE ($C_9H_{13}NO_3$)

Synonyms: Adrenalin, Suprarenin, adrine, norepinephrine (Arterenol).

Uses: Antihistaminic, hypertensive agent in acute circulatory collapse, with local anesthesia, bronchial asthma, and control bleeding (vasoconstrictor).

Properties: Sympathomimetic, slightly alkaline, short-acting. Mp 212°C. Slightly soluble in alcohol and water.

MLD: Approximately 50 mg (hypodermically) for a 70 kg person.

Symptoms: CNS stimulation, nausea, vomiting, fever, chills, nervousness, restlessnes, irritability, dilated pupils, blurred vision, tachycardia, twitching, convulsions, hyperglycemia, hypertension, pulmonary edema, coma, respiratory and cardiovascular difficulties, arrythmias, respiratory or cardiac failure.

Identification

Separated by an alkaline-chloroform extraction.

1. Mix 2 ml of test solution with 1 ml of sulfanilic acid solution, 2 ml of sodium bicarbonate solution, and 1 ml of phosphoric

acid (10%) → yellow color (which is proportional to concentration). Sensitive to 1:1,000,000.

2. Test solution plus:
   a. salicylaldehyde + sulfuric acid → yellow to flesh color
   b. sulfanilic acid + hydrochloric acid (5N) + sodium nitrite (10%) → deep rose-red, which quickly appears
   c. potassium hydroxoide (10%) → red → evaporates → gray residue with greenish cast

3. residue or solution plus 1 ml of sodium acetate (1%) + 4 drops of mercuric chloride (1%) + heat 40–50°C → rose-red color immediately (sensitive to 1:1,000,000)

4. residue or solution + potassium persulfate solution + heat → red color

5. residue or solution + phosphotungstic acid solution → blue color

6. UV spectrophotometry; TLC: See Section I.

7. In urine: determine catecholamine elevation (normal: less than 0.2 mg per diem).

Treatment

Control convulsions with Valium. Activated charcoal and gastric lavage, maintain vital signs. Maintain respiratory exchange, blood pressure, fluid and electrolyte balance.

Symptomatic and supportive measures.

ERGOT

Derivatives: Ergotoxine, ergotamine, egonovine.

Uses: In obstetrics to control uterine hemorrhage; migraine headaches.

Properties: Plant extract. Oxytocic. Fungus found on rye.

MLD: Approximately 1 gm/70 kg person. Derivatives are more toxic.

Remarks: Uterine contraction. Ergot extract may vary in intensity and properties due to variance of constituents.

Symptoms

ACUTE: In several hours: burning pain in abdomen, vomiting, great thirst, diarrhea. Delayed: edema of face and extremities, abnormal sensation of the skin, tonic contractions of muscles, slow weak pulse, tinnitus, miosis, blurred vision, intestinal and uterine contraction, loss of speech and inability to walk, convulsions and mania, skin gangrene after some time, death due to respiratory and cardiac failure.

CHRONIC: Spasmodic or convulsive type from ingesting food containing ergot. Indefinite pains, disturbed digestion, itching and numbness; anesthesia of arms, legs, toes and fingers; painful tetanic spasms, contraction of limbs, mental weakness, dementia. Limbs get cold and become dark in color; dry and gangrenous fingers and toes. Cataracts are common; internal organs become gangrenous. Kidney involvement.

Identification

1. The identification of ergot by isolating the coloring matter in the acid-ether extraction. The stomach contents are extracted with acidified alcohol and filtered. The filtrate is evaporated and the residue is again filtered and extracted with ether. The aqueous solution is drawn off and sodium carbonate solution added to the ether layer in the separatory funnel. On shaking, the ether layer will assume a red-violet color in the presence of sclererythrin. The color consists of three definite absorption bands: one in the yellow and two in the green.

2. Ergot alkaloids that are extracted by alkaline ether:
   a. Dissolve the residue in alkaline ether and stratify with sulfuric acid. In 2 hours an orange ring will appear that changes to violet and then blue, which persists for quite a few days before fading.
   b. The residue plus a few drops of sulfuric acid plus a trace of ferric chloride will give an orange color that changes to a deep red. The periphery of the drop will be colored bluish to greenish blue.
   c. The residue dissolved in glacial acetic acid plus a trace of ferric chloride or hydrogen peroxide is stratified with sul-

furic acid. A violet to intense blue color will be seen.

d. To the residue in ether, adding sodium bicarbonate and shaking produces a red-violet color.

e. To the residue in ether, adding 5 ml of 5% sodium oxalate produces a red color.

f. To the residue in *ether,* add 5 ml of potassium hydroxide (10%) ; heat gently and *cautiously* → fishy odor.

3. UV Spectrophotometry: See Section I.

4. TLC: $CHCl_3$:EtOH (95:5 or 90:10): See Section I.

Treatment

Withdraw drug; activated charcoal in half a glass of warm water. Emetics or gastric lavage, cathartic (sodium sulfate, 25 gm). Demulcents. Valium or short-acting barbiturates for convulsions.

Keep patient warm and quiet, in recumbent position. Maintain body fluid balance. Guard against kidney damage. Artificial respiration and oxygen therapy as needed. Supportive.

ESSENTIAL OILS

Members: Oils of absinthe, aloe, apiol, arnica, coriander, cottonroot bark, eucalyptus, juniper, garlic, lemon, menthol, mustard, nutmeg, parsley, pennyroyal, pine, rue, savin, tansy, thyme, turpentine.

Uses: Industry, volatile oils, flavors, spices, alleged abortifacient*.

MLD: Very toxic.

Symptoms: Severe gastrointestinal irritation, nausea, vomiting, abdominal pain, diarrhea, kidney involvement, hematuria, convulsions, pulmonary and cerebral edema, congestion, irregular respiration followed by depression, collapse.

Identification

Essential oils listed above are isolated by steam distillation and may be identified by characteristic odor. Volatile oils can be dis-

---

*Other alleged abortifacients: saffron, colocynth, soft soap, slippery elm bark, laburnum, lead, arsenic, mercury, quinine, oxytocin, petuitrin, ergot and derivatives, iodine paste, aminopterin.

tilled or extracted (NIR) , see Section I.

1. Essential oils can be isolated by adding sodium chloride to distillate. Extract distillate with ether; then slowly evaporate the ether → essential oil.

2. Oil of savin: Bp 208°C. Refractive index, 1.472 to 1.477 at 20°C. Colorless or pale yellow liquid.
   a. sulfuric acid → blood red color
   b. fuming nitric acid → explodes → red-orange color

3. Oil of turpentine (see under Turpentine) .

4. Oil of tansy: refractive index, 1.457 to 1.460 at 20°C; yellow liquid.
   a. sulfuric acid → brown color
   b. fuming nitric acid → violet color
   c. Mecke's reagent → brown color with violet rim
   d. iodine → violet → black precipitate

5. Oil of apiol (chief constituent of oil of parsley) may be crystallized by cooling. Mp 30°C.
   a. nitric acid → effervesces → brick red color
   b. fuming nitric acid → bright red color

6. Oil of pennyroyal: peppermint odor; refractive index. 1.482 to 1.487 at 20°C. Colorless or yellow liquid.
   a. sulfuric acid → orange color
   b. fuming nitric acid → no violence → deep yellow color

7. Pine oil + sulfuric acid → red (see Turpentine) .

Treatment

Gastric lavage with charcoal and much water; castor oil (1 oz) or sodium sulfate (30 gm) .

Demulcents. Valium or short-acting barbiturates for irritability or convulsions. Supportive and symptomatic treatment. Guard against kidney involvement.

ETHCHLORVYNOL (C_7H_9ClO)

Synonym: Placidyl.

Uses: Nonbarbiturate hypnotic.

Properties: Yellow liquid, sharp penetrating odor.

MLD: Approximately 10 gm/70 kg person.

Approximate Blood Levels: Therapeutic 0.5 mg/dl; lethal 10 mg/dl; half-life, 2 hours.

Remarks: Rapidly absorbed; largely metabolized by liver; maximum blood level in $1\frac{1}{2}$ hours.

Symptoms: Initial excitement is possible, CNS depression, GI upset is possible, dizziness, hypotension, pulmonary edema, respiratory depression.

Identification

(Finkle-Bath-Dal Cortivo-Matusiack)

1. Two (2) ml serum + 8 ml trichloracetic acid (10%) ; mix, filter, and centrifuge.   Two (2) ml clear filtrate + 3 ml diphenyl amine reagent.

   Reagent: DPA: 0.5 gm in 25 ml H_2SO_4, then carefully add to the mixture 25 ml H_2O and 25 ml glacial acetic acid.

   Positive test → pink to red color (read at 510 nm) .

2. TLC: See Section I.

Treatment

Gastric lavage or emesis.   Symptomatic and supportive measures for depression.   See under Barbiturates.

ETHER ($C_4H_{10}O$)

Synonyms: Diethyl ether.

Uses: Anesthesia, industry.

Properties: Very volatile, colorless liquid.   Definite odor, flammable, explosive.   Bp 35°C.

MLD: Approximately 25 ml orally for a 70 kg person.

Approximate Blood Levels: therapeutic, 100 mg/dl; lethal, 150 mg/dl.

Light anesthetic level: approximately 50–130 mg%.   Deep anesthetic level: approximately 130–150 mg%.   Respiratory failure: approximately 150–170 mg%.

Remarks: Usually absorbed by inhalation; deaths rarely due to anesthetic overdose (1:5000) .

Symptoms: Ethereal odor on breath, dilated pupils, loss of corneal reflexes, burning taste, vomiting, nausea, acidosis, cyanosis, apnea, coma, respiratory depression, possible pneumonia, slight renal damage, respiratory failure, death.

Identification

Separated by steam distillation and rectification. Distillate is very volatile, so catch with freezing mixture of dry ice and acetone bath.

1. By odor, history, flammability, volatility, strong characteristic odor in blood, tissue, and cavities.

2. Pure ether identified by boiling point (35°C) and reaction with iodic acid → ethyl iodide.

3. Positive Fehling's test for sugar in urine.

4. Blood or tissue homogenate is steam distilled into pure carbon tetrachloride. Read in the NIR and UV. See Section I.

5. GLC for anesthetics (Lowe). Flame ionization detectors are specific for volatile organic compounds and do not respond to fixed gases normally found in blood (oxygen, nitrogen, carbon dioxide) or water; nor does it respond to N_2O or ammonia. Hydrogen flame detectors are very much more sensitive than thermal conductivity detectors. About one part of organic vapor in one billion parts of hydrogen may be detected. The explosive factor is minimal and, in practice, the maximum sensitivity is obtained by using the lowest nitrogen (carrier gas) and hydrogen flows compatible with stability of the instrument. A small hydrogen generator is now preferable to the usual tank (always available and safer).

The use of electron capture detectors for the analysis of halogenated anesthetics is about one hundred times more sensitive than even the flame ionization detector.

Flame ionization detection (Lowe, H.J.: *Anesthesiology,* 25:808, 1964) :

1. methoxyflurane
2. halothane
3. ether
4. cyclopropane
5. chloroform
6. trifluoroethylvinyl ether

Column: 5 feet long; i.d., $\frac{1}{4}$ inch; 10% by weight polyethylene glycol 400 on Celite. Carrier gas, nitrogen. Cell voltage, 1 mv. Column temperature, 85°C; pack to very end so that injection needle enters packing (85°C) .

Head space: Finkle and Dubowski: See Section I; Table XXI.

Take 10 μl of blood plus 10 μl of *n*-propanol (or heptane) as internal standard. Mix and inject 1 μl. Finkle, Table XXI.

Treatment

Remove from exposure. Give artificial respiration and oxygen therapy. Vital to keep patient well-ventilated. Maintain body heat and fluid balance. Supportive.

ETHYL ALCOHOL (C₂H₅OH)

Synonyms: Grain alcohol, whiskey, alcohol, ethanol.

Uses: Beverage, medicinal vehicle, solvent, fuel, antiseptic.

Properties: Clear colorless liquid. Characteristic odor. Bp 78° C. Flammable.

MLD: One pint to 1 quart of whiskey taken within a very short interval.

Remarks: Whiskey = 40–50% alcohol; wines = 10–20%; beers = 2–6%. Whiskey proof = 2 × % (86 proof = 43%) .

Barbiturates, chloral hydrate, paraldehyde, anticonvulsants, morphine and derivatives, antihistamines, tranquilizers, or other CNS depressants are synergistic with alcohol.

Absorbed through all portals.

Death within 10 hours, but may be delayed more than 10 hours. If there is a delay between the last drink and death, the terminal blood-alcohol level may be low.

INTOLERANCE TO ALCOHOL: The presence of even small amounts of certain substances may interfere with the normal and safe breakdown of ethanol in man. Disulfiram (Antabuse) is one such compound. It stops the metabolism at acetaldehyde, which is now far more toxic than the original ethanol. There are other substances that may act in a similar fashion: *Coprinus atramentarius* (mushrooms) ; chlorpropamide (Diabinase) ; carbutamide (Nadisan; Invenol) ; Tolbutamide (Orinase, Rastinon) ; furazolidone (Furoxone); furaltadone (Altafur); thiuram derivatives (rubber industry); N-butyraldoxime (printing industry); cyanamide; and dithiocarbamate (ferbam, tiram, maneb, teneb, nabam).

Symptoms: Nausea, vomiting, vertigo, odor of alcohol on breath and in vomitus, slurred speech, dilated pupils, flushed face, sweating, noisy or quiet, poor reflexes, poor motor coordination, ataxia, poor judgment, loquaciousness, sleepiness, unsteady gait, delirium, personality changes, diuresis, hypoglycemia, weak rapid pulse, cerebral edema, dyspnea, cyanosis, acidosis, circulatory coldapse, coma, death from respiratory depression.

Identification
Isolated by steam distillation.
In pure form:

1. Put 1 ml of unknown plus 1 ml of acetic acid and 1 drop of sulfuric acid in a test tube and gently heat for 1 minute. A characteristic fruity odor of ethyl acetate is positive for ethyl alcohol.

2. Physical characteristics: distinct odor. Miscible with water in all proportions. Bp 78°C. Flammable (cold blue flame).

3. To 3 ml of unknown solution, add a few drops of 10% sodium hydroxide, then several drops of iodine until persistent yellow color appears. Gently heat for 1 minute and allow to cool. Appearance of yellow crystals (iodoform) may indicate ethyl alcohol. Methyl does not interfere but acetone does.

4. To 1 ml of unknown solution, add 10 ml of water and place in an 8-inch Pyrex test tube. Obtain a thick copper spiral with an insulated handle. Heat and then plunge this red-hot spiral into the unknown solution while test tube is being cooled under the tap. Repeat this mild oxidation eight to ten times, taking precaution not to lose drops adhering to copper spiral. This oxidized product may be:
   a. methyl alcohol → formaldehyde—pungent odor
   b. ethyl alcohol → acetaldehyde—sweet odor
   Further confirmation is made by adding 5 ml of Schiff's reduced fuchsine reagent. Both formaldehyde and acetaldehyde

will produce a pink-violet color on standing.   Add 2 ml of concentrated sulfuric acid; the color produced by acetaldehyde will decolorize. Pink-violet produced by formaldehyde (methyl alcohol) will persist. See Methyl Alcohol.

In blood, urine, spinal fluid, or stomach contents.

5. Modification of the microdiffusion technique (Feldstein-Sunshine-Conway microdiffusion cell.   Available from Bel-Art Products, Pequannock, New Jersey; item number 40941) .

Sealer: 2 ml of liberating agent (saturated K_2CO_3) is placed in small outer groove of rim.

Reactant: 2 ml of Ansties reagent is placed in center chamber.

One (1) ml of blood or urine is spread in the outer chamber. Spread 2 ml of liberating agent (saturated K_2CO_3) on top of blood and quickly put lid in place. To seal lid in place, gently twist to obtain a liquid seal. Then gently swirl entire unit to mix specimen and liberating agent. Diffusion is started. Allow to diffuse for 2 hours at room temperature (30°C). Early change of color suggests high levels. Ethanol standards should be used: 1 ml of 95% ethanol in 250 ml of water makes a stock solution.

Stock Solution		Approximate gm per 100 ml of blood	Color of Anties Solution
0.00 ml	0	0.00	yellow-canary
0.25	+	0.08 (under the influence)	yellow-yellow-green
0.50	++	0.15	yellow-green
0.75	+++	0.23	yellow-green-green
1.00	++++	0.30 (dangerous)	green
		Above 0.40 (coma)	blue (not reliable) repeat with 0.5 ml blood

Transfer the center Ansties solution that appears to be positive. This quantitative transfer is carefully diluted to 3.00 ml. Match color visually with standards, or measure absorbance (yellow) at 350 nm or at 450 nm, or measure absorbance (green) at 605 nm, or back titrate for the unreduced $K_2Cr_2O_7$ (see test 6 below).

Reagent: Ansties: Dissolve 3.70 gm of potassium dichromate c.p. in 150 ml of distilled water. Add slowly, with constant stirring, 280 ml of sulfuric acid c.p. Finally dilute to 500 ml with distilled water.

EVALUATION: Below 0.15% blood alcohol is not usually dangerous to life, except that this level *may provoke* a hazardous situation. Above 0.15% blood alcohol may be dangerous to life, especially in the presence of other depressant drugs such as morphine and derivatives or other narcotics, barbiturate derivatives, hypnotics, phenothiazine derivatives, other tranquilizers or antihistaminics, or anesthetics, etc. Above 0.30% blood alcohol may be dangerous to life by respiratory difficulties.

Methyl alcohol and isopropyl alcohol in the blood also give positive results with this test. These can be individually ruled in or out by history and further laboratory testing. Negative results conclusively rule out these three alcohols; cause for coma or depression must therefore be looked for elsewhere.

6. (Muehlberger): Simple steam distillation with a long-neck Kjeldahl flask (glass fitted joints).

Place 5 ml of picric acid into flask; then add exactly 3 ml of blood. The sides are washed down with 10 to 15 ml of water and flask is then tightly attached to the steam-distillation apparatus. Gently heat steam-generating flask and collect 10 to 15 ml of distillate directly into a 1 × 8 inch Pyrex test tube which has been previously charged with *exactly* 5 ml of 0.26N $K_2Cr_2O_7$ and *exactly* 6 ml H_2SO_4. Be certain that the condensor is cold to prevent ethanol loss. The distillate will collect dropwise on top of the dichromate solution; keep receptical cold with an ice pack. The distillate is then gently swirled into solution while cooled. Immerse total solution in a boiling water bath for about 10-15 minutes to complete the reaction.

The tube and contents are then cooled in a beaker of cold tap water, transferred quantitatively to a 500 ml Erlenmeyer flask, and then diluted to 150–200 ml with water. Two (2) gm potassium iodide is added and dissolved by swirling. After a minute or two, the liberated iodine (freed by the excess $K_2Cr_2O_7$) is titrated with 0.0274N $Na_2S_2O_3$ until the brown color changes to a very pale yellow. Then about 1 ml of starch solution is added and the titration with $Na_2S_2O_3$ is continued (usually 1 to 2 more ml) to a point where purple-lavender color of starch iodine changes to very pale apple green. This end point is sharp and easy to determine.

Record the milliliters of $Na_2S_2O_3$ required. If volume of distillate used is found to contain more than 12 mg of ethanol, repeat the titration using a smaller aliquot of distillate.

STANDARDIZATION OF SODIUM THIOSULFATE SOLUTION: Exactly 5 ml of 0.26N $K_2Cr_2O_7$ and 6 ml H_2SO_4 and 10 to 15 ml of water are gently heated in a test tube in the same fashion as in the determination. Then cool and titrate as above. This will require 47.5 ml $Na_2S_2O_3$ ($\pm$ 5 ml). This is the blank. A reagent blank should also be done on all fresh batches of solutions as prepared. This should not vary from above. Allow solution to "age" overnight.

Normal (nonalcoholic) blood may show a normal reaction, but this is below 0.01 percent. Stomach contents (nonalcoholic) may give somewhat higher results: about 0.03 percent.

SAMPLE CALCULATION: Three (3) ml of blood (equals about 3.15 gm) gives a $Na_2S_2O_3$ titration of 24.7 ml. The "blank" titration is 47.5 ml $Na_2S_2O_3$.

Ethanol in blood: $47.5 - 24.7 = 22.8$ ml $Na_2S_2O_3$

$$\frac{22.8 \times 15}{47.5} = 7.20 \text{ mg of ethanol in sample}$$

7.20 mg $= 0.00720$ gm

$$\frac{0.00720 \times 100}{3.15} = 0.228\% \text{ w/w} = 0.23\% \text{ ethanol}$$

Reagents:

* Picric acid saturated solution (about 16 gm per liter).
* Potassium dichromate solution 0.2607N (1 ml oxidizes exactly 3 mg of ethanol). Dissolve 12.78 gm of dry reagent-quality $K_2Cr_2O_7$ in sufficient distilled water to make 1000 ml. Keep in glass-stoppered bottle.

• *Sulfuric acid*—reagent grade.
• Sodium thiosulfate solution, 0.0274N. Dissolve 13.7 gm $Na_2S_2O_3$ crystals in sufficient water to make 2000 ml. Add 1 ml of chloroform as preservative. Allow to stand overnight before use.
• Soluble starch solution (0.5%). About 0.5 gm of soluble starch is made into a thin paste by shaking with 10 ml of distilled water. Then, while shaking, about 90 ml of boiling water is quickly added and shaking is continued. A clear solution should result. Keep in refrigerator and sensitivity is retained for about 1 week.

POSSIBLE INTERFERENCES:

A. Methyl or isopropyl alcohol or formaldehyde may give a similar positive test and should be ruled out either by history or a specific analysis (see test under each).

Analysis of 0.05 gm% of methyl alcohol, isopropyl alcohol, or formaldehyde by above test when compared with ethyl alcohol standards: methyl alcohol—0.09%; isopropyl alcohol—0.11%; formaldehyde—0.07%.

B. Chloroform, ether, chloral hydrate, or paraldehyde do not interfere in human blood sufficiently, even in extreme situations, to present an interference.

C. Acetone bodies, even in the most severe cases of diabetic acidosis and coma, do not interfere with this test if precautions are taken (use Scott-Wilson reagent).

D. For medicolegal purposes, urine is not as satisfactory as an analysis of blood, because equivalence is *not* reliable.

7. a. Breath Analysis with conversion factor (2300:1); several good instruments are available.
   b. Alcohol dehydrogenase test kits.
8. GLC (Dubowski: method of choice): Gas chromatography—Flame ionization detector. Stainless steel (or glass) column 6 feet by $\frac{1}{8}$ inch i.d. packed with Porapak S or Porapak Q (80–100 mesh). Typical operating conditions (Kurt Dubowski) for Varian 1860-3 GC.

Carrier Gases	Inlet pressure	Flow rate
Helium or Nitrogen	55 psig	45 ml/min
Hydrogen	20 psig	45 ml/min
Air	12 psig	330 ml/min

Temperatures: column, 165°C; injection port, 175°C; Detector; 2255°C.

a. Head space (internal standard *n*-propanol, acetonitrile, or ethyl methyl ketone)

Place 1.0 gm NaCl and 1.0 ml blood (well mixed) into a 15 ml screw-capped septum vial with a butyl rubber septum stopper. Swirl to mix well.

Porapak S absolute retention time is 2.00 minutes. Relative retention time:

    acetone   1.44
    acetonitrile 1.23
    ethanol   1.00 (Unity)
    isopropanol   1.80
    methanol   0.48

Place vials into a water bath maintained at 38°C ± 0.05°C and allow vials (immersed to just below screw caps) to equilibrate for 45 minutes.

Use a plastic 1 ml syringe and inject 0.25 ml of head space.

b. Direct injection: Dilute blood (1:9) with internal standard (*n*-propanol or ethyl methyl ketone) and make direct inject of 0.5 μl of mixture. Also see Section I; Table XXI.

Treatment

Treatment for the acute phase and the chronic alcoholic is different. Treatment for the acute phase (deep coma) is chiefly aimed at maintaining vital signs. Emergency measures are to keep a patent airway and maintain respiration. If blood alcohol content is above 0.5%, hemodialysis may be considered.

Maintain body heat, water and electrolyte balance. Avoid giving excess fluids. Avoid depressant drugs. If hypoglycemic, give glucose.

Prevent and guard against aspiration into lungs or strangulation with regurgitated food particles. Guard against secondary infection. Supportive measures.

Do not use paraldehyde, which will further depress. Do not use disulfiram (Antabuse); this will block oxidation and allow accumulation of acetaldehyde, which is far more toxic than ethanol.

If stuporous and even if "alcohol odor," rule out coexistence of cerebral injuries, toxic delirium, uremia, etc. Many die with alleged "alcoholic coma" from other undiagnosed conditions.

SOME COMMON FALLACIES

1. "Drinking black coffee in large amounts will help sober up"—only time (metabolism and elimination) will help.
2. "Stressful incidents such as hot then cold showers, exercise or running to work up a sweat, emotional shock such as an accident or arrest by police will help sober up"—none of these work. Although there may be a "momentary" improvement in the objective signs of depression, this is very temporary and, as a matter of fact, produces by rebound a further depression.
3. "You cannot get drunk on beer"—you just have to drink more; a 12 ounce bottle of beer is equivalent to about one ounce of whiskey.
4. "Alcohol acts as an aphrodisiac (sexual stimulant)"—it may accent the desire by "lack of inhibitions" but can also inhibit or minimize performance.
5. "Use of alcohol is a good method to keep warm on a very cold day"—this is actually dangerous. Alcohol may produce a dilation of peripheral blood vessels in the skin, which will increase perspiration and heat loss; this may give a rapid transient feeling of warmth when actually the body is rapidly losing heat. Furthermore, large amounts of alcohol depress the heat regulatory centers, and heat production by the body may now be impaired.
6. "Mixing alcoholic drinks such as whiskey, beer, or gin produces a marked potentiation or increase of action"—it may make one

sick due to congeners (the flavor or bouquet that is enhanced by "aging"); but it does not make one more intoxicated, except only in proportion to total amount of alcohol. Vodka is purified alcohol, has no odor or congeners, and is purest.

7. "After an overindulgence of champagne, upon drinking water the next morning one again may become intoxicated"—one may get sick but cannot become intoxicated without the actual presence of alcohol.

8. "A small amount of alcohol may improve normal driving abilities"—alcohol is a depressant and dulls the presence of tenseness, the sense of alertness, responsibility, and self-criticism. Drinking to any extent reduces self-control and reduces the driving ability of any person.

9. "Alcohol dilates the coronary arteries and is therefore good for atherosclerosis"—alcohol does not dilate the coronaries, although it gives a peripheral flushing. On the other hand, alcohol significantly increases the effects of hypoxia. This then makes alcohol a calculated risk in high altitudes (on mountains and in airplanes) and also in persons with cardiac or pulmonary conditions with borderline hypoxia. Even one cocktail can trigger a myocardial infarction.

MEDICOLEGAL EVALUATION OF BLOOD-ALCOHOL LEVELS

Actions: Ethyl alcohol is basically a central nervous system depressant, acting in a manner similar to that of the general anesthetics such as ether and chloroform.

Absorption: Alcohol requires no digestion, and absorption occurs apparently by simple diffusion from the stomach and intestines into the bloodstream. This diffusion is so rapid that from 80 to 90 percent of the ingested quantity may be absorbed in about 30 minutes, although *complete* absorption requires approximately $1\frac{1}{2}$ hours. Twenty percent is absorbed from the stomach and the remainder from the small intestine. A delay in gastric emptying time is an important factor in slowing the rate of absorption. Largely because of this, speed of absorption may vary between individuals and in the same individual at different times.

Ordinarily the most important factor in delaying absorption is the presence of food; carbohydrates and proteins being equally or possibly more effective than fats in this respect. The concentration and nature of the alcoholic beverage are also influencing factors; for instance, the alcohol in beer is more slowly absorbed than that in an equal concentration in water.

Fate: Approximately 95 percent of the alcohol absorbed is completely oxidized to carbon dioxide and water. The initial stage of this metabolism begins in the liver, hence the possible effect of liver disease on the intensity of the alcohol activity. The remaining 5 percent is eliminated unchanged chiefly by the lungs and kidneys. Normally the body destroys and eliminates alcohol at a rate equivalent to about one ounce of whiskey per hour. In terms of changes in the blood-alcohol percentage, this corresponds to a decrease of approximately 0.015–0.02 percent per hour (somewhat less if small amounts are ingested, and a little higher rate if larger amounts of alcohol had been imbibed).

Individual tolerance: This depends upon congenital or acquired tissue (brain) susceptibility, rate of absorption, rate of elimination, age, pattern of drinking, and general medical condition of the subject. Individuals in ill health, mentally or physically, are usually more profoundly affected by alcohol than those in a state of good health.

Usual methods of testing: Direct determination of the concentration of alcohol in the *blood* by chemical analysis is the most reliable practical method. Indirectly, blood-alcohol levels may be reasonably well determined by analysis of the expired air for alcohol.

Synergisms: Subjects taking depressant drugs such as the barbiturates, morphine or derivatives, chloral hydrate, paraldehyde, anticonvulsants, antihistamines, or tranquilizers or *any* CNS depressant drug, concomitantly with alcohol will be more *markedly* affected than otherwise. Such drugs should only be used with extreme caution in the presence of alcohol, if at all.

Physiologic Changes

Alcohol is basically a central nervous system depressant, acting in a manner generally similar to anesthetics such as ether or chloroform. The inhibitory centers (judgment) are depressed first, and now one feels euphoric, less tense, and under less social restraints, as though the "brakes" had been released. It acts as a "social lubricant" and shyness, prudence, self-criticism, and self-control are diminished.

Depression, if severe, often produces death by respiratory failure. There is an increased proneness to aspiration of food into the lungs, infections, or exposure to extreme weather. There is a marked proneness to violent death resulting from brawls, foolhardy stunts, or accidents because of a lack of judgment or a lack of ability to avoid or resist assault or accident.

Other findings are nausea, vertigo, characteristic odor on the breath, slurred speech, dilated pupils, flushed face, sweating, impaired reflexes, poor motor coordination, unsteady gait, clumsiness, loquaciousness, sleepiness, diuresis (increased urine output), weak rapid pulse, cerebral edema, dyspnea, cyanosis, mild acidosis, circulatory collapse, coma, respiratory failure, and death.

The pathological findings in fatal cases of *acute* alcoholism are not characteristic or striking except, perhaps, for an alcoholic (and congener) odor of the tissues. It is, therefore, difficult to make a diagnosis of fatal *acute* alcoholism without an adequate history and postmortem toxicological study.

Behavioral Changes

The effects of ethyl alcohol intoxication on people are fairly typical and, generally, are characterized by a release from usual social restraints and inhibitions. As a result, there may be the appearance, initially at least, of stimulation; actually this is pseudostimulation. Depending on the amount taken, there is a sense of security, feeling of being a "superman," a "nothing-matters-plenty-of-time" attitude, hilarity, and boisterousness. Judgment, vision, mental efficiency, concentration, reaction time, and motor coordination suffer. There is analgesia (insensibility to pain), general depression of all the five senses, mental confusion, slow and sluggish thinking, impulsive behavior, decreased efficiency in responding to an emergency situation, and an inability to perform simple tasks with normal speed and accuracy. All these vary somewhat with the individual.

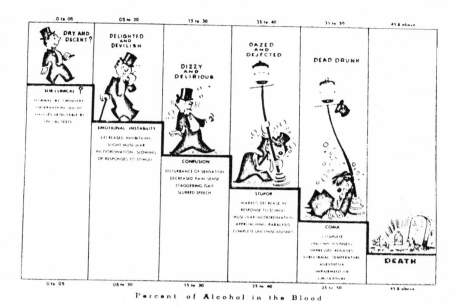

FIGURE 5. Modified from Bogen-Muehlberger.

Interpretation of Blood-Alcohol Values

The following material is taken largely from data furnished by the National Safety Council:

Less than 0.05 percent—prima facie evidence that the subject is not under the influence of alcohol.

From 0.05 to 0.10 percent—corroborative evidence to be considered with outward physical symptoms. In general, the nearer the level of 0.10 percent is approached, the more likely the subject is of being under the influence of alcohol.

Values of 0.10 percent and above—prima facie evidence that the subject *is* under the influence of alcohol insofar as the operation of a motor vehicle is concerned.

Values of 0.25 percent and above—the subject is markedly intoxicated.

Values of 0.40 percent and above—comatose levels of alcohol, which may lead to death.

Approximation of alcoholic beverages to reach given blood level: A 12 ounce bottle of beer (4%) contains approximately the same alcohol content as 1 ounce of whiskey (90 proof). For an average 70 kg individual* tested within 30 to 45 minutes after drinking, a *minimum* of—

$2\frac{1}{2}$ ounces whiskey = 0.05% alcohol in blood.
5   ounces whiskey = 0.10% alcohol in blood.
$7\frac{1}{2}$ ounces whiskey = 0.15% alcohol in blood.
10   ounces ($\frac{1}{2}$ pint) =0.20% alcohol in blood.

ETHYLENE GLYCOL ($C_2H_6O_2$)

Synonyms: Antifreeze; Prestone; permanent antifreeze.

Uses: Auto antifreeze, solvent, coolant, industry.

Properties: Colorless odorless liquid. Bp 197.5°C. Miscible with water and alcohol. Nonvolatile. Bitter sweet but pleasant taste. No hazard by inhalation or skin absorption.

MLD: Approximately 100 ml/70 kg. person.

APPROXIMATE BLOOD LEVEL: Lethal, 200 mg/dl.

Remarks: Twice as toxic as propylene glycol. Half as toxic as diethylene glycol. Ethylene and diethylene glycol metabolize to oxalic acid in the body, and symptoms are generally similar to each other.

Relative toxicity: Propylene glycol → diethylene glycol → ethylene glycol → dioxane. Toxicity (oral) increases as the chain polymerization decreases (Patty).

Symptoms

IMMEDIATE (1–2 HOURS) : Nausea, vomiting, abdominal pain, diarrhea; warmth in throat, mouth, and stomach. Signs similar to alcoholic intoxication: restlessness, irritability, talkativeness, ataxia, increase in pulse rate; depression, dyspnea.

THREE TO TWELVE HOURS: Deep depression, coma, increased pulse and respiratory rate, rise in blood pressure (systolic and diastolic) , generally an absence of reflexes, oliguria, capillary damage,

*Other things being equal, the greater body weight the larger the alcohol intake (in rough proportion) must be to achieve an equal alcohol value.

hematuria, acidosis, convulsions; hemorrhages in pleura, lungs, heart, kidney, and brain; anuria, nephrosis; calcium oxalate crystals in kidney tubules, urine, and brain. Ethylene glycol is distributed evenly in body; some formaldehyde may be found in urine in small amounts. Pulmonary edema and bronchopneumonia; within 2 hours prior to death, rales may appear in both lung bases and patient may expire from pulmonary edema; death usually occurs within 12 to 36 hours following ingestion. It is controversial whether death is due to oxalate poisoning or paralysis of respiration and/or circulatory failure.

DELAYED: Manifested clinically by an acute nephritislike state; hypertension; signs of renal insufficiency and uremia, which may or may not terminate in death; state is characterized by an absence of red blood cells in urine.

In all stages, the carbon dioxide combining power is low; there is increase of the blood urea nitrogen, sugar, and protein fraction. In all cases, a hemoconcentration with leukocytosis had been observed. However, the most specific findings are in the urine, in which always are found large amounts of oxalate crystals. Also, albuminuria is constantly present. The gastric lavage usually had been positive for occult blood. In many cases the spinal fluid had been tinged with blood, and the cell count showed an increase in the number of leukocytes.

Identification

Samples of choice are vomitus, gastric lavage, or residue of suspected fluid. Urine will contain the metabolite as the oxalate.

1. Add 5 ml of a dichromate solution → solution turns green-blue on standing (nonspecific). See Ethyl alcohol.

2. Identify by boiling point and derivatives; 3,5-dinitrobenzoyl derivative; Mp 169°C.

3. Kidney function tests may be of presumptive value.

4. Test for formaldehyde and/or oxalates in the urine. (See under Formaldehyde and under Oxalates.)

5. Fuchsine test (Harger and Forney) :
   a. *Blood:* Take 1 ml of blood with 7 ml of water and add 1 ml of 10% sodium tungstate. With vigorous shaking, add,

dropwise, 1 ml of $\frac{2}{3}$N sulfuric acid solution. Stopper the flask and shake well. Filter through a small dry filter paper.

Place in a small test tube 1 ml of the protein-free filtrate and then 4 ml of water. Next add 0.25 ml of the M/10 periodic acid solution and shake. Allow to stand 10 minutes. Introduce 2 ml of the fuchsine reagent and mix → violet. The color is allowed to develop fully and, after 25 minutes, the depth of color is read with a spectrophotometer set at wavelength 555 nm. Compare the result with the percent transmission curve for 10 to 70γ of ethylene glycol dissolved in water and run in the same way.

Concentration	Transmission
10 mg	96%
20	88
30	79
40	70
50	54
60	45
70	35

This curve does not follow the Beer-Lampert law. Comparison is made with standards.

Reagents:

• Periodic acid, M/10: Dissolve 2.28 gm H_5IO_6 (periodic acid) *or* 2.13 gm $NaIO_4$ in 100 ml of $\frac{1}{3}$N sulfuric acid.
• Fuchsine reagent (as described under Methyl Alcohol) .

b. *Urine:* Diluted urine may be analyzed directly, using the procedure for the protein-free filtrate of blood.

c. *Tissues:* Weigh out 50 gm of the tissue and add 200 ml of water. Make a uniform suspension of tissue and water by means of a Waring blender. Measure out 25 ml of the suspension. Add 15 ml of water, 5 ml of 10% sodium tungstate and, with shaking, 5 ml of $\frac{2}{3}$N sulfuric acid. Filter. The filtrate should be clear and free from protein. Continue analysis as the Protein-free filtrate of blood. Tissue gives a high blank.

Blanks may give results up to 30 mg%, but a *positive* case

(within 8 hours of exposure) will give levels at least ten times this value. Levels may disappear in tissue on standing.

Treatment

Gastric lavage, enemas, liberal administration of alkalis and fluids; sodium bicarbonate (IV) for acidosis; saline cathartics (sodium sulfate, 30 gm) ; Valium or short-acting barbiturates for convulsions. Oxygen therapy and artificial respiration as needed. Maintain body heat, body fluids, and electrolyte balance. Calcium gluconate for hypocalcemia.

Treat for kidney damage. Hemodialysis, if available, will hasten elimination. Support respiration and cardiovascular irregularities. Renal function test will indicate progress of patient and effectiveness of treatment.

Ethanol when given early has been reported to be effective to slow down oxalate formation.

ETHYLENE OXIDE

Use: Fumigant gas.

Symptoms: Gastrointestinal upset, vertigo, cough; irritant to nose, eyes, and lungs. Bradycardia, extrasystole. Acts as vesicant locally and internally. Narcosis. Converts to ethylene glycol by metabolism.

Identification: Test for ethylene glycol in urine.

Treatment: As immediate measures, treat as a vesicant; delayed and secondary, treat as ethylene glycol. Supportive.

FERROUS SULFATE (FeSO$_4$)

Synonyms: Green or iron vitriol; iron protosulfate, copperas; Feosol. Also as the ferrous fumarate, gluconate.

Uses: Medicinal, hematinic, astringent, deodorant. Industry, inks, dyes, pigments, tanning, photography, disinfecting.

Properties: Pale bluish green crystals. Soluble in water; insoluble in alcohol. Easily oxidized to ferric.

MLD: Approximately 10 gm/70 kg person; 0.5 gm is dangerous for an infant. Ferric is more toxic.

APPROXIMATE BLOOD LEVELS: Normal serum, 0.15 mg/dl; lethal, 0.8 mg/dl.

Remarks: Relatively nontoxic in small doses but is a strong corrosive in large doses.

Symptoms: Metallic taste, gastrointestinal irritation and corrosion, nausea, vomiting, abdominal pain, bloody diarrhea, pallor, drowsiness, dehydration, tarry stools, cyanosis, possible liver damage, acidosis, elevated serum iron, shock, cardiovascular collapse, death.

Death by collapse may occur from 1 to 4 hours after exposure. Occasionally, fatal collapse may follow apparent recovery.

Identification

Gastric content is specimen of choice.

1. Gastric contents may be bloody or may have a pale blue-green color.
2. Ferrous sulfate may be extracted from stomach contents by dialysis, or may be diluted with water, and the following tests performed:
   a. Potassium ferricyanide plus H_2SO_4 (10%) → dark blue precipitate
   b. The precipitate of iron in test a is insoluble in dilute hydrochloric acid but is decomposed by sodium hydroxide (10%)
   c. ferrous salts + sodium hydroxide (10%) → green-white precipitate → green → brown (when shaken)
   d. ferrous salts + dilute ammonium hydroxide → brown precipitate + hydrogen sulfide → black precipitate
   e. sulfate + barium chloride (10%) → white precipitate, which is insoluble in either nitric or hydrochloric acid
   f. sulfate + lead acetate (10%) → white precipitate, which is soluble in ammonium acetate solution
   g. ferrous sulfate partially change to ferric ions. Ferric salts + ammonium thiocyanate → wine-red color
   h. ferric salts + potassium ferrocyanide (10%) → dark blue precipitate
   i. serum iron levels are elevated above 0.15 mg/dl.

3. Evaporate 10 ml of urine to dryness in a silica basin (4.5 inch). The residue is then ashed. The carbonaceous mass may be cooled, a few drops of concentrated nitric acid added, and the ashing continued. By this means, a white ash may be obtained in a very short time. The ash is dissolved in 10 ml of N-hydrochloric acid with the aid of heat. The final volume is adjusted to 10 ml with water. An aliquot containing about 0.1 mg of iron is diluted to 10 ml with water. Two drops of thioglycolic (thiolacetic) acid is added, followed by 22 ml of ammonia (SG, 0.88). The resultant purple color is read against an appropriate blank at 560 nm. Iron (0.1 mg) in 10 ml of N-hydrochloric acid will serve as a suitable standard.

Treatment

Immediately given milk as demulcent and also to slow absorption; gastric lavage, with caution, with milk. Use plasma expanders to maintain normal blood pressure. Maintain body fluid and electrolyte balance. Sodium bicarbonate for acidosis. Milk and/or bismuth subcarbonate to relieve irritation. Support against shock. Support against secondary infections. Oxygen as needed. Desferal (deferoxamine) selective for iron elimination. Read package insert.

Hemodialysis will hasten elimination. Support against possible kidney damage; support against possible liver involvement, with low-fat, high-carbohydrate diet and B complex vitamins.

Fatal collapse sometimes may follow apparent recovery. This may be due to ferritin (iron protein compound normally stored) escaping into circulation. Ferritin is reported to be a vasodepressor material (VDM) producing low blood pressure and shock.

Guarded prognosis for about 48 hours. Support against possible shock, and general supportive measures.

FLUORIDES

Derivatives: Sodium fluoride; calcium fluoride; sodium fluoroacetate (1080); hydrofluoric acid (HF).

Uses: Insecticide, rodenticide, erusticator, roach and ant killer.

Properties: White crystalline, strongly alkaline.

MLD: Approximately 1 gm/70 kg person.

APPROXIMATE LEVELS: Normal urine, 0.05 mg/dl; normal blood, 0.005 mg/dl; lethal blood, 0.02 mg/dl.

Remarks: Commercially distributed as a blue powder. HF more toxic; cryolite much less toxic.

Symptoms: Gastrointestinal irritation, corrosion of gastric mucosa and irritation of skin, nausea, vomiting, abdominal pain, watery diarrhea (which may occur within 30 minutes), salivation, perspiration, low blood-calcium level, convulsions, tetany, dyspnea, collapse, shock, coma. Death due to cardiovascular collapse, or respiratory failure, or ventricular fibrillation.

Identification

Gastric contents or urine is better suited than tissue.

1. Ash specimen (500–600°C) with calcium hydroxide in a porcelain or platinum dish. With water, transfer ash to a distilling flask. Add a pinch of silver sulfate, a pinch of silica, and several milliliters of 72% perchloric acid. Distill with caution between 135 and 140°C. Distillate is delivered into a 10% sodium hydroxide solution with a few drops of phenolphthalein. Adapter is dipped into alkali to allow no loss. As the distillation proceeds, some acid may come over and decolorize the phenolphthalein. Add more alkali; alkalinity must be maintained. Titrate with sodium alizarin sulfonate and carmine as the indicator and thorium as the standard.
   Reference: Anal Chem, 31:105, 1959.

2. Place 5 ml of urine, gastric lavage, or vomitus plus a pinch of calcium hydroxide in a small crucible. Heat gently to dryness, then ignite to a white ash to destroy organic material. Add a pinch of purified sand (SiO_2) and mix well by stirring and scraping the sides. Add 1 ml of sulfuric acid and *quickly* cover with a glass slide containing a hanging drop of 5% sodium chloride. Apply gentle heat for several minutes. The slide is kept cool with a *small* beaker of ice on it. The volatile silicon tetrafluoride will dissolve in the suspended drop to form sodium silicon tetrafluoride. Examine with a microscope at low power and

dim lighting; typical tiny hexagon crystals are visible at the periphery as the water evaporates (with microscope light heat). These typical crystals appear before the large square sodium chloride crystals. The hexagons are approximately one-tenth the size of the chloride and may show a pinkish hue (Gettler-Ellerbrook).

3. Urine or vomitus (20 ml) is ignited and fused with calcium hydroxide. Mix fusion with purified sand; add sulfuric acid and then quickly aspirate and distill the volatile silicon tetra-fluoride into 5 ml of zirconium oxychloride (pink). In the presence of even traces of fluoride, the pink color changes to yellow. This color change can be quantitated.

Reference: Icken and Blank: *Anal Chem, 25:*1741, 1953.

4. *Etch test:* Material is dried as described above, then transferred to a lead dish. Concentrated sulfuric acid (5 cc) is added and quickly covered with a slide painted with paraffin on which is scratched a symbol that exposes a small portion to glass. Allow the hydrogen fluoride to generate and attack the exposed glass for about 20 minutes. Remove the paraffin with xylol or toluene and examine for evidence of glass etching. This test is specific for fluorides.

5. Fluorides by microdiffusion: Spectrophotometer: Beckman DU or equivalent. Millipore No. PD10 04700 petri dish.

Distribute 0.1 ml of 0.5N sodium hydroxide solution by successively touching the pipette tip to the inside of the plastic Petri dish cover. The individual spots dry rapidly. One (1) ml of urine, or other prepared sample, is measured by pipette and transferred to the lower section of the dish. To the urine droplet is added 0.3 gm of solid silver sulfate. Add 2.0 ml of 66% sulfuric acid beside the urine sample; the vessel is tilted to make contact between acid and sample, and the dish is immediately covered with a previously prepared lid, taking care to maintain the Petri dish assembly horizontal at all times. The dishes are placed in an oven at 50°C for 20 hours. At the end of this period, the covers are removed carefully and the sodium hydroxide absorbent is transferred to a 10 ml volumetric flask with successive washings of distilled water applied from a 5 ml pipette. Add 3 ml of Belcher's reagent to the flask; the contents are made up to volume with distilled water and carefully mixed. The absorbance is read in the spectrophotometer at 622 nm and referred to a standard amount of fluoride put through the diffusion procedure.

Reagents:

- *Sodium hydroxide* (0.5 M) : Reagent-grade sodium hydroxide (20 gm) is dissolved in 500 ml water and diluted to 1 liter with absolute alcohol.
- *Silver sulfate:* Reagent-grade powdered silver sulfate.
- *Belcher reagent:* Dissolve 8.2 gm of sodium acetate in 6 ml of glacial acetic acid and sufficient water to effect solution. Transfer quantitatively to a 200 ml volumetric flask. Dissolve 0.0479 gm of alizarin complexone (obtained from Hopkin and Williams, Chadwell Health, Essex, England, under the name 3-aminomethylalizarin-*NN*-diacetic acid, catalogue no. 1368.4) in 1.0 ml of 20% ammonium acetate with the assistance of 0.1 ml of ammonium hydroxide and 5 ml of water. Filter this solution through Whatman No.1; filter into the 200 ml volumetric flask. Wash the filter with a few drops of water and discard. Add 100 ml of acetone to flask slowly with swirling. Dissolve separately 0.0612 gm of lanthanum chloride (obtained in a purity of 99.9 percent from Kleber Laboratories) in 2.5 ml of 2M hydrochloric acid, warming gently to aid solution. Add this to the contents of the flask, with swirling. Dilute to 200 ml with water; mix well; cool contents to room temperature; adjust volume to 200 ml mark. (Teichman, Dubois, and Monkman) .

Treatment

Induce vomiting with emetics. Gastric lavage with limewater, cream, or milk. Calcium gluconate (4–10 ml of 10% solution IV); repeat as necessary. Combat collapse and shock. Large amounts of milk, cream, or limewater demulcents. Valium or short-acting barbiturates with caution for convulsions.

Keep patient quiet and warm; maintain body calcium and fluid balance. Sodium glycerol monoacetate (monacetin) in (0.25 gm per pound, IM) for several hours. Artificial respiration, oxygen therapy as needed. Cardiac monitor and supportive. Avoid digitalis. Guard against ventricular fibrillation.

FLUOROACETATE SODIUM (CH₂FCOONa)

Synonyms: 1080; sodium monofluoroacetate.

Uses: Rodenticide, very toxic.

Properties: White crystalline.

MLD: Approximately 50 mg/70 kg person.

Remarks: Very toxic, odorless, tasteless. Death may occur within 5 hours. Latent period of 30 minutes to 2 hours before symptoms appear. Some accumulation occurs. This is an organically bound fluoride.

Symptoms: Predominantly cardiac symptoms and central nervous system stimulation. Tart sour taste. Agent is very toxic, fast-acting. Causes vomiting, tingling sensation in nose; face becomes numb; tingling spreads to arms and legs; excitability, spasmodic contraction of muscle, epileptiform convulsions followed by severe depression, respiratory failure and/or ventricular fibrillation, cardiac arrest. Children are more susceptible to cardiac arrest than to ventricular fibrillation.

Identification

Do tests 3 and 4 as given under Fluorides.

Treatment

Induce vomiting with emetics, and do gastric lavage immediately with limewater, cream, or milk. Induce purging with oral sodium sulfate (30 gm). Calcium gluconate (4–10 ml of 10% solution IV) ; repeat as necessary. Sodium glycerol monoacetate (monacetin) (0.25 gm per pound, IM).

Sedation with short-acting barbiturates or Valium.

Complete rest for cardiac symptoms. Guard against ventricular fibrillation. Cardiac monitor. Supportive.

Recovery from convulsive seizures may occur, only to be followed by a sudden attack of ventricular fibrillation and cardiac arrest. Guarded prognosis for 48 hours. See Fluoride above.

FOOD POISONING

Synonyms: Botulism; *Clostridium botulinum.*

Uses: Potentially in warfare because of high mortality and toxicity.

MLD: Very toxic, estimated at 0.01 mg.

Remarks: A spore-forming, anaerobic, gram-positive rod: Types A, B, C, D, E, and F. Man is never affected by C or D; mainly affected by types A and E; Less frequently affected by types B and F.

Case fatalities vary from 20% to 70%—this depends upon type and quantity of toxin ingested.

Leading source in the United States is improperly canned string beans, also meat and fish; onset of symptoms may be delayed 12 to 100 hours after ingestion of the toxin.

Symptoms: Sudden intense vertigo, later followed by difficulty in swallowing; nausea, vomiting, foul breath, severe abdominal pain, diarrhea, hyperpyrexia, dysphagia, mydriasis.

Neurologic symptoms and sensory disturbances usually overshadow the above gastrointestinal symptoms. Spasm of the jaw and continued difficulty in swallowing saliva, and difficulty in speech and breathing. Blurred vision and difficulty to move the eyes or facial muscles, followed by general weakness, especially in the arms then the legs. Severe respiratory difficulty, general muscular paralysis worsens; collapse and death is usually due to respiratory paralysis or from secondary pneumonia. Recovery is very slow; weakness persists for months.

Identification

Inject mice with suspected serum. If positive, the mice will develop progressive muscular paralysis, which will produce death, except those mice that were given a specific "type" botulism antitoxin. This test then can also suggest which specific botulism antitoxin may be helpful.

Treatment

Slow down absorption with activated charcoal if toxic food is still in the stomach, and if the spasm of the jaw and difficulty in swallowing has not yet occurred. A cautious attempt to remove by gastric lavage may also be considered. Saline cathartics and enemas may also help to eliminate unabsorbed toxins.

Maintain a patent airway and respiratory exchange. Guard against respiratory and secondary infection complications.

Suspected cases should be given A, B, and E antitoxin until tests demonstrate which toxin is responsible; then only that particular type is given.

These antitoxins can be obtained by phoning the National Communicable Disease Center (CDC) in Atlanta Georgia [(404) 633-2176 (night) or (404) 633-3311 (day)] or consultation and antitoxin may also be obtained at the state or city health department center.

Reference: Smith, J.W.: Resident & Staff, 17:35, 1971.

FORMALDEHYDE (CH₂O)

Synonyms: Formalin; embalming fluid; formol.

Uses: Fixing tissue, preservative, disinfectant, embalming, industry.

Properties: Sharp penetrating odor. Colorless liquid, 40% solution: lacrimating, volatile; Bp 21°C.

MLD: Approximately 30 ml/70 kg person.

Remarks: Symptoms are immediate and severe. In severe cases, death usually occurs within 10 hours. In milder cases, recovery is rapid. Prognosis is good, with little systemic effect, except occasional scar formation of stomach and esophagus.

Symptoms: Strong odor of formaldehyde on breath, vomitus, and body cavity; lacrimation, irritation of eyes, severe local respiratory irritation, pulmonary edema, difficult breathing, possibly secondary pneumonia. Later nausea, vomiting, throat and mouth irritations; pallor, clammy skin, vertigo, abdominal pain, increased gastrointestinal peristalsis, diarrhea, edema, convulsions, stricture of throat, kidney damage, hematuria, anuria, possible cardiovascular collapse, shock, acidosis, coma, death. If patient survives 48 hours, prognosis is good.

Identification

Volatile steam-distillation separation or by microdiffusion.

1. Place 1 ml of suspected solution or 10 ml of steam distillate in a small test tube. Add a small pinch of chromotropic acid powder (1,8-dihydroxynaphthalene-3,6-disulfonic acid) and shake gently. Add 3 ml of concentrated sulfuric acid, tilting the tube and allowing the acid to flow down the sides of the tube so that it forms a separate layer underneath the solution. At this point, carefully examine the junction between the aqueous solution and the underlying sulfuric acid. If formaldehyde is present, a purple ring will be seen at the junction. Mix the contents of tube by gently swirling. If formaldehyde is present, a diffuse violet color will be produced, the intensity of which will be proportional to the concentration of formaldehyde present (specific test). See test 1 under Methyl Alcohol.

2. To 1 ml of solution, add 5 ml of water and 5 ml of Schiff's reagent (reduced fuchsine) → pinkish violet color, which is directly proportional to concentration. See Methyl alcohol.

3. To 1 ml of solution, add 10 ml of dichromate-sulfuric acid (5% potassium dichromate in 50% sulfuric acid) → green color (any reducing agent may also be positive).

4. To 10 ml of distillate, add 10 drops of phenylhydrazine hydrochloride (5%), plus 3 drops of sodium nitroprusside (0.5%), plus 10 drops of sodium hydroxide (10%) → blue color (acetaldehyde gives a red color).

5. A few milliliters of unknown is added to 5 ml of a 10% solution of either tannic or gallic acid in sulfuric acid and then heated on steam bath → green or blue-green.

6. Refer to tests for Methyl Alcohol. *Omit* step oxidizing methyl alcohol → formaldehyde.

   Note: Methenamine breaks down to formaldehyde in humans.

7. GC: See under Glue Sniffing, following section.

Treatment

INHALATION: Carefully inhale *dilute* ammonia fumes. Guard against pneumonia.

ORALLY: Gastric lavage with 0.1% ammonia; use demulcents such as olive oil, pectins. Morphine for pain. Artificial respiration, if indicated, or oxygen therapy. Combat shock or collapse. Combat acidosis with sodium bicarbonate intravenously. Alkaline diet. Supportive measure for possible kidney damage; and stricture of esophagus. Supportive.

GLUE SNIFFING

Abused Compounds: Plastic cement solvent fumes (airplane glue), which may contain ethylene dichloride or toluene, acetone, cyclohexane, chloroform, carbon tetrachloride, etc. Leather cement or paint or lacquer thinner, which may contain benzenes, toluene, xylene, or ethanol. Gasoline, lighter fluid, and other petroleum distillates.

Remarks: The common practice is to saturate a handkerchief and occasionally take a sniff, or to put it into a large paper bag and submerge the head and breathe.

Symptoms: May be mild (a "jag" or exhilaration, euphoria, red eyes, flushed face, excitement closely resembled effects of whiskey). Ataxia, slurred speech, diplopia, drowsiness, stupor, and even coma may develop. Constant users may have nasal irritation, running nose, and cough; nausea, anorexia and weight loss, irritability, lack of concentration in school. Symptoms can be more severe and can result in brain, liver, or kidney damage and blood changes—depending upon the ingredient and duration of exposure. See under individual solvent.

Identification

GLC: Varian Aerograph 600-D; FID; stainless steel column 6 feet by $\frac{1}{4}$ inch; 30% Carbowax 20M on 60-80 mesh Chromosorb W. N_2—35 ml/minute; H_2—28 ml/minute; O_2—100 ml/minute. Injection port temperature: 160°C. Blood: direct injection of mixture of 0.5 μl H_2O + 0.5 μl blood or urine Internal standard: n-propyl acetate.

Retention Time (Minutes) at Column Temperature

	100° C	130° C
acetaldehyde	2.56	1.25
acetone	2.38	1.62
benzene	4.31	2.81
chloroform	5.62	3.25
ethanol	3.50	2.12
formaldehyde	1.81	1.38
isobutanol	7.25	3.94
isopropanol	3.19	2.06
methanol	3.25	2.06
methyl ethyl ketone	3.38	2.19
propyl acetate	4.50	2.75
toluene	6.94	4.06
xylene	11.38	6.38

Reference: Jain: *Clin Chem, 17:*82, 1971.

GOLD (SALTS)

Compounds: Chrysarobin; gold chloride.

Uses: Treatment of rheumatoidal arthritis, lupus erythematosus. Chrysotherapy.

Properties: Yellow salts.

MLD: Undetermined.

Remarks: Cumulative, especially toxic to susceptible persons.

Symptoms: Increased capillary permeability, gingivitis, agranulocytosis, acute yellow atrophy of liver, ulcerative colitis, skin rash, exfoliative dermatitis, stomatitis, albuminuria, hematuria, aplastic anemia, loss of hair, kidney damage.

Identification

1. In slightly acid solution (hydrochloric), gold will deposit with heat onto a copper spiral (Reinsch test).
2. Spectrographic analysis or atomic absorption.
3. Dithizone titration at pH 1–2. See under Mercury.

Treatment

Discontinue gold therapy.

Antibiotics prophylactically in cases of agranulocytosis or aplastic anemia. Supportive and symptomatic treatment. Guard against kidney and liver damage.

BAL by instramuscular injection should be started within a short time after symptoms are evident.
See Arsenic.

HEXACHLOROPHENE ($C_{13}H_6Cl_6O_2$)

Synonyms: Soy–Dome Cleanser; hexachlorophane.

Uses: Dermatological detergent, bacteriostatic skin cleaner. 3% solution; antiseptic.

Properties: White crystalline; Mp 164°C; turn yellow-brown; soluble in ether, chloroform, or ethanol; extracted from acid or alkaline solution.

MLD: 75 ml (3% solution) for 70 kg person.

Symptoms: INGESTION: anorexia, nausea, vomiting, abdominal cramps, diarrhea, dehydration, convulsions, oliguria, hypotension and shock, lethargy, stupor.

SKIN ABSORPTION: Infants have developed dermatitis, irritability, generalized muscular contractions, and decerebrate rigidity.

Identification

1. UV spectrophotometry:
   a. In 0.5N NaOH: Maximum density, 320 nm; $E_{1cm}^{1\%}$, 315.
   b. In ethanol: Maximum density, 298 nm; $E_{1cm}^{1\%}$ 150.
2. $FeCL_3$ (0.5%) → purple color

Treatment

Emesis, gastric lavage, fluid and electrolyte balance, anticonvulsant therapy. Symptomatic and supportive measure.

Reference: Dome Laboratories (Miles Laboratories) Report Sept. 20, 1973.

HYDROCHLORIC ACID (HCl)

Synonyms: Muriatic acid; spirits of salts.

Uses: Metal cleaner, bowl and toilet cleaner, saniflush, flux for soldering. Industry. Medicine.

Properties: Colorless liquid.   Fumes have acid penetrating odor.

MLD: Approximately 3 ml/70 kg person.

Remarks: Normally found in stomach (0.2%).

Symptoms: Burns on mouth and on lips, sour acrid taste, white eschars on skin and mouth, severe gastrointestinal irritation and corrosion, nausea, vomiting, abdominal pain, diarrhea, charred stomach contents, thirst, difficult swallowing, acidosis, convulsions, collapse, shock.   If inhaled, irritation of respiratory tract, pulmonary edema, laryngeal spasm, possible pneumonia, collapse, shock, death.

Identification

In stomach contents:
1. Pungent odor; white fumes (sharp and penetrating).   Colorless liquid.
2. Turns litmus paper pink.
3. Place open bottle of concentrated ammonia near unknown solution, stomach contents, or vomitus; will produce white copious fumes of ammonium chloride.
4. Several milliliters of unknown plus 1 ml of 10% silver nitrate plus 1 ml of 10% nitric acid will produce a white precipitate of silver chloride, which dissolves with ammonia.
   Caution: Normal stomach contents contain very dilute hydrochloric acid (0.2 to 0.5%) .
5. Quantitative determination by titration with standard sodium hydroxide solution.

Treatment

Do not use stomach tube or emetic if severe corrosion is evident.   Dilute with water with caution.   Neutralize with milk of magnesia, lime-water, soap suds.   Amphojel, Cremalin, or other mild antacid.   Do not use sodium bicarbonate or other carbon dioxide forming compounds.   Milk, cream, or white of eggs as demulcent.   Keep patient warm and quiet.   Morphine for pain.   Sedatives, antibiotics, and combat shock as necessary.   Crushed ice to relieve thirst.   If there are signs of asphyxia, tracheotomy may be indicated.   Protect against respiratory obstruction, perforation, or stricture formations.

Guard against secondary infection. Corticosteroid therapy has been recommended in persistent shock. Supportive measures.

If burns are external, wash with plenty of water and apply a paste of sodium bicarbonate.

HYPOCHLORITE (NaOCl; HOCl)

Derivatives: Sodium or calcium salts of hypochlorous acid.

Synonyms: Bleaching solutions; Clorox; Purex; Sani-Chlor, HTH.

Properties: Sodium salt is *strongly alkaline;* liberates chlorine.

MLD: Approximately 15 ml for a child.

Symptoms: Severe gastrointestinal irritation, nausea, vomiting, abdominal pain, diarrhea; mouth, throat, and lung irritation; edema of glottis, respiratory depression, shock.

Identification

1. Easily releases chlorine gas; reacts as alkaline to litmus.
2. plus silver nitrate solution → white precipitate
3. plus iodo-starch paper → blue
4. See under chlorine.

Treatment

Immediately give either milk or egg white, starch paste, aluminum hydroxide gel, or magnesium trisilicate gels; avoid sodium bicarbonate because of possible release of carbon dioxide gas. Do not use acid antidotes, which may release more hypochlorous acid. Cautious gastric lavage with 2% sodium thiosulfate. Some milk of magnesia may be left in stomach as a demulcent. Opiates for pain and fluid for shock; guard against secondary infection. Keep air passages open; oxygen and artificial respiration if needed. Treat as for chlorine gas and mild alkali. Supportive measures.

INSECT BITES

In order of severity of sting: fire ants, honey bees; bumble bees; wasps, hornets (yellow jackets) ; black widow spiders.

Effects on man: Usually a local reaction that appears rapidly at site of sting.   Pain, redness, and swelling; toxic systemic action due to venom.   Anaphylactic shock may be produced in hypersensitive persons.

Mann's Classification of Characteristic Effects

1. Hemolytic—May produce hemoglobinuria.
2. Hemorrhagic—Responsible for uterine bleeding, which sometimes follows stinging, by preventing formation of thrombokinase.   Venom increases coagulation time of blood.
3. Neurotoxic—Accounts for paralysis that sometimes occurs.
4. Histamine—Most common effect of venom.   Venom contains histamine and also stimulates the body to release more histamine.   The histamine produces the redness, flare, and wheal seen at site of the bite.

   Sometimes, a person receives sufficient venom to produce systemic poisoning.   The clinical findings resemble that of a hypersensitivity reaction with an increase in the frequency of gastrointestinal upsets such as diarrhea and vomiting.   Patients usually recover in 24 hours, but an urticarial attack may occur at the end of a week.
5. Anaphylactic—May have fatal results.   In many cases, symptoms immediately follow the sting or bite arise within 20 minutes.   Symptoms usually reach the peak of severity within 30 minutes, with the victim suffering acutely for an hour or so with recovery in 3 to 4 hours.   The main symptoms are due to the reaction of histamine on smooth muscle.   Respiratory distress: faintness with partial or complete loss of consciousness occurs, frequently followed by some form of an itching rash.   If fatal, death usually ocurrs within 15 to 20 minutes after the sting, or as early as 2 minutes.

Treatment

Depends upon severity of the sting.

Remove stinger.   The stings of bees and wasps should be scraped out rather than pulled out to prevent more venom being squeezed into the wound.

Apply an antiseptic locally.   Guard against anaphylactic reactions.

If acute systemic symptoms occur, give intravenous adrenalin or antihistamine. If adrenalin and antihistamine fail, give corticosteroids. Intravenous calcium gluconate has also been beneficial.

Secondary reactions may sometimes be prevented with oral antihistamine and local application of antipuritic agents. Cold compresses may relieve pain. Sedation and supportive measures.

Specific antivenin, if available, from health department or CDC.

Black widow spider, see under Spider Bite.

INSULIN

Derivative: Protamine zinc insulin; NPH.

Uses: Diabetes mellitus treatment.

Properties: Hormone. Colorless solution.

MLD: Varies, but is low.

Remarks: Hyperinsulinism is usually due to incorrect medication and may also be the result of pancreatic adenoma. The resulting symptoms are produced by the hypoglycema.

Symptoms: Hunger sensation, dizziness, cramps, palpitation, mydriasis, weakness, fatigue, tremors, apprehension hypoglycemia (low blood sugar, below 60 mg%), mental distress, delirium, profuse sweating, shock, hypotension, coma, death.

Identification

1. Determine normal blood sugar of a rabbit; then give intravenous injection of unknown into rabbit ear. Reduces blood sugar from original normal level.
2. Do blood sugar determinations on patient. Normal values are 80 to 120 mg%.
3. Radioimmuno Assay: Kits are available.

Treatment

Orange juice, glucose, or candy will partially increase blood sugar. If regular insulin was the causative agent, the patient will recover promptly with the above treatment without relapse.

However, in cases of protamine zinc insulin, or any other long-acting insulin, the patient must be watched carefully after initial recovery; further treatment is necessary periodically.

IODIDES

Synonyms: Inorganic and organic iodides.

Uses: Medicinals, reagents, industry.

Properties: White or yellow crystaline. Water-soluble.

MLD: Approximately 20 gm/70 kg person as NaI; 2 gm as iodoform.

Remarks: Acute poisoning very rare; chronic more likely.

Symptoms: Yellow staining of skin and mouth, gastrointestinal irritation, nausea, vomiting, diarrhea, increased capillary permeability (increased secretions), fluid exudate, headache, swelling of lips and eyelids, skin rash, catarrhal swelling, mouth and throat irritation, rales, pulmonary edema.

Identification

Vomitus, gastric lavage, original drugs are best specimens. Urine may also be used.
1. To 10 ml of specimen, add 10 ml of chlorine water plus 10 ml of chloroform and gently shake → purple chloroform layer (specific).
2. To 10 ml of specimen, add 10 ml of chlorine water plus 2 ml of starch solution → blue-black (specific).
3. To 10 ml of specimen, add 1 ml of silver nitrate (10%) plus 1 ml of nitric acid → yellow precipitate, which is insoluble in ammonia.

   chlorides → white precipitate (soluble in ammonia)

   bromides → brown precipitate (insoluble in ammonia)

Treatment

Remove source of drug. Gastric lavage with solution of soluble starch. Replace fluids and electrolytes. Symptomatic and supportive measures.

IODINE

Synonyms: Lugol's (5% free iodine); tincture of iodine; iodine crystals.

Uses: Antiseptic (2% aqueous is most effective).

Properties: Purple, glittering, flat, volatile, odoriferous crystals Mp 114°C.

MLD: Approximately 2 gm/70 kg person.

Remarks: Powerful irritant and vesicant.

Symptoms: Mouth, skin, mucosal, and intestinal irritation; nausea, vomiting, diarrhea, edema of mucous membranes, running nose and eyes, chest rales, yellow-brown stains on skin and mouth, thirst, kidney damage, albuminuria, hematuria, anuria, cardiac depression, twitching, collapse, death.

Identification

1. Purplish fumes and characteristic odor.
2. Stomach contents or vomitus in a beaker is gently heated; iodine will sublime on a cold surface (watch glass placed on top of beaker with piece of ice).
3. To 10 ml of specimen, add 1 ml of starch solution → blue-black.
4. To 10 ml of specimen, add 5 ml of chloroform and gently shake → violet chloroform layer.

Treatment

EXTERNALLY: Wash with 20% alcohol.

INTERNAL: Administer starch and water or dilute sodium thiosulfate (3%). Gastric lavage with starchy water or dilute sodium thiosulfate (3%). Demulcents such as white of egg, milk, or mineral oil. Morphine for pain; keep air passage open.

Give abundant fluid and sodium chloride (isotonic). Prevent shock. Maintain electrolyte balance. Supportive measures for corrosion, stricture of esophagus and kidney damage.

ISONIAZID ($C_6H_7N_3O$)

Synonyms: INH; isonicotinic acid hydrazide; Pyrizidin; Rimifon; Nydrazid; Niconyl.

Use: Tuberculosis treatment.

Properties: White crystalline. Soluble in water or chloroform.

MLD: Approximately 1 gm for a 4-year-old child; 10 gm/70 kg person.

Remarks: Absorption is rapid, and symptoms appear within several hours.   About 80 percent is eliminated in urine in the first 24 hours.   Inhibitor of mono amino oxidase.   Potentiates effects of alcohol and barbiturates.

Symptoms: Tachycardia, muscular twitching, exaggerated reflexes, convulsions, tinnitus, vertigo, weakness, vomiting, constipation, electrolyte imbalance (hyperkalemia, metabolic acidosis), hyperglycemia, acetonuria, sudden drop in blood pressure, apnea, cyanosis, arrhythmia, coma, death from respiratory or cardiovascular difficulties.

Identification: See UV, Table X.   Maximum density, 267 mm.

Treatment

Induce emesis with ipecac prior to onset of CNS stimulation. Gastric lavage only after convulsions are controlled.   Maintain respiratory exchange and electrolyte balance.   Maintain control of convulsions with Valium.   Supportive and symptomatic treatment as needed.   Hemodialysis have been reported of some help when very large doses were ingested.

ISOPROPANOL (CH₃-CHOH-CH₃)

Synonym: Isopropyl alcohol.

Uses: Antiseptic, alcohol rubs, in perfumes and colognes, window cleaner, Nylon-Nu.

Properties: Colorless liquid, Bp 82°C, pleasant odor resembles acetone.

MLD: Approximately 250 ml/70 kg person.

Remarks: Lethal dose in blood about 0.30 gm/dl.

Symptoms: Gastric irritation, nausea, vomiting, diarrhea, bradycardia, hypotension, pulmonary edema, dizziness, headache, confusion, coma, shock, death by respiratory failure.

Symptoms generally similar as for ethanol but the nausea, vomiting, and danger of aspiration is more pronounced.   Acidosis due to acetone metobolite is mild but kidney and liver involvement is more likely.

Identification

1. Microdiffusion test for ethanol and isopropanol. See Section I.
2. Five (5) ml of blood, urine, or tissue is steam distilled with 1 ml of tartaric acid (Sat.). Five (5) ml of clear distillate is transferred to a calibrated centrifuge tube; then add 10 ml of Deniges' reagent and heat in water bath for 15 minutes.

   A white or yellow-white precipitate (which settles) indicates the presence of isopropyl alcohol, acetone, or tertiary butyl alcohol. Centrifuge and compare precipitate with standards similarly prepared.

   Reagent: Deniges': 2 gm of yellow mercuric oxide plus 16 ml of water; slowly add and mix with 8 ml of sulfuric acid; stir and dissolve with an additional 16 ml of water.
3. Test for acetone in urine and/or blood; see under Acetone.
   ACETONE OR ISOPROPYL ALCOHOL
4. Steam distill vomitus, blood, organs, or urine (1 gm equivalent to 1 ml of distillate) :

   Add 4 ml of distillate to each of two test tubes. Oxidize one with 3 drops of potassium permanganate; allow to stand 5 minutes and decolorize excess $KMnO_4$ with a pinch of sodium bisulfite; add 1 ml of 10% sodium hydroxide and 1 ml of 5% furfural (purified). Filter both test tubes, using Whatman No. 42 filter paper, into test tubes each containing 2 ml of concentrated hydrochloric acid. A pink ring in the oxidized test tube indicates presence of isopropyl alcohol. A pink ring in the unoxidized test tube indicates presence also of acetone. Sensitive to 0.05 gm/dl.

   Reagent: Potassium permanganate: 3 gm $KMnO_4$ and 15 ml of 85% H_3PO_4 in 85 ml H_2O.
5. One (1) ml of blood or stomach contents plus 2 ml of 20% trichloracetic acid are mixed thoroughly and then filtered through Whatman #1 filter paper.

   Transfer 1 ml of this clear filtrate to a test tube and add several drops of $KMnO_4$ until a pink color persists. Wait 8 minutes and then decolorize with several mg of $NaHSO_3$.

   Add one pellet of NaOH followed by 3 ml of 30% NaOH and 1 drop of salicylaldehyde reagent. Heat in a boiling water bath for 4 minutes; then cool. A red color is positive for iso-propyl alcohol or acetone.

For low concentration the early appearance of a red color around the NaOH pellet is positive for this test. Sensitivity: 0.05 to 0.35% (Cardona).

Visually compare with standards prepared in a similar manner. Does not follow the Beer-Lampert Law.

6. Gas liquid chromatography (GLC): See Section I.

Treatment

Gastric lavage before depression (if possible). Treat generally similar as ethanol. *Guard against* dehydration, aspiration pneumonia, pulmonary edema, hypotension. Maintain a patent airway and a respiratory exchange. Maintain heat, fluid, and electrolyte balance. Symptomatic and supportive measures. Support against liver and kidney involvement.

KEROSENE

Synonyms: Coal oil; petroleum by-product; Varsol; Viosol.

Uses: . Solvent for insecticides; diluent; fuel; cleaning agent.

Properties: Liquid. Characteristic odor. Volatile flammable, oil soluble. Bp range, 150–300°C.

MLD: Approximately 100 ml/70 kg person.

Remarks: Absorbed through all portals including skin. Similar to gasoline, naphtha, benzene, charcoal igniting fuel, mineral seal oil, mineral spirits, spindle oil, Stoddard solvent, and other petroleum distillates in symptoms and treatment.

Symptoms: Strong odor on breath, gagging and coughing, irritation to eyes and hands, fullness of the head, headache, blurred vision, inebriation. May resemble alcoholic intoxication: dizziness, unsteady gait, nausea, vomiting, diarrhea, dilated pupils, cyanosis, dyspnea, thirst, nervous twitching, drowsiness, hyperpyrexia. Narcotic depressant that may or may not be preceded by excitement stage, visceral congestion, respiratory embarrassment. Aspiration usually produces rapid pulmonary edema, chemical pneumonitis, and may result in rapid coma and death.

CHRONIC STATE: Marked malnutrition, pallor, low hemoglobin values with anorexia and nervousness, liver and kidney involvement.

Identification

1. Characteristic odor. Bp range, 150-300°C.
2. X-ray, liver and kidney function tests may be of some presumptive value.
3. Place 1 drop on a piece of paper → translucent.
4. Burns with a smoky flame.
5. Gasoline or kerosene may show distinct UV absorbance due to trace impurities characteristic to a particular "brand" product. Read in UV range; also read in NIR. See Section I.
6. Kerosene in blood: Place 35 ml of 0.1N hydrochloric acid and 5 ml of blood in a small glass-stoppered bottle.   Invert and gently mix; add 5 ml of carbon tetrachloride; mix and shake vigorously.   Carefully remove the upper layer with suction. Centrifuge and separate the CCl_4, which is transferred to a colorimeter test tube.   Add 5 ml of Marquis' reagent.   Cap the tube with a polyethylene stopper and shake for 2 minutes. Centrifuge for 5 minutes at 2000 rpm.   Compare with standards: 5, 10, 15, 20, 25, 50, ppm.   Also positive for benzene, toluene, and xylene.

    Reagent: Marquis':   1 ml of formaldehyde in 100 ml H_2SO_4.
    Reference: Gerard, *Clin Chem, 6:*327, 1970.
7. *kerosene,* benzene, toluene, or gasoline, plus Marquis' reagent → red
8. Conway Microdiffusion (Hensel) :   Also see Section I.

    14 drops H_2SO_4, inner chamber
    14 drops H_2SO_4, outer chamber
    1 drop formaldehyde, inner chamber (Marquis' reagent)
    1 ml H_2SO_4 for sealing well
    2 ml of urine + 2 ml of ether + 2 gm of $(NH_4)_2SO_4$

Shake and separate; then centrifuge and transfer the ether layer to another tube containing Na_2SO_4 (anhydrous) and quickly again shake, separate, and centrifuge.   Transfer the ether very quickly → outer chamber Conway cell.

Ether is soluble in H_2SO_4, and vapor tension is reduced so that only kerosene, benzene, toluene, and gasoline diffuse. Allow to diffuse for 1 hour at room temperature (30°C).

Red color positive for all (Marquis' reagent in inner chamber).

Can make a semiquantitative estimate by comparison with standards.

Very sensitive reaction: 0.004 ml/ml blood for kerosene; 0.001 ml/ml blood for others.

Treatment

Emetics or indiscriminate gastric lavage should be avoided for fear of aspiration. Very careful gastric lavage may by performed when large amounts have been ingested, as a precaution against regurgitation and aspiration due to involuntary gagging or coughing. Oxygen therapy and artificial respiration if indicated; prevent secondary infection. Avoid fats or oils; demulcents such as crushed bananas or white of egg should be used instead. Saline cathartics (30 gm of sodium sulfate). Alcohol rub or sponge baths to reduce elevated body temperature. Supportive measures against possible liver or kidney involvement.

Low-fat and high-carbohydrate diet, B complex vitamins, calcium gluconate (4–10 ml of 10% solution IV).

Kerosene is also eliminated from blood through the lungs and may present continued irritation during this process. X-ray the chest even in absence of chest signs because this may still reveal an extensive chemical pneumonitis.

Kerosene may be aspirated into the lungs; even small amounts are dangerous. This can rapidly produce a severe pulmonary edema and chemical pneumonitis. Steroids may be used as an anti-inflammatory drug. Guard against secondary infection.

Do not give epinephrinelike drugs.

Symptoms and treatment are generally similar for benzene, benzine, gasoline, some chlorinated hydrocarbons, and 2,4D, 2,4,5T.

Supportive and symptomatic treatment as needed.

LEAD

Derivatives: Sugar of lead, lead tetraethyl; all soluble lead salts—lead nitrate and lead acetate are the most common. Lead carbonate, hydroxide, and oxide are soluble even in dilute acids. Metallic lead as recovered from used or old auto batteries is also a source of lead intoxication.

Uses: Outside paints, storage batteries, gasoline additives, ceramics, chinaware (especially unglazed), alloys, printing type, insecticides, vulcanized rubber; bloom talc for rubber, plumbing, etc.; lead toys, solder, foil wrapper, bullets (projectile), etc. Lead exposure is very common due to its many uses.

Properties: Toxic heavy metal, usually white crystalline, lead tetraethyl (liquid); even some insoluble salts (carbonates and oxides may be dissolved by gastric juice). Metallic lead (battery plates) gives off its toxic fumes when melted. Inhalation may produce symptoms within a week.

MLD: Soluble lead salts, approximately 10 gm/70 kg person. Lead tetraethyl, 100 mg/70 kg person (very toxic).

Remarks: Lead poisoning is not usually an acute emergency *except,* of course, after exposure to lead tetraethyl, when even adults develop encephalopathy. Lead is usually a *slow chronic exposure.* It is cumulative, and children are especially susceptible. This cumulative poisoning or intoxication occurs when absorption exceeds elimination and, since elimination is slow, typical signs and symptoms develop. Lead is absorbed through all portals, especially if soluble or in fumes. Since children are especially susceptible, they usually show signs of encephalopathy (convulsions), which occur in adults very rarely. Following absorption, lead is stored in the bones as phosphate and carbonate. High calcium tends to favor storage; low calcium releases lead into the bloodstream. Also, acid-base shift similarly affects mobilization storage. Lead stored in bones is always potentially dangerous because it depresses the hemepoetic system and at any time, even mild acidosis would put lead into circulation and produce symptoms. Sunlight (vitamin D), sweating, fevers, or drinking alcohol can also do this.

Symptoms

ACUTE: Metallic taste, gastrointestinal irritation, nausea, persistent vomiting, abdominal pain (lead colic), diarrhea, malaise, anorexia are all evidence in the acute stages.

CHRONIC: *Delayed stages or chronic exposure* may show avitaminosis, loss in weight, foul mouth odor with possible stomatitis, blue-black (Burton) gum line, severe colic, anemia, increase in reticulocytes, basophilic stippling, jaundice, coproporphyrin III in urine, constipation following initial diarrhea, possible hepatic or kidney damage, central nervous system damage, mental retardation, arthralgia (especially at night), wrist or foot drop, encephalopathy (especially in infants but also in adults with lead tetraethyl), peripheral neuritis, partial paralysis, collapse, coma, death.

AIDS IN EARLY DIAGNOSIS IN INFANTS

1. Vomiting and gastrointestinal upset
2. History of pica or other exposure
3. Elevated lead level in blood and urine: above 40 μg/dl blood.
4. X-ray shows opaque material in gastrointestinal tract
5. X-ray lead line in long bones at metaphyseal ends
6. Central nervous system manifestations
7. Anemia
8. Positive coproporphyrin in urine (chronic exposure)
9. Basophilic stippling (chronic exposure)
10. Encephalopathy (convulsions)
11. Delta-aminolevulinic acid (ALA) in urine elevated
12. Free erythrocyte porphyrins

Occasionally, an elevated lead level in urine (up to 300 μg per diem) may be chronic without clinical signs or symptoms of poisoning.   In these few cases, a high exposure increases urinary output without associated signs or symptoms, but this is rare.

Identification

In blood, urine, or ground tissue.*

1. Urine or blood is the specimen of choice.   A 24 hour urine specimen or a 10 ml sample of blood (without anticoagulant or

---

*Modified from U.S. Public Health Service method. (Mixed-color method when bismuth is absent.)

any foreign material) is collected in a Pyrex container. Use a glass stopper or a cork *(rubber stoppers contain lead, as do soft glass).*

Determination of lead requires many precautions against contamination. Urine specimens are preferable over blood; a 24 hour specimen may reflect a better estimate of degree of intoxication; however, since it is not easy to collect an uncontaminated true 24 hour specimen, blood is a satisfactory alternate. When the lead levels are just slightly elevated (if at all), and lead poisoning is still suspected, the administration of one-fourth the therapeutic dose of disodium calcium EDTA *(Versenate)* will, within 2 to 3 hours, *markedly* elevate the blood-lead level, if lead is present in the bones. This is proof of lead storage in bones and soft tissues.

All glassware and separatory funnels must be Pyrex or lead-free. Stopcock grease must be lead-free or use glycerine. Glassware must be washed with nitric acid and rinsed with re-distilled water. Use glass stoppers or corks: rubber stoppers contain lead; also soft glass is contaminated. All reagents must be highest purity with low lead.

Check the phenol red indicator to be certain that EDTA was not used in its preparation. The presence of even small traces of EDTA would nullify the determination.

a. *Slow Digestion:* Measure the total urine volume (24 hours). Collect in a 2 liter glass-stoppered Pyrex bottle and then transfer a 50 ml aliquot to an appropiate-sized Phillips beaker; or measure 5 ml of blood, as the case may be.

To this, add 5 ml of nitric acid and 5 ml of 10% K_2SO_4 and evaporate at low heat. Avoid spattering when solution is dry; add 3 ml more of nitric acid and put watch glass on lid. Evaporate carefully to dryness.

To the ash, add 1 or 2 ml of nitric acid and increase heat on the hot plate to moderate temperature, while swirling to dislodge and dissolve the ash. Continue to heat until dry. Cover the beaker with a watch glass and continue to heat for about an hour. Allow to cool and again add 1 ml of nitric acid and repeat as above. Continue this nitric acid addition, each time gradually increasing the hot plate temperature, inducing as much charring as possible. Cool between each addition. Avoid overheating, which may produce spattering and loss. After three or four such additions, the hot plate should be about 400°C. It is while dry that the residue is most violently oxidized by production of red fumes of NO_2 at high temperatures of the hot plate. The final development of a white ash indicates destruction of the organic materials. To be certain of complete oxidation, an additional 1 ml of nitric acid is used and oxidation and heating repeated. The ash is then white and ready for extraction. An alternate aid in oxidation of the organic material is the use of perchloric acid (72%). This will greatly reduce the time. Only a few drops of perchloric acid (72%) *with nitric acid* is very effective. Use with caution because this may be explosive with large amounts of organic material in the absence of nitric acid (nitric acid: perchloric acid 4:1).

b. *Rapid Digestion:* Transfer 5 ml of blood or 50 ml of urine (aliquot of a measured per diem output) to a Kjeldahl flask with several glass beads. Add 50 ml of nitric acid and 4 ml of sulfuric acid. Heat gently at first to minimize foaming; then slowly increase heat until actively boiling. Continue to heat until volume is reduced to approximately 25 ml. Remove flame and add 50 ml more of nitric acid and *carefully* and slowly add 4 ml of concentrated perchloric acid (72%). Heat again until all nitric and perchloric acid is driven off. If residual solution does *not* turn black, the digestion is complete in one step. If the residual solution (approximately 3 ml) *starts* to turn dark black (carbon), immediately remove the flame and add 15 ml more of nitric acid; again heat and digest until solution is clear and white copious SO_3 fumes are evolving. Continue to heat for 2 or 3 minutes to remove all nitric and perchloric acid. The specimen is completely digested and the residual sulfuric acid is about 3 ml. Do not allow the complete removal of sulfuric acid. If necessary during the digestion, add 1 or 2 ml of additional sulfuric acid. Allow to cool and add 10 ml of water. Carefully neutralize with ammonium hydroxide while rotating the flask under cold tap water to keep cool.

This digestion method is very rapid and efficient, but caution must be taken with the use of perchloric acid (can be dangerous and explosive). Nitric acid contains traces of lead and must be redistilled. With the use of these large amounts of acid, a blank is necessary. However, this is not a valid objection since it is advisable to always parallel a blank reagent run with every series of analyses to subtract the lead contamination introduced by the reagents.

The solution from either method of digestion (slow or rapid) is now completely digested and should be clear and free from nitric and perchloric acids. Add 15 ml of water and 10 ml of 25% sodium citrate to the digest and then swirl to dissolve salts. Add 4 ml of 20% hydroxylamine and 2 drops of phenol red indicator. Adjust the pH of this solution to 9–10 with the addition of ammonium hydroxide. (Yellow in weak acid → red in alkaline.) Check the pH with pHydrion test paper to verify that the pH is above 9, to allow for the complete extraction of lead. Transfer with double-distilled water to a 125 ml Squibb separatory funnel containing 5 ml of 10% KCN. Shake for 1 or 2 minutes with 5 ml portions of dithizone for extraction until a definite green extract indicates all the lead has been removed (generally two times). If more is required, this is an indication of elevated lead. The addition of the chloroform at this point initiates precipitation of calcium and magnesium phosphates; therefore, once the extraction is begun, it should be completed without delay. Combine all the extracts quantitatively in a second separatory funnel containing 30 ml of 1:99 nitric acid.

The extracted lead is then stripped from the dithizone chloroform layer by shaking the second separatory funnel for 2 minutes, and the chloroform layer is discarded. The aqueous layer is then washed by shaking with an additional 5 ml of chloroform, which is discarded with as close a separation as possible. The last drop of chloroform floating on the surface is evaporated by blowing air gently into the funnel.

Add 6.0 ml of ammonia-cyanide solution and exactly 15 ml of standard dithizone; shake for 2 minutes. Allow layers to separate, then transfer and drain the chloroform layer into a dry test tube. Be certain that all water droplets are absent. Read the optical density at 510 nm, using the reagent blank as a reference, with a 22 mm or 10 mm light path. Refer to *your* standard curve for lead (10 mm cuvette: $8 \mu g$ = o.d., 0.12).

Standard curves should be prepared individually by each analyst. Quantities of lead from 0 to 25 μg in 30 ml of 1% nitric acid are run through the procedure, omitting the digestion and the first extraction with dithizone. The zero standard is used as the reference blank, and optical densities are plotted against micrograms of lead.

Report all results (in μg) per 24 hours of urine or per dl of blood.

NORMAL LEVELS FOR LEAD: Blood, less than 40 μg per 100 ml. Urine, less than 40 μg for 24 hour output. Anything above these levels may be regarded as a suspected lead poisoning.

To further confirm this, a *partial* therapeutic dose of edathamil is given, and about 4 hours later another blood specimen is taken (or another 24 hour urine specimen is collected). These will show a *very marked increase of lead* over the previous determinations if lead poisoning is present; 2–4 hours is peak time.

Other metals which also give color with dithizone at specific pH are listed below:

	Adjusted pH	*Color Change*
Mercury	2	orange-peach
Copper	4	red
Zinc	5.5	orange
Gold	2	rose-purple
Bismuth	4	cherry red
Lead	9	cherry red

Reagents:

Water: Double distill in all Pyrex still.
• Nitric acid: Redistill in all Pyrex still, or use low lead.

- Ammonium hydroxide: Distill 3 liters into $1\frac{1}{2}$ liters of water chilled in an ice bath; the delivery should be deeply submerged in the water to cut down loss. Distill volume increases to about 2 liters. Can also be prepared from tank ammonia in a similar fashion, or use low lead reagents.

- Sodium citrate: Use 125 gm of the $5\frac{1}{2}$ water hydrated salt in redistilled water to make almost 500 ml. Add some phenol red indicator and a few drops of sodium hydroxide until a red color (pH 9–10) appears. Extract with strong dithizone until a green extract is obtained. Add a small amount of citric acid until an orange color (pH 7) appears, and extract the excess dithizone with chloroform until a colorless extract is obtained. Discard the chloroform.

- Hydroxylamine · HCl: Use 20 gm in water to make 65 ml. Add a few drops of *m*-cresol purple indicator and then add ammonium hydroxide to a yellow color (pH 3). Add sufficient 4% solution of sodium diethyl dithiocarbamate to combine with metallic impurities. After a few minutes, extract with chloroform until excess reagent is removed. (The absence of a yellow color in the chloroform, when a portion of the extract is shaken with dilute copper solution, indicates that this point has been reached.) Add distilled hydrochloric acid until the indicator turns pink and adjust the volume to 100 ml with water.

- Dithizone for extraction: Dissolve 16 mg of diphenylthiocarbazone (dithizone) in 1 liter of redistilled chloroform. Keep in brown bottle in the refrigerator.

- Standard dithizone: Dilute equal parts of above dithizone with equal parts of redistilled chloroform (8 mg per liter). Keep in a brown bottle and in the refrigerator. Always allow to come to room temperature before using; also, age 1 to 2 days before use.

- Potassium cyanide: Prepare a saturated solution (a weaker solution will not have the proper pH) with about 50 gm KCN. Extract with dithizone (30 mg dithizone per liter) until a green color is obtained; then extract excess dithizone with chloroform. Dilute with redistilled water to 500 ml.

- 1:99 nitric acid: Dilute 10 ml of nitric acid HNO_3 to 1 liter with redistilled water.
- Ammonia-cyanide solution: Mix 200 ml KCN and 150 ml of ammonium hydroxide and dilute to 1 liter with distilled water.
- Standard lead: Use 1.5984 gm of lead nitrate in 1 liter of 1:99 nitric acid to make a stock solution of 1 ml = 1 mg of lead. A working stock of 1 ml = 2 μg is prepared by diluting with 1:99 nitric acid.

2. Coproporphyrin III, acid ether soluble (Blanke)

To 5 ml of freshly voided urine add 2–5 drops of acetic acid and 5 drops of 3% hydrogen peroxide and 5 ml of diethyl ether. Cork and gently shake. Allow layers to separate and discard lower aqueous level. To ether add 1 ml of 1.5N HCl and gently shake. Examine under UV lamp (wood filter).

Blue or blue-green fluorescence is *normal*.

Pink or red fluorescence is *positive*.

Positive for intoxication with lead, arsenic, mercury, bismuth, copper, iron, gold, silver, zinc, phosphorus; barbiturates, sulfonal, sulfonilamides, alcohol, TNT, chloroform, carbon tetrachloride. Also hepatitis, blood dyscracias, hypovitaminosis.

This simple rapid test can be a presumptive test for *chronic lead poisoning*. It is sensitive and appears sooner than the basophilic stippling of the erythrocyte.

3. Quick urine test by ALA for lead exposure:

Delta-aminolevulinic acid (ALA) is closely associated with excessive lead exposure. ALA levels remain high even up to 1 year after lead exposure. Random urine samples are used.

Simple, inexpensive, prefilled, disposable ion-exchange columns are supplied by BIO-RAD Laboratories. Complete setup, including reagents, is available.

This test for ALA first requires a preliminary separation of urea and porphobilinogen from the urine. Two simple disposable "piggy back" ion-exchange columns do this and then eliminate the urea and allow the porphobilinogen to be eluted with sodium acetate. This is collected and condensed with acetyl acetine to form a pyrrole, which develops a strong red color on adding fresh Ehrlich's reagent.

Negative		
Trace	+ —	
Small	+	(1 mg%)
Moderate	++	
Large	+++	
Very large	++++	
Very very large	+++++	(10 mg%)

This test will even detect (1 year after exposure) those asymptomatic patients (under treatment) with lead immobilized in the bones.

Reference: Davis and Andelman: *Arch Environ Health, 15:* 53, 1967.

4. Lead exposure estimated by "free erythrocyte protoporphyrins":

Turner model III fluorometer with standard lamp #110-850; sample holder high sensitivity #110-865; primary filter #110-812 (405); secondary filter #110-820(25); cuvettes 12 by 75 75 mm Pyrex.

Blood by finger prick is collected into one heparinzed micro tube and into two heparinized microhematocrit capillary tubes. Place in ice; stable for four hours. Determine blood hematocrit.

0.1 ml sample by disposable micropipette is added to a Pyrex (12 by 75 mm) tube containing 1 ml of ethylacetate and 0.25 ml of glacial acetic acid. Stopper and shake tube vigorously 40 times (about 15 seconds). A reagent blank of 0.1 ml. of 5N HCl and a standard 0.1 ml of 0.5 μg coproporphyrin per ml in 1.5N HCl is also carried through the entire procedure parallel to unknown.

Add 3.5 ml of 1.5N HCl and shake each tube vigorously 40 times (about 15 seconds).

Centrifuge for 2 minutes and read the HCl layer in the fluorometer versus the blank. The standard is read at both 10× and at 30×. *Take care* to exclude the upper ethylacetate layer and the bottom precipitate when reading in the fluorometer.

CALCULATIONS

Hematocrit reading is divided by 100 to be used in following formulas e.g., hematocrit of 35 is expressed as 0.35.

For readings at 30× slit:

$$\frac{50 \ (\mu g/100ml)}{\text{Standard reading at } 30\times} = 30\times \text{ factor } (\mu g/100 \text{ ml})$$

$$\frac{(\text{sample reading at } 30\times) \ (30\times \text{ factor})}{\text{Hematocrit}} = \begin{array}{c} \mu g \text{ coproporphyrin} \\ \text{per } 100 \text{ ml} \\ \text{of packed RBC} \end{array}$$

For readings at 10× slit:

$$\frac{50 \ (\mu g/100 \text{ ml})}{\text{Standard reading at } 10\times} = 10\times \text{ factor } (\mu g/100ml)$$

$$\frac{(\text{sample reading at } 10\times) \ (10\times \text{ factor})}{\text{Hematocrit}} = \begin{array}{c} \mu g \text{ coproporphyrin} \\ \text{per } 100 \text{ ml} \\ \text{of packed RBC} \end{array}$$

μg coproporphyrin in 100 ml of packed RBC	*Interpretation*
0—60	normal
60—120	indicates exposure to lead
> 160	further work-up indicated

Reagent: Coproporphyrin standard 0.5 μg/ml in 1.5N HCl. A 5 μg coproporphyrin vial (sigma) is reconstituted with 10 ml of 1.5N HCl. Stable in refrigerator for 2 weeks.

Reference: Nelson, Town, Kim, Fields, Clark, and Batayras: *Traces, 9:2,* 1976 (G. K. Assoc).

5. *Lead in blood—Delves Sampling Cup,* Atomic Absorption.

Atomic Absorption Spectrophotometer: Perkin-Elmer, model 403 or equivalent equipped with Delves sampling cup accessory and a three-slot burner head.

Instrument settings: Wavelength—217 (line 283 can also be used but greater sensitivity and repeatability with line 217). Slit—4. Lead current 12 ma or that required in the lamp specifications. Range: UV. Full scale: 0.5 A (can be changed depending on concentration of lead in the sample and the sensitivity desired). Response: 1. Chart speed: 120 mm/min. Flame: Air acetylene.

Alignment of the quartz absorption tube: Place the absorption tube between the brackets on the burner head so that the circular opening in the tube wall is facing the burner head slots. Position the burner with the absorption tube on, so that the optical beam is passing through the absorption tube. To complete the alignment procedure, slowly adjust the burner position (rotational, vertical, and horizontal) to obtain the minimum value on the read-out display of the instrument. The alignment of the absorption tube may need slight readjustment after the system has reached thermal equilibrium with the flame on.

Alignment of the Delves assembly: Position the sample holder assembly directly beneath the absorption tube aperture. Lower the sample holder assembly so that the loop is about 5 mm below the quartz tube. Place the cup position spacer in the loop and slide the loop and spacer under the hole in the quartz tube. Raise the loop until the spacer makes minimum contact with the tube (2–3 mm below the aperture). Remove the spacer and replace with Delves cup. It may be necessary to adjust the sample cup position so that it is directly under the tube hole. This may be done by using the insertion rod locking nuts in and out adjustment and the rotational stop adjusting screw for rotational adjustment. When adjustment is completed the Delves cup will be in the same position each time a new sample is inserted for analysis. Lower the heat shield into place.

Determination (Method of additions): Ignite the flame and after allowing about 5 minutes for thermal equilibrium, condition and clean the cups by inserting into the flame for 20–30 seconds. (Before igniting the flame, be sure to have deionized distilled water constantly aspirated through the burner-nebulizer system; this will keep burner head at a constant temperature.)

Place the heat control plate on the hot plate and bring the temperature to about 100°C.

Pipette 10 μl of blood sample to be analyzed into each of six previously conditioned sample cups using a suitable micropipet such as the Eppendorf micropipet. Arrange the sample cups in the sample tray with the tweezers using the position numbers on the tray for cup identification. Dry the blood samples by placing the tray on the heat control plate. Remove for cooling.

To two of these sample cups, add 10 μl of the 0.4 μg Pb/ml calibration standard and to two other cups add 10 μl of the 0.8 μg Pb/ml calibration standard. Again dry the samples to which the standard was added until completely evaporated. Remove for cooling.

Add 20 μl of 30% hydrogen peroxide to each of the six cups prepared. Dry again on the heat control plate until a creamy yellow residue is obtained (as the sample oxidizes, a white froth will extend above the rim of the cup and then collapse back inside). Remove for cooling.

Insert each cup into the flame for measurement, obtaining peak in the recorder. Measure the recorder peak height and take the average of each pair. *(Note:* The recorder trace will show a peak representing smoke and combustion products of the sample before the peak for lead absorption.) Prepare a calibration curve for each blood specimen to be analyzed, and from this, determine the lead content of the sample by extrapolating on the x axis.

Reagents:

* Stock standard, 1000 μg Pb/ml: 1.598 gm lead nitrate [Pb (NO$_3$)$_2$] dissolved in 1 L of 1% nitric acid (HNO$_3$).
* Working standard, 10 μg Pb/ml: 1 ml stock standard diluted to 100 ml with 1% HNO$_3$.
* Calibration standard, 0.4 μg Pb/ml: 0.4 ml working standard diluted to 10 ml with distilled water.
* Calibration standard, 0.8 μg Pb/ml: 0.8 ml working standard diluted to 10 ml with distilled water.

References

H.T. Delves: A micro-sampling method for the rapid determination of lead in blood by atromic absorption spectrophotometry. *Analyst, 95:*431, 1970.

F. Fernández and H. L. Kahn: The determination of lead in blood by atomic absorption spectrophotometry with the Delves sampling cup technique. *Atomic Absorption Newsletter, 10:1*, 1971.

J.D. Kerber and F. Fernández: The Determination of trace metals in aqueous solution with the Delves sampling cup technique. *Atomic Absorption Newsletter, 10:78*, 1971.

F. Fernández: Some observations on the determination of lead in blood with the Delves cup method. *Atomic Absorption Newsletter, 12:3*, 1973.

Perkin-Elmer 990-9889 (1973): Instructions Atomic Absorption Microsampling System for Double Beam Instruments.

6. *Identification of residues* or contents in container found at scene (simple and presumptive):

If an insoluble lead sulfate, first dissolve a small trace in hot saturated ammonium acetate. If a soluble salt (nitrate or acetate), dissolve in water. If acid is required to dissolve the residue, do so. The now-soluble solution is made alkaline with ammonium hydroxide and is divided into aliquot portions.

Acidify with hydrochloric acid → lead chloride, a white precipitate, which dissolves when heated. Lead precipitates as lead chlorides only when large amounts are present (over 100 mg). Alkalinize with sodium hydroxide following the acidification described → lead hydroxide (white precipitate).

To another portion, add 0.5 ml of sulfuric acid and 5 ml of ethanol; allow to stand about an hour. A fine white precipitate of lead sulfate appears.

To another portion (alkaline with ammonia), reacidify with acetic acid; then add 0.5 ml of acetic acid in excess. Add 5 drops of saturated potassium chromate, and lead chromate is a yellow precipitate. (Test is sensitive to about 0.02 mg.)

Treatment

In the acute phase, eliminate as much of agent as possible by induced vomiting or gastric lavage. Purge with sodium sulfate (30 gm) in one-half glass of warm water. Keep bowels open with saline laxative; exercise, massage, and adequate diet. Demulcents such as white of egg, cream, or milk.

Demobolize lead from circulation into the bones and soft tissue with an alkaline diet, milk, calcium gluconate.

Supportive measures for possible liver or kidney involvement.

Barbiturates may be ineffective or even unsafe. Valium may be more effective for the convulsions.

Specific treatment of choice is EDTA as the disodium calcium salt (Edatate; edathamil; Versenate) IV; oral is ineffective and may be even dangerous.

Dilute contents of vial according to directions of manufacturer and drip slowly. See package insert.

In severe cases or with encephalopathy BAL may also (in addition) be given to improve effectiveness of treatment.

Lead elimination is peaked at about the third or fourth hour after EDTA treatment. Analysis of urine and blood lead will show very high levels. This will further confirm the diagnosis, and efficacy of treatment and lead elimination. Analyze urine and blood for residual lead. If still elevated, proceed again with an additional 5-day therapy, after a 10-day rest.

Analyze urine or blood at intervals to evaluate treatment. Normal lead should be below 40 μg in 24 hours of urine. Prompt improvement usually follows and, in children, the encephalopathy subsides and usually does not recur.

Treatment for chronic lead is the same as described above. If treated promptly and brain or nerve damage has not occurred, prognosis is favorable.

EDTA has been reported (*under rare* circumstances) to be nephrotoxic. Its course of therapy should therefore be short; a patient's renal status should be evaluated before, during, and after therapy. These adverse reactions are, however, *very rare.*

D-LYSERGIC ACID DIETHYLAMIDE, ($C_{20}H_{25}N_{30}$)

Synonyms: *N,N*-diethyl-D-lysergamide; Delysid; LSD-25.

RELATED COMPOUNDS: Seeds of some morning glory varieties *(Oloiuqui, Rivea corymbosa; Ipomoea violaceus)*, the active principle of which is closely related to LSD.

Other hallucinogens have been available much longer: peyote (dried top of cactus) ; mescaline is a purified extract (phenethylamine) present in the small button (seeds) in small cacti; psilocybin (Indocybin) is found in a mushroom *Psilocybe mexicana;* dimethyltryptamine (DMT) is a synthetic indole, also found in seeds of the South American plants *Piptadenia peregrinia* and *Prestonia amizonica*.

Other hallucinogens are STP (methyl dimethoxy methyl phenylethylamine) and DET (*N,N*-diethyltryptamine).

Derivation: A naturally occurring constituent of the parasitic fungus, ergot; unlike the amino acid alkaloids of ergot, it produces only slight vasoconstriction. LSD is a semisynthetic derivative of ergonovine.

Properties: MW, 323. Prisms crystallized from benzene Mp 80–85°C. *D*-tartrate derivative $(C_{20}H_{25}N_{30})_2 \cdot C_4H_6O_6 \cdot 2\ CH_3OH$. Elongated prisms from methanol. Mp 198–200°C.

MLD: 14,000 μg, or even higher (Hoffer). Half-life about 3 hours.

Remarks

Antagonizes serotonin, and this may have a potent effect on the brain. Rapidly metabolized in the liver (almost completely). Only negligible amounts may be found in the urine. Alcoholics or drug habitués require higher initial doses to get a "reaction."

LSD, sometimes called "acid," is a very powerful hallucinogenic drug. It probably has no safe or satisfactory uses, and can be dangerous. A "trip" is not always pleasant (terror). Some LSD users have reported sudden "flashbacks," unwanted, months later. LSD may be unpredictable; may trigger mental illness in some susceptible-persons; may alter or injure hereditary genes.

Tolerance to hallucinogens develops rapidly but is usually lost in several days. Some users have built up LSD dose to 2,000 μg over a period of days. The average dose for a "trip" is about 200 to 400 μg, but only 25 μg may produce effects on some susceptible individuals. Initial dose is usually about 100 μg, which may be built up.

An LSD trip usually lasts about 12 hours and onset is usually fairly gentle, whereas, a DMT trip lasts about 2 hours and has a sudden or "rough" onset.

Symptoms: Pupillary dilation, nausea, palmar sweating, erection of hair (goose pimples), tachycardia, and rise in body temperature. *Perceptual changes:* distance change; objects seem to disintegrate and then reconstitute into different shapes; walls seem to close in, expand, or pulsate, inanimate objects appear to move and change size; designs, tiles, or pictures on the wall take on new shape or design. User may become unaware of his body—feels free as a bird floating on air. Numbness and paresthesia may be experienced. Time may stop, slow up, become fast, or even reverse itself.

Sleep, deep coma, and even death can occur.

Euphoria is perhaps the first sign that the LSD is beginning to work. Some users act silly; others are in a state of contentment—relaxed, supremely happy even though for no apparent reason. Some are fearful, anxious, feel alone and abandoned; hyperventilation.

Identification

1. Pure LSD requires no extraction or clean up, but when mixed with sugar, starch, talc, or NaHCO$_3$, extraction is necessary. Tests are sensitive to about 100 μg.

   A sugar cube with LSD, placed under UV light, exhibits a definite blue fluorescence.

2. Dissolve the sugar cube powder, talc, etc. (containing about 1 mg LSD) in 15 ml of 1% tartaric acid. Add 10 ml CHCl$_3$ (redistilled) and then make basic with 1N NaHCO$_3$ solution. Shake and extract; allow layers to separate, then filter organic layer through glass wool (previously moistened with CHCl$_3$) into a 25 ml volumetric flask. Re-extract with additional portions of CHCl$_3$ to bring final volume up to the 25 ml mark. If LSD is too dilute, bring CHCl$_3$ volume down to 4 ml with a current of air (keep below room temperature). Scan in UV spectrophotometer: maximum peak is at 310 nm; minimum at 273 nm. Compare with known standards taken through entire procedure; sensitive to 25 μg.

3. Column chromatography. Mix 3 gm of acid-washing Celite 545 and 3 ml of 1N NaHCO$_3$ with sample preparation. Transfer to glass chromatographic column containing a 1 inch plug of acid-washed Celite 545 packed firmly but not too tightly on top of a plug of glass wool. Later, elute LSD from column

using 25 to 50 ml of $CHCl_3$. Bring to volume and scan in UV spectrophotometer as above.

Reference: Martin and Alexander: *JAOAC, 50:*1236, 1967.

4. Pure sample of LSD is dissolved in 3 ml of 10% tartaric acid and is read in the UV spectrophotometer: maximum density is at 312 nm (100 μg is at 68 T) ; minimum density is at 269 nm. This is more sensitive than reading in chloroform.

5. TLC (Martin and Alexander) : LSD shows bright blue fluorescent spots under UV light. If deteriorated by heat, air, or light, several additional spots will be demonstrated.

   a. *Plate:* Silica gel G.

   Developing solvent: $CHCl_3$:methanol (1:4) . Examined under UV light, shows an intense fluorescence.

   Spray: *p*-dimethylaminobenzaldehyde.

   DMBA reagent: Carefully mix 65 ml H_2SO_4 with 35 ml of water. Allow to cool and then add 125 mg of *p*-dimethylaminobenzaldehyde.

   Shake vigorously, then add 2 drops of 10% $FeCl_3$. Spot turns dark blue and is sensitive to about 0.2 μg.

       Rf about 0.7: LSD

       Rf about 0.4: LSD-25 (iso)

   b. *Plate:* Coated with silica gel G and aluminum oxide, each prepared as separate slurries and then mixed half and half.

   Developing solvent: Acetone (only) . Examine under UV; shows a fluorescence (less intense than above) .

   Spray: As above.

   Rf as above.

   Small tails, color lighter than in test a above; sensitive to about 1 μg.

6. a. Take 20 drops of LSD, a fragment of sugar cube, 20 drops of water, 20 drops of 1% tartaric acid, and 1 ml of reagent. Swirl, let stand for 10 to 20 minutes. Blue color is positive for any lysergic acid derivative.

   Reagent: 12 mg of *p*-dimethylaminobenzaldehyde, 6 ml H_2SO_4, 3 ml of water.

   b. TLC 30 gm of silica gel G and 0.1N sodium hydroxide (60 ml) .

Solvent: CHCl₃:methanol (9:1).

Spray: *p*-dimethylaminobenzaldehyde reagent (0.5 gm in 5 ml of hydrochloric acid and 95 ml of ethanol).

LSD and ergot alkaloids: blue-violet, intense in 10 minutes.

Compound	Rf
LSD	0.60
ergonovine maleate	.18
ergometrine	.43
ergotamine tartrate	.52
ergotamine	.72
lysergic acid	.05
dihydroergotamine	.35
heroin	.48
morphine	.10
codeine	.30
amphetamine	.16
methamphetamine	0.17

c. Spot test material on another plate; then irradiate with UV light for about 2 hours. Spray as above.

Compound	DMBA Spray Rf	UV Fluorescence Rf
LSD	0.61 & 0.38	0.80 GB—0.73Y—p.0.61B—0.47YB
ergotamine	0.72 & 0.52	0.72 Gy—0.52 Or — 0.20 Gy — 0.17 ol
heroin	0.48	0.48B—0.13 B

Reference: Genest and Farmilio: *J Pharm Pharmacol, 16:* 250, 1964.

7. Dissolve sugar cube in water; add some NaHCO₃ and then extract with methylene chloride.

TLC yielded two spots: One was fluorescent under UV light and gave a yellow color with *p*-dimethylaminobenzaldehyde in ethanol acidified with hydrochloric acid. The other spot was not fluorescent and gave a deep blue color with above reagent.

Reference: Radecka and Nigam: *J Pharm Sci, 55:*861, 1966.

8. GC. Methanol:CHCl₃ (3:1) adjusted to pH about 8.5 with

NH_3. Extract with above chloroform, filter, collect, and concentrate $CHCl_3$ extract in the cold under vacuum to very small volume.

a. Inject into gas chromatograph: 2% SE-30 column 250°C.

b. Add cold trifluoroacetic anhydride to the cold original $CHCl_3$ extract dropwise until original volume is double. Allow to stand at room temperature and inject into GC. Retention time is 12 minutes (6 minutes less than original parent compound).

Reference: Lerner, Mills, and Mount: *J Forensic Sci, 8:*126, 1963.

9. Fluorimetry.

a. Bile, plasma, liver, brain (in order of concentration). Saturate 5 ml of bile or plasma with sodium chloride in a 60 ml glass-stoppered bottle that contains 25 ml of *n*-heptane plus 0.5 ml of isoamyl alcohol plus 0.5 ml of 1N sodium hydroxide and about 3 gm NaCl (enough to just saturate the solution mixture).

Shake and extract mechanically for about 30 minutes and then centrifuge. Transfer 20 ml of the heptane to a 40 ml glass-stoppered centrifuge tube containing 3 ml of 0.004N hydrochloric acid, and shake for 10 minutes. Read the acid phase in a quartz cuvette by measuring its fluorescence. Activate at 325 mμ and read at 445 mμ. (All solvents used must be purified by successive washing with 1N NaOH followed by water.) This method is highly sensitive.

Reference: Axelrod *et al.: Ann NY Acad Sci, 66:*435, 1957.

b. Separate by TLC as above. Develop spot and then scrape it off and elute LSD with hydrochloric acid and methanol mixture. This is activated at 325 nm and read at 430 nm.

Reference: Dal Cortivo.

10. a. Mescaline (peyote cactus). Extract by Soxhlet apparatus; crystallized as SO_4.

    i. *Weak* alkaline pH 8; chloroform extraction (ether is not satisfactory): Read in 0.5N H_2SO_4 in the UV—maximum density, 268 nm.

    ii. Ethanol solvent (sensitive); extract with ethanol and

read in UV—maximum density: 270 nm; $E_{1cm}^{1\%}$ 75; shoulder at 225 nm. Methanol solvent—Maximum density: 268 nm; $E_{1cm}^{1\%}$ 27; minimum density: 230 nm.

  iii. Color, precipitate, crystal, or color tests: See alkaloids.

      Iodoplatinic chloride → negative

      Gold chloride → positive

      Wagners → positive

      Picric acid → positive

      Marquis → orange

      NH_4MoO_4 → green → blue

b. STP, DOM—4 methyl 2,5-dimethoxy amphetamine: Mp 70°C; HCl salt: Mp 188°C. Water-soluble compound. Read in UV; in water or 0.5N H_2SO_4.

Maximum density: *288*, 220 mμ in H_2SO_4

Minimum density: 252 mμ

c. DMT (dimethyltryptamine). Dissolve in 20 ml of 10% sodium bicarbonate. Extract 5 × 20 ml of chloroform. Separate and evaporate the chloroform layer to dryness (gently with an air current). Pick up the residue with a minimal amount of ethanol and read in with a UV spectrophotometer with an ethanol reference blank.

Maximum density: 290, *282*, 276 nm

Minimum density: 287, 278 nm

Part of the chloroform extract is spotted onto a TLC plate. DMT, DET, and LSD standard are included.

Developing solvents: NH_4OH:EtOH (1:4).

Spray: 40% Formaldehyde:3N HCl:EtOH (10:10:20). Spots show under UV light → yellow → orange → green. Heat plate at 100°C for 5 minutes → yellow → brown.

Compound	Rf
DMT	0.60
DET	0.45
LSD	0.75

Test is sensitive to about 1 μg.

DMT may be extracted from parsley leaves by extracting with 3 × 30 ml of benzene. Pour each portion through a florisil column and collect. Evaporate gently on a steam bath with a current of air. Pick up residue in ethanol and read in UV with ethanol reference blank.

d. *p*-dimethyl amino benzaldehyde (1 gm in 25 ml ethanol + 25 ml HCl conc) :

LSD → blue

DMT → blue

DET → blue

psilocybin → blue

psilocin → blue

any ergot alkaloid → blue

Reference: Martin and Alexander: *JAOAC,* 51:159, 1968.

Treatment

Valium has shown some effectiveness in treating LSD patients. Bed rest, fluids; reassurance, sympathy, psychologic support, and general supportive measures.

MARIHUANA

Synonyms: Indian hemp; *Cannabis sativa L* is the genus with geographic varieties, i.e. Indica, Americana, Africana, and others; resinous material is known as hashish, kif, ganja, dagga, bhang, or charas. Tetrahydro cannabinol (THC) is the active ingredient of marihuana (Δ9 THC).

Uses: Hemp, fiber, homespun; behaves as a mild hallucinogen. No known or accepted medicinal use.

Properties: Both male and female plant contains THC; only female produces seed. Resin from flowering tops is the main source of THC. Marihuana is a crude preparation of the whole plant including the flowers, leaves, seeds, and stem and is about $1/_{10}$ less potent per weight than hashish.

MLD: Not known but has very low toxicity. Deaths are rare.

Remarks: Effects are produced rapidly, but vary with individuals and specie (geographic) differences; rarely fatal; psychologic compulsion, no apparent physiologic dependency.

Symptoms: Vary with individual differences of the plant variety and also biopsychologic differences between people.

Vertigo, dreamy state, apathy, fatigue, sluggish and confused medical and physical responses; increased pulse rate; euphoria, vivid dreams, dry mouth and throat, thirst and hunger, reddening of eyes, increased sensitivity, time slowed down, increased libido, depression or stimulation, lack of concentration, poor social judgment; after depression, delirium; acts of violence and other psychological and behavioral disturbance in unstable persons or particularly susceptible individuals.

Chronic users may have anxiety and guilt complex; irritability, insomnia, apathy, dullness; impairment of judgment, concentration, and memory.

Identification

Directly on plant material.

1. Suspend some small leaf fragments in several drops of 10% chloral hydrate on a microscope slide and examine under low power for characteristic cystolith-type hairs. These look like bear claws (elephant tusks). At the base of these claws is a wartlike cluster, which is a calcium carbonate deposit. Add a drop of 20% hydrochloric acid and note the effervescent evolving of carbon dioxide gas in tiny bubbles. Plant stems and rough underside of leaf (sometimes the resin) have these cystoliths. The odor, color, and form of cannabis is usually quite distinctive from materials commonly used as substitute or diluent.

2. Duquenois-Levine: Extract specimen with petroleum ether and filter into a small white porcelain dish. Evaporate down to dryness on a water bath. To the residue, add 2 ml of Duquenois reagent. Swirl and mix specimen residue and reagent, then add 2 ml of hydrochloric acid. Color changes from green to blue to dark violet. Allow to stand for about 5 minutes, add 2 ml of chloroform and shake. The violet color developed by marihuana will be extracted readily by the chloroform. Some coffee extracts may also give these positive results (Winek) but resulting colors are not identical to marihuana in shade or persistence; coffee furthermore has no cystoliths. Confirm by TLC.

Reagent: Duquenois: 0.4 gm vanillin, 5 drops acetaldehyde in 20 ml ethanol; prepare fresh.

3. Thin layer chromatography (TLC) for cannabinol: Preliminary extraction: Petroleum ether, evaporate, pick up in methanol.

Absorbant:
* 50 gm silica gel G in 100 ml 0.1N NaOH.
* 6 gm AgNO$_3$ in 38 ml H$_2$O; then suspend 18 gm silica G.

Developing solvents:
* 1,1,1-trichloroethane:methanol (9:1) (Phillips & Shupe)
* benzene (dry) (Turk et al)
* n-hexane:diethyl ether (4:1)

Spray:
* 3 gm vanillin in 100 ml absolute ethanol plus 0.5 ml sulfuric acid.
* Naphthanil diazo blue B, 0.15% aqueous.
* Duquenois followed by HCl fumes.

a. Phillips & Shupe: Grind hashish (conc) and extract with 2 ml of methanol; decant and spot on plate; develop to 10 cm; dry plate at 52°C → large reddish at Rf 75 → then three or four blue spots at 40, 50, 69, and 88. Immediately remove from hot plate and the blue (green) colors fade. Many plant extracts develop various colors but only the blue (green) suggests a cannabinol; old or weak hashish may show only two or three spots.

b. Turk et al.:
cannabidiol—0.16 → violet-red
tetrahydrocannabinol—0.36 → pink
cannabinol—0.63 → purple
synthetic (THC) —0.36 → pink
Sensitivity of 0.05 μg.

4. (Beckstead H.D. and French, W.N.: Food and Drug Directorate, Canada) :
Extract and purify with petroleum ether, methanol, or n-hexane. Evaporate at 40°C under reduced pressure; and then pick up oil in minimal amount of methanol or choloroform.

Flame ionization: 6 feet ($\frac{1}{8}$ or $\frac{1}{4}$ inch. Columns: 3% SE-30 on Chromsorb W-HMDS treated; 60/80 mesh *or* 3% QF—1 on Chromsorb W-HMDS treated; 60/80 mesh.

Column temperature, 180°C isothermal. Carrier gas flow: 30 ml/minute. Hydrogen gas flow: 20 ml/minute. Injection temperature: 275°C. Detector temperature: 275°C.

Treatment

Removal of drug exposure. Symptomatic treatment. There are no withdrawal symptoms (physiologic). It has been reported that phenothiazines (chlorpromazine) is contraindicated. Diazepam (Valium) may be useful for hyperexcitability.

References

Fochtman, M.S. and Winek, C.L.: *Clin Tox, 4:*287, 1971.
Halikas, J.A., Goodwin, D.W., and Guze, S.B.: *JAMA, 217:*692, 1971.
Kolansky, H. and Moore, W.T.: *JAMA, 216:*486, 1971.
Phillips, D.K. and Shupe, L.M.: Crime Laboratory, Div. of Police, Columbus, Ohio.
Tennant, F.S. and Groesbeck, C.J.: *Arch Gen Psych, 27:*133, 1972.
Turk, R.F., Dharir, H.I., and Forney, R.B.: *J Foren Sci, 14:*389, 1969.

MEPROBAMATE ($C_9H_{18}N_2O_4$)

Synonyms: Equanil, Miltown, 2-methyl-2-propyl-1,3-propanediol dicarbamate.

Uses: Tranquilizing drug, skeletal muscle-spasm relaxant.

Properties: White crystals, bitter taste. Insoluble in water; soluble in alcohol, acetone, or ether. Extracted from urine (best) or blood or tissue in neutral or alkaline solution with ether. Ten percent eliminated unmetabolized in urine. Acid-ether extracts only its metabolite.

MLD: Approximately 15 gm/70 kg person.

APPROXIMATE BLOOD LEVELS: Therapeutic, 1 mg/dl; lethal 15 mg/dl; half-life, 8 hours.

Symptoms: Sleepiness, stupor, coma, areflexia, lowered blood pressure, pinpoint pupils, respiratory and cardiovascular collapse.

Identification

Extract urine with alkaline (NH_4OH) ether; evaporate and purify.

1. Mp 104–106°C.
2. Acetic anhydride + 2 drops $H_2SO_4 \rightarrow$ diacetyl derivative (Mp, 125-130°C).
3. Add 3 ml of sulfuric acid; heat gently to develop orange-red color. Sensitive to 1 μg (McBay). Compare with blank at 450 nm.
4. 25 ml urine made alkaline with NH_4OH is extracted with 50 ml of ether or chloroform. Allow to settle, separate, filter to remove droplets of water, then gently evaporate to dryness. Reconstitute with about 1 ml of ether and transfer by spotting onto a small filter paper. Stain spot with 1 drop of furfural (make fresh; 10% in ethanol). Dry spot at room temperature, then expose spot to HCl fumes. Carbamates $\rightarrow$ blue-black.

    Run a negative blank and a positive control at the same time.
5. Extract 25 ml of urine as above. To the residue add 1 ml of sulfuric acid to reconstitute. Heat on a water bath at about 90–100°C for about 20 minutes. After cooling, bring volume up to 3 ml with water; the absorbance is read at 450 nm.
6. Make 25 ml of urine alkaline with 2 ml of NH_4OH and extract with 100 ml of ether. Separate, wash ether with water, and evaporate ether. Dissolve residue with 5 ml of 95% ethanol. Add a few drops of alcoholic KOH; then evaporate *nearly* to dryness. Carefully neutralize with glacial acetic acid dropwise. Add 1 ml of acetone and 1 drop of cobalt acetate (2% in glacial acetic) $\rightarrow$ blue color. Color fades on standing. (Test is sensitive to 0.1 mg.)
7. TLC: After a basic ether extraction from urine, the ether is carefully evaporated and the residue picked up with alcohol and spotted on a TLC plate. Use one of the following solvent developers:

    Developers:
    - cyclohexane:ethanol (85:15)
    - cyclohexane:acetone:diethylamine (20:20:10) or (30:10:10)
    - dioxane:benzene:NH_4OH (25%) (40:50:10)
    - $CHCl_3$:acetone (9:1). (Rf 0.24.)
    - $CHCl_3$:ether (85:15)

- CHCl$_3$:ethanol (9:1)
- CHCl$_3$:ethanol (8:2)
- CHCl$_3$:diethylamine (9:1)
- cyclohexane:acetone:diethylamine (7:2:1)
- CCl$_4$:acetone (7:3)

Detection spray. First examine under UV light; then spray lightly with one of the following:
- fluorescein 0.2% in ethanol; view under UV light.
- H$_2$SO$_4$
- Hydroquinone (0.2%) in H$_2$SO$_4$
- Furfural (10% in ethanol) then HCl fumes

8. Reagents must be reagent-grade, and solvents purified.

One (1) ml of serum, plus 2 drops of ammonium hydroxide, 2 drops of (sat.) potassium chloride, and 25 ml of mixed solvent are added and extracted for 5 minutes in a 40 ml glass-stoppered centrifuge cone. Centrifuge and carefully remove and transfer the organic layer, which is filtered into another centrifuge cone. Rinse filter through with 5 ml of mixed solvent. Combine and evaporate to dryness by immersing tube in an oil bath at about 80°C. Rinse tube down with several milliliters of acetone and continue heat until dry.

To dry residue, add 0.2 ml of AAA followed by 0.2 ml of DMB; mix. Add 1 ml of ATA and mix; tubes are stoppered and placed immediately in a 50°C water bath for exactly 10 minutes. Remove, quickly cool, and dilute with 1 ml of benzene. Measure color developed with Beckman DU spectrophotometer in 550 nm. Color is constant for about an hour. A blank (1 ml of distilled water) must be run concurrently and is used as reference blank. Standards of 0.5 to 10 μg of meprobamate are prepared. Absorbance of a 1 cm cell at 550 ml of 10 μg = 0.755.

Urine contains higher concentrations of meprobamate. Urea interferes; therefore, dilute 1:5 or 1:10 prior to extraction. Also, the residue on first evaporation of mixed solvent extract is heated for 15 minutes at 50°C with 1 ml of 0.2N hydrochloric acid. Then, again make it alkaline with ammonium hydroxide and potassium chloride and proceed as above.

Reagents:

- Mixed solvent: Equal volumes of carbon tetrachloride and chloroform.

- AAA (Acetic acid-acetone) : Three volumes acetone and 1 volume glacial acetic acid.

- ATA: (Antimony trichloride and acetic anhydride) Stock solution: Saturated $SbCl_3$ in chloroform (approximately 20% w/v). Warm mixture on hot plate to solution; cool; filter through Whatman 41 H filter paper.

  ATA: Four volumes of stock solution added with 1 volume of acetic anhydride. This is stable for 2 days when kept in refrigerator.

- DMB (*p*-dimethylaminobenzaldehyde) : 1% w/v solution in benzene. Stable for 1 month in refrigerator.

Reference: Hoffman and Ludwig: *J Am Pharm Assoc, 48:* 740, 1959.

9. GC Column 6 feet glass; 6 mm o.d., 2.5 i.d. packed with 2.5% S.E. 30 on 80/100 Chromosorb G (AW-DMCS). Temperature, 195°C; inlet, 225°C; detector 210°C. Carrier gas, nitrogen, at flow rate about 50 ml per minute. Detector hydrogen, flame ionization.

   Extract 3 ml of blood or urine or 1 gm of homogenized tissue with 50 ml of chloroform. Filter $CHCl_3$ layer through anhydrous Na_2SO_4 supported by glass wool plug in a small funnel. Evaporate to a low volume, then transfer to a 2 ml centrifuge tube and evaporate to dryness. Pick up residue in 25 μl of internal standard. Inject 1 μl in gas chromatograph. Evaporate the remainder of dissolved residue to dryness and pick up in 25 μl chloroform:ethanol (50:50). Now make another 1 μl injection.

   Retention times: glutethimide, 5.8 minutes; meprobomate, 4.5 minutes; internal standard, 1.8 minutes.

Reagent: Internal standard: 100 mg of *p*-dimethylaminobenzaldehyde in 50 ml of chloroform and 50 ml of ethanol.

Reference: Finkle: *J Forensic Sci, 12:*509, 1968

Treatment

Gastric lavage, cathartics.   Oxygen therapy and artificial
respiration as needed.   Symptomatic and supportive measures.
See Barbiturates for generalized support.

MENTHOL

Remarks: Produces phenollike muscular disturbances that
may last several weeks. Test for phenols in the urine; see under
Phenols. Treat as for phenols.

MERCURY (Hg)

Synonyms: Quicksilver, liquid elemental mercury.

Derivatives: Bichloride of mercury (corrosive sublimate) is
the most common (blue coffin-shaped tablet) ; mercuric cyanide
or nitrate; organic antiseptics (Merthiolate: sodium ethyl mercuri-
thiosalicylate) ; organic mercurial diuretics; bivalent organic
mercury (anti-mildew) ; methyl mercury (very toxic) .

Uses: Disinfectants, antiseptics, diuretics, antiluetics, amal-
gams (dentistry) , cathartics (calomel) , insecticides ($HgCl_2$ especially for ants) , fungicide (ethyl mercury phosphate—EMP;
methyl mercury dicyandiamide; phenylmercury acetate; Ceresan;
methyl or other alkyl) ; other bivalent mercury compounds are
also used to preserve seeds, grains, etc; also to process wood,
plastics, and papers. Mercury is also found in laboratory instruments (manometers, barometers, thermometers) , paints, pre-
serving specimens, fingerprint (police) , treating furs and "hatter's" felt hats, dry-cell batteries, long-life batteries (in pace-
makers) , mercury arc lamps, automatic thermostats, fabric soften-
ers, mercury solder, fulminate for detonators in bombs, silent
electric switches, preparation of chlorine gas, etc.

Properties: Metallic mercury is a liquid, silvery, heavy globule;
thirteen times heavier than water. It is insoluble but can vaporize
sufficiently at room temperature to reach toxic levels *in time*.
$HgCl_2$ is a very corrosive white crystalline salt, sparingly soluble
in water (1:13) . MW-200 (Hg) . Organic bivalent mercury compounds are very volatile and can be absorbed through all portals
including skin; these are strong skin irritants. Methyl mercury is

water soluble and can pass the brain barrier and is the most toxic.

MLD: Approximately 500 mg/70 kg person ($HgCl_2$) ; other inorganic mercury compounds vary in toxicity, depending upon their solubility. Organic mercury compounds vary widely, are more toxic than $HgCl_2$, but are less corrosive.

Remarks: Known since the first century. Metallic mercury was believed to be nontoxic until recently, when experience showed that high exposure to its vapors may produce CNS symptoms. Air saturated with metallic mercury vapors at 20°C contains about 15 mg per cu m and at 40°C saturated air contains 68 mg/cu m (Dreisbach).

Maximum allowable concentration (MAC) : 0.1 mg/cu m (inorganic) (*Arch Envirn Health, 19*:891, 1969) ; 0.01 mg/cu m (organic) ; 0.5 ppm (in food) (Food and Drug Administration).

Mercury is not a normal trace metal in man. Normal levels are below 1 μg in 100 ml of blood, and below 30 μg per liter of urine, depending upon environment, occupation, and food.

Exposure can be by all portals including metallic inorganic vapor inhalation; mercury is cumulative. If exposure is low grade and chronic, kidneys may eliminate mercury in urine for many months (after last exposure) without any apparent damage.

In the acute phase, symptoms are produced very rapidly (in minutes) and can be life-threatening. All forms of mercury can kill or injure.

Mercury combines with sulfhydril groups in the cell and depresses the enzymatic mechanism.

Symptoms

The action and symptoms of mercury on man depends upon the type and nature of compound. Inorganic versus organic mercury compounds produce different symptoms:

a. Inorganic mercury of the bichloride of mercury (oral) : acute; rapid onset; corrosion and severe kidney damage.

b. Metallic vapors of elemental mercury (lungs) ; least toxic, usually requires long exposure; CNS symptoms (least severe).

c. Bivalent organic mercury (antifungal) (oral or lungs) : intermediate toxicity; CNS symptoms (severe).

d. Methyl mercury (most toxic) (oral) : most toxic; very severe CNS symptoms.

ACUTE SYMPTOMS: *(HgCl₂) oral early phase:* Very quickly there is a sensation of burning in the mouth and throat, nausea, vomiting, edema of glottis, corrosion, eschars on mouth and lips (ash gray), severe gastrointestinal irritation, severe abdominal pain, profuse vomiting and diarrhea, extreme thirst and salivation, loss of fluids and electrolytes, rapid weak pulse, pallor, cold moist skin, slow breathing, shock; sudden death by corrosion, hemorrhage, or vascular circulatory collapse. If much vomiting occurs and fluids are replaced, the patient may survive for several days and even recover if the amount of absorbed mercury compound was less than 500 mg.

Delayed action (after several days) : Large bowel is more injured than stomach; ulcerative colitis in about 24 hours. Salivary glands swollen, stomatitis, excessive salivation, astringent metallic taste, foul breath, soft spongy gums, loose teeth, blue-black (Burtonian) gum line. Initially urine volume increases; later there is oliguria, anuria, uremia, acidosis, tubular nephrosis (kidneys badly damaged). Central necrosis of the liver is possible. Death is usually due to renal failure (uremia).

CHRONIC SYMPTOMS: Exposure by all portals of entry including the *breathing* of metallic mercury, which may vaporize sufficiently at room temperature to be dangerous. Brushing of mercury salts onto furs or hats is a well-known exposure (mad hatter). Usually low grade but continuous dangerous exposures may bring the following triad of symptoms and signs, which are mainly nervous (CNS) :

(1). Inflammation of the mouth, swollen salivary glands, soft bleeding spongy gums, loose teeth, blue-black (Burton) gum line, excessive salivation, stomatitis, numb tongue and fingers, metallic taste, foul breath. Blurred vision, sleeplessness, loss of speech, weight loss.

(2). Muscular tremors: Trembling when patient knows that he is observed, stops while sleeping or when not observed. "Hatter's shakes" (trembols). On accustomed job, he does fine; under pressure, observation, or in new job he will shake violently. As condition develops and gets worse, tremors spread to arms and legs. Severe pain; unable to dress self, difficulty in walking, staggering. Trembols, cannot write legibly, cannot even sign name (signature).

(3). Mental and nervous symptoms: Behavioral changes (Kussmahl called it erethism, Greek for irritant). Patient stammers; is shy, disturbed easily, anxious, restless. Has insomnia, loss of self-confidence, fear of losing job, loss of concentration and memory; loss of drive, energy or interest. Is forgetful; has melancholia; irritable. "Nervous timidity, loss of joy of living." With *low-grade exposure,* excretion of small amounts of urine may go for a long time without any apparent damage.

With an *increased* regular exposure, the above symptoms may be intensified.

Mental and nervous symptoms are rare in the single acute (inhalation exposure) phase of low levels.

Chronic mercury poisoning as a result of exposure to inorganic mercury vapors is difficult to diagnose because urine analysis is not reliable: Results may vary widely in the same patient from day to day. Results may vary on the same specimen when "shipped" to another laboratory. Normal levels have not been clearly established. For example: 300 μg/24 hours usually shows some symptoms, but symptoms are not always present even when higher levels are excreted (Ganley and Porteus) ; 100 μg/24 hours has been established as high "normal" by some reports, but this also may sometimes show symptoms; correlations of mercury levels of blood and urine in the same patient is poor; urine levels may show increase with increased exposure. There is very little evidence of correlation of blood and urinary mercury content with *clinical* signs of poisoning (Hamilton and Hardy).

Hg in urine 300 μg/l—probable poisoning with symptoms present. Hg in urine 100 μg/l—environment (exposure) requires correction. Hg in urine below 50 μg/l—probably safe (Dreisbach).

The severe damage to the kidneys that is characteristic of bichloride of mercury poisoning is not seen in industrial cases. Apparently the kidneys can eliminate mercury at low levels for a long period without damage (Hamilton and Hardy, 1975).

ORGANIC MERCURY COMPOUNDS: Organic mercury compounds of the diuretic type have been no great problem in the past. Recently this group have become of much interest because of massive accidental exposure to the fungicidal organic mercury type or methyl mercury. These cases are more of a repeated exposure to very toxic compounds producing severe neurologic symptoms. They do not respond to the usual inorganic mercury treatment with dimercaprol (BAL).

Bivalent organic mercury compounds that are usually used as fungicides (antimildew include ethyl mercury phosphate or phenylmercury acetate or cyanomethyl mercury guanidine, ethyl mercury *p*-toluene sulfonanilide, methyl mercury dicyandiamide, and other similar mercury derivatives.

Exposure is usually accidental by eating the mercury treated "bright pink" colored grain seed intended for planting. Poisonings have occurred by eating hogs that were fed with these seeds, and by eating bread accidently made with these grain seeds.

Symptoms resemble the "blind staggers." Symptoms may be delayed days, weeks, or several months (continuous eating of small amounts of mercury contaminated food).

Symptoms then start to develop such as fatigue, headache, irritability, delirium, tremors; numbness of mouth, tongue, and limbs; blurred vision; loss of coordination, weight, concentration, and memory. Symptoms may get worse and produce severe brain damage with deafness, blindness, inability to walk or talk; mental retardation; loss of control of bodily functions, paralysis of limbs (like a paraplegic), mental retardation, even coma. Children born during an exposure may exhibit (delayed) similar symptoms and may also show birth defects.

Absorbed though all portals including skin and inhalation of dusts; highly volatile; strong skin irritant; and highly toxic in any form. However, when exposure is small, symptoms may be mild and transient.

BAL (dimercaprol) may be contra-indicated and dangerous; it also may help to transport mercury to the brain. *N*-acetylated DL penicillamine have been reported of some benefit.

METHYL MERCURY (MOST TOXIC): Insoluble metallic mercury

refuse, when dumped into rivers or lakes for disposal, sinks and penetrates the mud beds where microorganisms (anaerobic) convert it (in time) to soluble methyl mercury. This in turn is easily assimilated by other microorganisms, which in turn enters the food cycle of the sea until accumulated in large amounts in large fish including the tuna or swordfish and other sea predators. This may now be toxic when eaten in large or in continuous small amounts by man.

Methyl mercury very easily crosses the brain barrier and is the *most* toxic known form of mercury. Symptoms are mostly CNS-related and are even more severe than described above for organic mercury compounds.

Identification

For the acute phase of large amounts of mercury salts.
1. Reinsch modification: Place a small strip of clean copper sheet (about 5 × 5 mm) in 20 ml of urine, gastric contents, vomitus, or ground homogenate of kidney or liver. Add 5 ml of hydrochloric acid and gently heat in a suitable size Erlenmeyer flask for about 1 hour. Heat gently and try to maintain volume with a watch glass on top. If mercury is present (sensitivity about 0.030 mg), the copper strip would be silver-coated. This silver coating can be estimated fairly well in ranges 0.05, 0.10, 0.15, 0.25 mg per 20 ml by visual inspection.

The silvery deposit can be confirmed specifically by placing the copper and deposit on a piece of filter paper and overlaying several drops of a suspension of cuprous iodide. Cover with a watch glass; within 1 to 2 hours, a distinct salmon pink indicates mercury (HgI_2) (sensitive to about 0.020 mg/20ml).

The intensity and distribution of this pink color are proportional to the quantity of mercury on the copper strip.

Reagent, Cuprous iodide: Dissolve 5 gm $CuSO_4$ and 3 gm $FeSO_4$ in 10 ml of water. Seven (7) gm of KI in 50 ml of water is then slowly added while stirring. Allow to stand and settle and then decant. Wash the settled precipitate (Cu_2I_2) with small amounts of water and again carefully decant. Repeat until the washing is relatively free of excess iodine (yellow washings). The light tan Cu_2I_2 is then transferred with minimal water (to make a suspension) to a small brown bottle with a tight stopper. This is used in the form of drops or emulsion.

2. S-diphenylcarbazone (EK #4459) : Ten (10) ml of filtered stomach contents, vomitus, or residue plus 1 ml of reagent produces an intense blue color with even traces of mercury (presumptive). Sensitive to 1 mcg. Blue color due to Hg^{++} dissolves in benzene; color due to Hg^+ does not dissolve.

Reagent: S-diphenylcarbazone: 100 mg dissolved in 100 ml of 95% ethanol.

3. Natelson (modified for trace amounts) :
To 10 ml of urine (if only a trace of mercury is suspected, use 50 ml of urine) in 300 ml round-bottom flask, while cooling under tap water, add 1 ml of sulfuric acid. Mix and add 2 ml of nitric acid. Connect with water condensor or watch glass cover and heat gently to barely a simmer for about 5 minutes. Remove from heat and add 5 ml of 5% potassium permanganate a little at a time to minimize foaming. MnO_2 will start to precipitate out. When all is added, heat gently again for about 10 minutes at barely simmering. Swirl gently from time to time.

Allow to cool to room temperature; then add 3 ml of hydroxylamine reagent in small portions to dissolve the MnO_2 and to remove excess oxidizing agents. Now test for absence of oxidizing agents with KI starch paper (colorless). Transfer to a small Pyrex separatory funnel and shake with 5 ml of carbon tetrachloride to remove fats. Continue the extraction with dithizone *without delay*. First make certain that pH is below 2 (1–2). Adjust if necessary with dilute NH_4OH or H_2SO_4 (as required) using pH test paper.

Mercury dithizonate is photosensitive; carry out the following titration and reading procedure as rapidly as possible away from direct light.

Add 5 ml of dithizone *dilute* solution (1:2) and shake extract vigorously; yellow to peach-orange indicates mercury. Settle, separate, and collect the bottom dithizone extracts. Add an additional 5 ml of dithizone and again shake extract vigorously. Allow to settle, combine, and collect extracts. Repeat with another 5 ml if necessary until all the mercury is extracted as indicated by a final persistent green dithizone. Calculate how much dithizone was required to reach this point. All the combined dithizone extracts are now shaken with 25 ml of 9N NH_4OH to remove excess dithizone.

Quickly separate and filter the dithizone through filter paper to remove droplets of water. Read rapidly; color may fade.

Read at 490 nm in a spectrophotometer, with a dithizone reference blank, even though it appears to be negative.

To rule out possible bismuth interference, add 50 mg of potassium cyanide to the residual 9N NH_4OH and return a sample of the mercury dithizone and shake. The color will instantly disappear. If bismuth is present, the orange color will persist.

Using 10 ml of urine, and if only one 5 ml of dithizone is required, with a Beckman DK-2A recording spectrophotometer and a 10 mm light path, the following optical density is obtained (F. Matos) with added mercury standards.

Hg	*OD (watch glass cover)*	*OD (water condensor)*
2 μg	—	0.0915
4 μg	0.130	0.194
6	—	0.260
8	0.270	0.362
12	0.390	—

Reagents:

• Mercury standards: Stock standard 0.1354 gm $HgCl_2$ (or 0.1668 gm Hg $(NO_3)_2 . \frac{1}{2} H_2O$) is diluted to 100 ml with 0.25 N HCl producing 1 mg/ml. Working standard: Dilute stock standard 1:100 which will produce 10 μg/ml. Store all standards in plastic coated containers.

• Hydroxylamine · HCl: 50 gm in 50 ml of water. Purify with dithizone.

• Dithizone: 25 mg per liter of redistilled chloroform. Dilute 1:2 before use with redistilled $CHCl_3$.

• Ammonium hydroxide (9N) : 100 ml NH₄OH + 60 ml of water. All distilled water is redistilled through Pyrex glass apparatus. Copper is the most common interference (especially in HNO₃). Fisher reagents have been low in copper.

4. Atomic absorption (cold, flameless, for trace amounts) :

Atomic absorption spectrophotometer: Perkin Elmer Model 403, or equivalent, equipped with Hg hollow cathode lamp and gas flow-thru cell, 25 mm i.d. by 11.5 cm long with quartz windows cemented in place. Instrument setting: left front panel to wavelength 253.7 nm; slit setting at 4; lamp current at 6 ma, range UV. Setting right panel: absorbance, repeat, 10 average.

Diaphragm pump: Neptune Dyna-Pump or equivalent. Coat diaphragm and internal parts of the pump with acrylic-type plastic spray (the first time before using it).

Gas Inlet Adapter: Outfitted with Vacutainer stopper and ⅙ inch i.d. Teflon tubing.

Reaction vessel: 100 × 16 mm Pyrex digestion tube or (127 × 16 mm B-D Vacutainer test tube may be used).

Make all connections with tygon tubing so that the passage of air is in the following order: from the pump to the gas inlet adaptor and through the reaction vessel to the dessicant tube, and then to the cell; from the cell to a three-way stop-cock that directs the air either to the pump again (for absorbance reading, closed system) or to the atmosphere (extractor) toward the flusing system (open system).

Sample Preparation: Pipet duplicate 1 ml of fresh urine samples into 100 × 16 mm Pyrex digestion tubes. If the urine contains much precipitate, mix it thoroughly, pipet 10 ml of the sample into a Pyrex flask and carry out the digestion as described below with ten times the amount used for a 1 ml sample. After digestion use 3 ml of solution for the mercury determination.

Place the digestion tubes in a wire stand and cool them in a vessel containing water. To each tube add 1.5 ml of the

---

*Fresh urine is submitted in plastic containers because Hg may adhere to wall of glass containers.

digestion solution. Shake cautiously and leave the tubes loosely stoppered overnight at room temperature (Parafilm may be used to cover the tubes). After standing, reduce the excess of permanganate by adding hydroxylamine hydrochloride dropwise until solution is clear (2 or 3 drops are enough).

Analysis: Add 10 drops of the stannous chloride solution and immediately connect the tube to the flowing system.

Calculations: Prepare a calibration curve using the maximum absorbance values obtained for a range of Hg standard solutions and the reagent blank (absorbance obtained for the reagent blank may be subtracted from that of the standards and samples). Determine the content of mercury in the samples from this curve.

Reagents:

- Digestion Solution: Mix 150 ml of potassium permanganate solution (6% w/v in deionized water) with 20 ml concentrated H_2SO_4 immediately before use.
- Hydroxylamine hydrochloride ($NH_2OH \cdot HCl$): 50 gm in 100 ml deionized water.
- Stannous chloride ($SnCl_2$): 20 gm anhydrous $SnCl_2$ in 1 liter deionized water containing 40 ml concentrated H_2SO_4.
- Hg Stock Standard Solution (100 μg Hg/ml): Dissolve 0.1354 gm $HgCl_2$ in 100 ml 1N H_2SO_4 (dilute 27.7 ml concentrated H_2SO_4 to 1 liter with deionized water). Use plastic bottles.
- Hg standards: Dilute the stock standard solution with 1N H_2SO_4 to prepare a 10 μg Hg/ml standard solution. From this, prepare standards with a range of 0.005 to 0.05 μg Hg/ml in deionized water. Use standards of higher concentration if the range of the samples to be analyzed is higher. The dilute standards should be analyzed immediately. Use plastic bottles.

References

G. Lindstedt and I. Skare: Analytical methods for atomic absorption spectrophotometry BC-10. *Analyst, 96:*223, 1971.

Atomic Absorption Newsletter, 13(1): Jan. 1974; Perkin-Elmer Corp.

Interpretation: Jacobs analyzed 1,107 normal urines from non-exposed healthy persons in fifteen different countries. These "apparent" normal urines ranged from a high of 221 μg Hg/liter; 95 percent of all tests were below 20 μg Hg/liter of urine. There can be a great fluctuation from day to day; in some cases, there were levels as high as 1000 μg Hg/liter with no apparent symptoms. It was also noted that some patients showing 200 μg Hg/liter did show typical symptoms of mercury poisoning.

Urine screening may be useful to indicate magnitude of exposure.

Perhaps 0.1 mg/cu m air $\rightarrow$ 100–300 μg Hg/liter. When exposure is cut by one-half $\rightarrow$ urinary mercury drops one-half.

Mercury is cumulative and may continue to be eliminated in the urine up to 6 months or more after the last chronic exposure.

Normal levels in humans should be near zero, but may be up to 2μg in 100 ml of blood or 30 μg/liter of urine.

Treatment

Vomiting helps to remove some of the (oral) poison quickly; use syrup of ipecac to stimulate vomiting. Gastric lavage (oral) (if early) with milk, water, or water and sodium formaldehyde sulfoxalate. Egg white, milk, and cream or albumin are good demulcents. Morphine for pain. Atropine may help to control excessive salivation; alkaline fluids. $NaHCO_3$ to correct acidosis. Maintain body heat, electrolytes, and fluid balance. Be alert for shock and early signs of kidney involvement. Supportive.

BAL is a specific antidote for the oral acute phase (of $HgCl_2$). Intramuscular doses slightly higher than for arsenic. Evaluate patient. Analyze urine for mercury levels and, if levels are still high, consider giving another series. Follow insert directions wrapped with antidote.

BAL has an objectionable odor and is painful on injection; it may also give side reactions. Antihistamines prior to BAL may help minimize side reactions.

N-acetyl-DL-penicillamine has also been used in mercury poisoning with good results; can also be given orally.

Hemodialysis is excellent for renal insufficiency, even though it may be ineffective in removing any appreciable amounts of mercury. Chelation prior to dialysis improves elimination rate.

Prognosis is poor if there is oliguria or anuria.

Sometimes there is a hypersensitivity (rare) to organic mercurial diuretics leading to renal failure.

BAL is very useful during the acute phase ($HgCl_2$) but is contraindicated when patient is having renal failure because it may aggravate the renal damage. BAL is also of doubtful use (perhaps even dangerous) for the bivalent *organic* mercury compounds.

References

Bakir, F., Damluji, S.E., Amin-Zake, L., Murtadha, M., Khalidi, A., Al-Rawi, N.Y., Tikriti, S., Dhahir, H.I., Clarkson, T.W., Smith, J.C., Doherty, R.A.: Methyl mercury poisoning in Iraq. *Science, 181*:230, 1973.

Christensen, H.: personal communications.

Clarkson, T.W.: personal communications: Clarkson, T.W.: In G. Norborg (Ed.): *Dose Response Relationship with Heavy Metals.* Amsterdam. Elsevier.

Curley, A., Sedlak, V.A., Girling, E.F., Hauk, R.E., Barthel, W.F., Pierce, P.E., and Likosky, W.H.: Organic mercury identified as the cause of poisoning in humans and hogs. *Science, 172*:65, 1971.

Dreisbach, R.: *Handbook of Poisonings: Diagnosis and Treatment,* 7th ed. Los Altos, Cal, Lange Medical Publ, 1971.

Faulkner, W.R., King, J.W., and Damm, H.C.: *Handbook of Clinical Laboratory Data,* 2nd ed. Cleveland, Chem Rubber Co.

Hamilton, A. and Hardy, H.: *Industrial Toxicology.* Action, Mass, Publishing Science Group Inc. (Harvard), 1974.

Jacobs, M.B., Ladd, A.C., and Goldwater, L.J.: Absorption and excretion of mercury in man: VI significance of mercury in urine. *Arch Envirn Health, 9*:454, 1964.

NIOSH (National Institute), USPHS: *Criteria for a Recommended Standard—Occupational Exposure to Inorganic Mercury.* Washington, D.C., US Govt Print Office, 1973.

Threshold limit values of air-borne contaminants (1968), adapted at the 30th annual meeting of the Am Conf of Govt Ind Hygienists, St. Louis, May 13, 1968.

Various world experts: Maximum allowable concentration of mercury compounds. *Arch Envirn Health, 19*:891, 1969.

METALDEHYDE

Remarks: Polymer of acetaldehyde.

Symptoms: May be delayed an hour or more. Gastrointestinal irritation, disorientation, loss of memory, salivation, fever, somnolence, irritability, convulsions, coma, respiratory difficulty, possible kidney and liver involvement if recovery is delayed.

Treatment

Gastric lavage with charcoal; demulcents such as aluminum gels; Valium or short-acting barbiturates for excitement or convulsions. Convulsions may persist 24 to 48 hours, keep sedated. Symptomatic and supportive.

METHADONE ($C_{21}H_{27}NO$)

Synonyms: Amidone, Dolophine; Miadone; Hoechst 10820; Adanon; Diaminon; Physeptone; Polamidon, Butalgin.

Uses: Analgesic; treatment for morphine and heroin addiction.

Properties: Basic synthetic alkaloid. Bitter taste. Soluble in ethanol, chloroform, benzene, acetone, or petroleum ether. Less toxic than morphine but is also addicting.

MLD: Approximately 100 mg/70 kg person. Addicts can tolerate five times as much.

APPROXIMATE BLOOD LEVELS: Therapeutic, 0.05 mg/dl; lethal, 0.5 mg/dl.

Symptoms: Generally similar to morphine. Miosis, nausea, vomiting, collapse, coma, respiratory difficulties, death.

Identification

1. Make 100 ml of urine plus 50 ml of water alkaline, with calcium hydroxide; steam distill into a receiver containing 5 ml of 1% hydrochloric acid. Collect about 100 ml of distillate. Transfer to a separatory funnel and make alkaline with NH_4OH. Extract with 50 ml of chloroform and again with 25 ml of chloroform. Combine extracts, add 3 drops of concentrated hydrochloric acid and very carefully evaporate on a water bath. Pick up with 3 ml of 0.1N hydrochloric acid and read in UV spectrophotometer:
   Maximum density, *292*, 265, <u>259</u> 251 nm $E^{1\%}_{1cm}$ 19; minimum density, *274,* 262, 257, 250 nm.

2. Make 50 ml of urine alkaline with NH_4OH; directly extract with chloroform (2 times 50 ml). Alkaloidal precipitants all yield crystals (see Alkaloids).

3. Alkaloidal color tests (see Alkaloids).
4. TLC; GLC: See Section I.
5. Dissolve residue in minimal water; add 3 drops of reagent (1 gm of cobalt acetate and 1.5 gm KSCN in 90 ml of water and 10 ml of glacial acetic acid). Shake. Blue precipitate indicates methadone.

Treatment

Withdrawal of drug. Artificial respiration and oxygen therapy if needed. Activated charcoal; gastric lavage with (1:10,000) potassium permanganate. Symptomatic and supportive measures similar to morphine.

SPECIFIC TREATMENT: Naloxon (Narcan), follow the package insert instructions. It is a specific narcotic antagonist to morphine and its derivatives, as well as to Demerol and methadone. In these cases, it will rapidly relieve respiratory depression.

METHAQUALONE

Synonyms: 2-methyl-3-*o*-tolyl-4(3H)-quinazolinone; Quaalude, Optimil; Sopor, Parest, Somnafac; and Biphetamine T in USA. Melsedin, Mandrax in England. Revonal; Tuazolone; Sedanoct in Europe.

PREPARED DOSE: 40–400 mg.

Properties: Nonbarbiturate; sedative; produces high tolerance and dependency (physiologic and psychologic); cross tolerance with short-acting barbiturates and withdrawal symptoms are similar.

MLD: Approximately 8 gm/70 kg person.

APPROXIMATE BLOOD LEVELS: Therapeutic, 0.3 mg%; toxic, 2 mg%; lethal, 3 mg%. Half-life, about 3 hours.

Symptoms: Nausea, vomiting, delirium, restlessness, also behaves as a CNS sedative—hypnotic type, euphoria, ataxia; paresthesia of legs, arms, fingers, lips, and tongue. Mild poisoning is indistinguishable from overdose with other CNS depressants. There may also be hallucinations and agitation. Severe poisoning will produce unconsciousness. Neurologic signs may include positive Babinski sign, myolonia, tonic-clonic spasms and convulsions. Cardiovascular complications may include tachycardia, acute cardiac failure, and increased vascular permeability.

Identification

Separate by neutral ether or chloroform extraction (ether is best for urine); acid (6N HCl) hydrolysis of urine for about 5 minutes on a boiling steam bath increases recovery.

1. Five (5) ml blood is extracted vigorously with 35 ml of $CHCl_3$; separate, wash, filter, and then evaporate to dryness. Pick up with 5 ml of ethanol and read in UV spectrophotometer. Maximum density, 225, 265, 305, 316 nm; at 265, $E_{1cm}^{1\%}$ 314 (Bogan). (Does not form salt.)

2. TLC (Silica gel G):
   Solvent: Chloroform:methanol (3:1)
   Spray: Iodoplatinate
   Rf: 0.78

3. TLC: other developing solvents (Heyndrickx and Leenheer)
   • $CHCl_3$:acetone (9:1)
   • $CHCl_3$:acetone:NH_4OH (50:50:1)

4. GLC: $CHCl_3$ extract; retention time, 2.4 minutes for 5% SE on Chromosorb W at 200°. Flow rate, 30 ml/minute, nitrogen; 30 ml/minute, hydrogen. See Section I.

5. Positive reactions with Wagner's Mayer's, and picric acid.

Treatment

Support all vital signs, similarly as for barbiturates overdose; forced diuresis is ineffective and also is contraindicated because of danger of congestive heart failure. Guard against convulsions; gastric lavage to minimize absorption only when dangers of convulsions are removed. In conscious patients activated charcoal followed by careful gastric lavage; sodium sulfate catharsis to hasten elimination. General treatment as for barbiturate. Guard against pneumonia. Supportive.

METHYL ALCOHOL (CH_3OH)

Synonyms: Carbinol; methanol; wood alcohol; wood spirits; wood naphtha; Columbian spirits; Colonial spirits; Solox; Eagle spirits; Freezone.

Uses: To make formaldehyde; auto antifreeze (temporary-type) ; to denature alcohol; degreaser, organic solvent, organic dyes, fuel, paints, varnishes, enamels, paint remover, windshield washer, embalming fluid, rubber accelerants, canned heat (Sterno).

Properties: Colorless, clear, liquid, pleasant odor, bp 64°C, flammable, miscible with water.

MLD: About 75 ml/70 kg person; may vary widely (tolerance).

Remarks: Can be absorbed thru all portals; shellacking (painting) in an enclosed area (submarine) , inhalation, also skin absorption; poisoning is more serious when ingested. Although it is *acutely* less toxic as an *initial* CNS *depressant* than is ethanol, it is in fact far more toxic to man because of its metabolites, formaldehyde and formic acid (methanol $\xrightarrow{\text{ADH}}$ formaldehyde $\xrightarrow{\text{oxidase}}$ formic acid) , which cannot slip into the Kreb cycle as do ethanol metabolites. Can persist for many days. Elimination may take five to ten times longer than ethanol. Death may be within 5 hours (rapid) if massive quantities are taken (profound CNS depression) ; more usually it is the delayed *severe metabolic acidosis* (formic acid depletes the alkaline reserve, several days later) .

Symptoms

ACUTE: *Mild exposure* from inhalation or ingestion of small amounts; headache, nausea, vomiting, irritation to all membranes, roaring and ringing in the ears, tiredness, insomnia, vertigo, diplopia.

Severe exposure causes all above but more profound, abdominal pains, colic, GI irritation, diarrhea, constipation, lethargy, profound CNS depression, sleepiness, stupor, dizziness, dilated pupils, diplopia, cerebral edema, pulmonary edema, delirium, coma, profound delayed metabolic acidosis due to metabolite formic acid. Edema of the optic nerve and entire retina with temporary blindness, which can develop into permanent blindness if not promptly corrected. Imbalance of electrolytes with its serious complications; CNS degenerative changes, liver and kidney involvement.

CHRONIC: Prolonged chronic environmental exposure may produce pulmonary edema, diplopia; possible involvement of CNS, liver, and kidney.

Identification

Separated by steam distillation.

1. In blood, urine, or steam distillate: To 2 ml of blood, to which an anticoagulant has been added (except EDTA or heparin), add 4 ml of 20% trichloroacetic acid; shake to precipitate proteins. Filter and collect filtrate.

   To 0.1 ml of filtrate in a test tube, add 2 drops of potassium permanganate reagent. Wait exactly 2 minutes and decolorize excess potassium permanganate with a pinch (size of a pinhead) of sodium bisulfite. Add a pinch (size of a match head) of chromotropic acid (EK #P 1613), and mix into a solution by swirling. Then carefully underlay with 3 ml of sulfuric acid by allowing it to run down the inclined side of the test tube. A purple ring at the interface is positive for methyl alcohol; mix and diffuse the purple color. Allow to stand for 20 minutes to fully develop color and then read in a spectrophotometer at 570 nm. With sulfuric acid as the reference blank and a 1 cm light path, the following calibration curve may be approximated. Each should prepare his own calibration curves with sulfuric acid as reference blank and a reagent control blank.

Methyl alcohol (gm%)	Transmission
0.025	55% T
0.050	36%
0.075	25%
0.100	17%

Reagent: Potassium Permanganate: 3 gm $KMnO_4$ + 15 ml H_3PO_4 + 85 ml H_2O.

NOTES ON THE METHOD

This test is very sensitive (when water is omitted from test) and will even pick up trace amounts of methyl alcohol in the blood (0.01 gm%). Low levels may not be clinically significant; however, trace amounts should be reanalyzed using a larger specimen (1 ml of filtrate).

Always parallel a reagent blank at the time of testing the unknown. Occasionally, the blank will give a strong positive test, especially when the test is performed in a laboratory where formalin is used. An open bottle of sulfuric acid has a great affinity for traces of formalin in the atmosphere.

Formalin, heparin, methenamine, and EDTA also give a positive test. Heparin or EDTA therefore cannot be used as the anticoagulant for blood. Autopsy tissue also can become contaminated in the autopsy room. Maximum precaution must be taken.

To prove that the reaction is due to formalin, omit the (oxidation) potassium permanganate step and the test will still be positive, whereas methanol requires this (2 minute) $KMnO_4$ oxidation to be positive (for formaldehyde).

Large amounts of ethyl alcohol may sometimes give a brown interface ring, but this is distinctly different from the deep purple of methyl alcohol. This difference becomes even more apparent when the color is diffused by swirling.

The presence of any amount of methyl alcohol above 0.05 percent must be further studied and correlated with signs, symptoms, and history. It is imperative to perform the determination for carbon dioxide combining power of blood. It is the degree of acidosis that is of primary consideration in treatment.

Since methyl alcohol is metabolized and eliminated slowly, it may be found in the blood as long as 6 days later. Traces may also be found when large amounts of wine have been consumed.

2. Into 10 ml of distillate, plunge a red-hot copper spiral* eight times. (Gettler)

   a. To 5 ml of this oxidized solution, add 10 drops of 0.5% (fresh) phenylhydrazine hydrochloride, then 2 drops of 0.5% sodium nitroprusside, and then 10 drops of 20% sodium

---

*Twist a thick copper wire around a pencil up to about 6 spaces. Use cork or rubber stopper to insulate for handling.

hydroxide. Blue → green → yellow → red-violet color indicates presence of formaldehyde (oxidized methyl alcohol).

b. To 5 ml of this oxidized solution, add 2 ml of sulfuric acid and 5 ml of fuchsine solution. A violet color is developed in a couple of minutes. This color can be quantitated.

Reagent: Fuchsine solution: 0.2 gm of basic fuchsine is added to 150 ml of boiling water. Dissolve and then cool with running water. Two (2) gm of sodium bisulfite (meta) in 20 ml of water is added and mixed. Then add 2 ml of hydrochloric acid and 60 ml of water. Mix and store in a glass-stoppered dark bottle. This solution should be stored in a refrigerator and will be stable for several months. (Gettler)

3. Microdiffusion as for Ethanol.
4. Gas liquid chromatography: See Section I.

Treatment

Immediate gastric lavage with sodium bicarbonate, or emetics for quick evacuation, if patient is not comatose. Cathartics such as sodium sulfate (25 gm). Keep patient warm and quiet. Protect eyes from strong light. Maintain electrolyte and water balance. Acidosis is to be prevented or corrected if treatment is to be successful. The carbon dioxide combining power and electrolytes should be determined initially and then repeated at intervals to evaluate response to treatment.

Sodium bicarbonate intravenously, slowly until acidosis is corrected. Treatment with bicarbonate should be continued for several days, with careful evaluation.

Hemodialysis if available would materially hasten elimination of both methyl alcohol and formic acid (in severe cases).

Ethyl alcohol 50% orally (5-20 ml) every 2 to 4 hours may help slow down conversion of methyl alcohol to the more toxic formic acid by competing for the same metabolic enzymes.

Supportive measures to maintain vital signs; glucose and fluids; vitamin B_1 for visual disturbances; guard against secondary infections if patient is comatose. Symptomatic and supportive measures.

Massive ingestion can bring blood levels up to as much as 1,000 mg/dl within several hours. In these cases, treatment is directed to maintain all vital signs and counteract the powerful CNS depression (supportive and symptomatically) ; death can be rapid. Death several days later is due to the formic acid (acidosis); methanol levels are then low in the blood.

METHYL BROMIDE

Uses: Refrigerant, insecticide, fumigant.

Symptoms: Nausea, vomiting, gastric pain, dizziness, headache, anorexia, disturbed vision, confusion, mania, tremors, convulsions, pulmonary edema, acidosis, collapse, coma broncho-pneumonia, pulmonary lesions, kidney damage. These symptoms seem to subside in 2 weeks if patient survives.

Identification

1. Test for traces of methyl alcohol and bromides in blood or urine.
2. Positive for pyridine test; see under Chloral Hydrate.

Treatment

Valium or short-acting barbiturates for convulsions; sodium bicarbonate for acidosis. Guard against pulmonary edema, renal shutdown, secondary infection. Acute crisis for at least 48 hours. Symptomatic and supportive measures.

METHYL SALICYLATE ($C_8H_8O_3$)

Synonyms: Oil of wintergreen; betula; sweet birch.

Uses: Counterirritant, flavoring agent, antirheumatic, antipyretic, liniment (Ben Gay) .

Properties: Insoluble in water; soluble in chloroform, ether, or alcohol.

MLD: Approximately 10 ml/70 kg person.

Remarks: Corrosive and irritant, usually dispensed as a weak solution in alcohol. Absorbed through all portals.

Symptoms: Similar to aspirin plus severe gastrointestinal irritation, nausea, vomiting, aromatic vomitus (possibly blood) , abdominal cramps, bloody diarrhea, alkalosis followed by acidosis, hyperpyrexia, increased thirst, profuse sweating, dehydration. Urine colored (dark brown), burning sensation in mouth and throat, skin rash, initial hypernea followed by respiratory failure, stupor, tonic and clonic convulsions, coma, death.

Identification

1. Oily, odorous, colorless liquid. Smells like wintergreen.
2. Bp 220–224° C.
3. Stomach contents, vomitus, or urine (5 ml) is directly tested for salicylates with 1 ml of 10% ferric chloride → violet.
4. UV spectrophotometry: See Section I.
5. See tests described under Acetylsalicylic Acid, and methanol.

Treatment

Gastric lavage with warm water. Fluids to maintain urinary output. Do not use fats or oils. Sodium bicarbonate to combat acidosis and sodium loss.

Artificial respiration and oxygen as needed. Keep patient warm and quiet; maintain body heat, fluids, and electrolyte balance. Demulcents to ease pain and irritation (avoid oils). Supportive and symptomatic treatment as for aspirin; see under Acetylsalicylic Acid. Supportive against corrosion and shock.

METOL

Symptoms: Dermatitis, eczema; ulcers may develop that are slow healing; cyanosis; dark urine.

Treatment: Symptomatic. Treat as for Aniline.

METRAZOL ($C_6H_{10}N_4$)

Synonyms: Cardiazol; pentamethylenetetrazol; Leptazol.

Uses: Stimulation, analeptic.

Properties: Neutral crystalline. Soluble in water MP, 58°C. Bitter taste.

MLD: Approximately 2 gm (IV) or 10 gm (oral) for a 70 kg person.

Remarks: Central nervous system stimulant, alkaloidal.

Symptoms: Preconvulsive anxiety, pallor, tonic convulsions (epileptiform), unconsciousness. Blood pressure rises during convulsion. After convulsion, patient is confused and drowsy with mild convulsions following this period of restoration.

Identification

Separated by alkaline-chloroform extraction. Agent cannot be detected in urine. (It is rapidly detoxified by liver.)

1. To the residue, add:
    a. a few drops of hydrochloric acid (10%) plus 1 ml of cadmium chloride (20%) → agitate gently → white crystalline precipitate
    b. a few drops of sulfuric acid (10%) plus a few drops of potassium dichromate (10%) plus a few drops of hydrogen peroxide (3%) → violet-blue color, which quickly fades
    c. a few drops of sulfuric acid (10%) plus 1 ml of potassium ferricyanide (10%) → let stand overnight → transparent crystals
    d. a few drops of sulfuric acid (10%) plus 1 ml of cupric chloride (1% in 10% hydrochloric acid) → white precipitate → crystalline on standing
2. Metrazole is ammonia-chloroform soluble and on spontaneous evaporation (do not use heat) forms typical crystals.
3. Refer to Alkaloids.

Treatment

Gastric lavage with potassium permanganate (1:10,000). Valium or short-acting barbiturates for convulsions. Avoid morphine.

Protect patient during convulsions to prevent injury. Keep patient quiet and warm. Artificial respiration and oxygen therapy. Symptomatic and supportive measures.

MORPHINE ($C_{17}H_{19}NO_3$)

Homologues: Dried resinous fluid (opium) of the unripe poppy seed may contain approximately 10% morphine and 0.5% codeine. Laudanum and Brown's mixture are elixers of crude opium. Heroin (diacetylmorphine); hydromorphone hydrochloride (Dilaudid); oxymorphone hydrochloride (Numorphan);

Metopan (methyl dilaudid) ; codeine (methylmorphine) .

Uses: Analgesia, sedation, hypnotic, and narcosis.

Properties: Basic, alkaloid, white crystalline, bitter taste, mp 254°C. Slightly soluble in ethanol or chloroform:isopropanol (3:1) , at buffered pH 8.5–9.5.

MLD: Morphine approximately 200 mg/70 kg person; codeine is about one-fourth as toxic; heroin is about four times more toxic.

BLOOD LEVELS: Therapeutic, 0.01 mg%; lethal, 0.1 mg% (nonaddict) ; half-life, 4 hours.

Remarks: Death may occur within 2 hours but more often within 8 hours; occasionally is delayed 24 hours. If patient survives 48 hours, prognosis is good.

Symptoms:

ACUTE: Pinpoint pupils, powerful CNS depressant, decreased mental concentration, euphoria, elevated pain threshold, stimula-

TABLE XXX
APPROXIMATE COMPARISON

	Meperidine	*Morphine*	*Methadone*
Synonyms	Demerol; Pethidine; isonipercaine	......	Adanon; Amidone; Dolophine
Source	synthetic	natural	synthetic
Pupils	normal or dilated	pin-point	pin-point (moderate)
Euphoria	moderate	marked	rare (oral)
Dose (therap)	50–100 mg	5–15 mg	5–10 mg
Route	oral; IM	all routes	oral
MLD (nontolerant)	1 gm	200 mg	100 mg
MLD (tolerant)	4 gm	2 gm	500 mg
Antagonist	Naloxone or Nalorphine	Naloxone or Nalorphine	Naloxone or Nalorphine
Duration of action to prevent withdrawal sx	8 hours	8 hours	24 hours
Dependency liability	moderate	marked	moderate
Tolerance*	moderate	marked	moderate

*Tolerance is lost after a period of abstinence. This is a frequent cause of death due to "accidental" overdose.

TABLE XXXI
NARCOTICLIKE

	Approx. MLD/70 kg person*
alphaprodine (Nisentil)	100 mg
anileridine (Leritine)	500
apomorphine	100
diphenoxylate (Lomotil)	200
ethyl morphine (Dionin)	500
di hydromorphine (Dilaudid)	200
meperidine (Demerol)	1000
methadone (Dolophine)	100
nalorphine (Nalline)	200
omnopon (Pantopan)	300
opium	400
pentazocine (Talwin)	500
phenazocine (Prinadol)	200
propoxyphene (Darvon)	1000
morphine	200
mono methyl morphine (codeine)	800
diacetyl morphine (heroin)	50
	(for non addict)

*Dreisbach & others

tion of imagination and freedom from anxiety; sweating, loss of senses to time and space, no hunger sensation, nausea and vomiting, constipation, itching of skin, dry mouth, slow shallow respiration, cyanosis, pulmonary edema, cardiovascular depression, shock, marked respiratory depression (Cheyne-Stokes) until anoxia occurs, face markedly congested and cyanotic, deep coma, areflexia, respiratory failure, death. Pupils may dilate as death approaches.

WITHDRAWAL (ABSTINENCE SYNDROME) (CHRONIC): May start to appear about 4 to 8 hours after the last dose, reaching peak intensity between 36 and 72 hours. Lacrimation, rhinorrhea, yawning, and sweating appear early, followed by a restless sleep. At about 20 hours, gooseflesh, dilated pupils, agitation, and tremors may appear. The peak of distress during the second and third day may include insomnia, chills, weakness, intestinal cramps, nausea, vomiting, diarrhea, violent yawning, muscular aches in legs, severe low back pain, elevated blood pressure and pulse rate, sweating, dehydration that may become severe and serious by producing cardiovascular irregularities. This withdrawal episode may last up to 10 days; at any time during this period if an opiate (or related drug) is given, the symptoms disappear dramatically.

DEPENDENCY, TOLERANCE AND COMPULSION: This is a true physiologic *dependency* and although withdrawal symptoms are quite severe, death is a rare consequence.

Tolerance is rapidly acquired; it now requires many times the original dose to satisfy, or to hold off withdrawal symptoms. This tolerance is lost following abstinence for several weeks.

Compulsion is powerful to seek satisfaction and/or to abort the impending ugly withdrawal symptoms. The degree of compulsion (and compliance) varies widely. Much depends upon the socioeconomic, psychological, and mental make-up of each individual.

Identification

Heroin (diacetylmorphine) is metabolized in man almost completely to morphine. Codeine (methylmorphine) is metabolized only partly to morphine. The morphine metabolite then conjugates (90%) almost entirely to its glucuronide.

Acid hydrolysis may increase the chances of detecting trace amounts many hours after exposure. Specimens of choice are urine and bile. Bile contains much more morphine per unit volume but is very troublesome to extract. Chloroform:isopropanol (3:1) is the solvent of choice.

Separation by adsorption is not as effective as direct solvent extraction, but absorption, however, lends itself to multiple sample analysis. Separation technics in order of effectiveness: (a) Solvent of chloroform:isopropanol (3:1) (best) ; (b) Amberlite XAD extraction cartridge (Brinkmann) ; (c) Norit charcoal; (d) Reeves cation paper extraction—Reeve angel grade SA-2 ion exchange resin loaded paper cut in 6 × 6 cm square (least) .

The mere finding of morphine in urine or bile, if not supported by a good history and supporting pathology, *is not* sufficient proof of death due to overdose. An addict with high tolerance can have quite high urinary morphine levels and yet not be "over dosed." On the other hand, negative findings do not always rule out death due to overdose because some nonaddicts are very sensitive to small amounts; also, metabolism during a long survival period, or a rapid death following injection, may not always permit easy detection.

1. Fifteen (15) ml of urine with 5 ml of hydrochloric acid is hydrolyzed on a water bath for 5 minutes.

   Cool the hydrolysate and (while cool) carefully neutralize with 50% sodium hydroxide. Fix pH at 9 with 3 ml of buffer. Extract with 2 × 30 ml chloroform:isopropanol (3:1).

   Allow layers to separate and then filter solvent through small filter paper. Collect the solvent into a test tube to which is added one drop of 1N HCl; evaporate (carefully) to barely dryness at about 85°C. Pick up residue of free morphine in 50 μl of methanol.

   Reagent: Buffer—Saturated NH_4Cl adjusted to pH 9 with NH_4OH. Or pH 8.5: dissolve 53.5 gm of NH_4Cl in 950 ml of H_2O. Add 18 ml of NH_4OH. Check the pH and adjust as necessary to pH 8.5 with either dropwise NH_4OH or HCl.

   a. Thin Layer Chromatography (TLC): Spot the TLC plate parallel with standard references, controls, and unknown. Place 200 ml of developing solvent in a TLC developing chamber (solvent tank). Insert plates after the chamber atmosphere is saturated with vapors. See section I.

      When the solvent front reaches (in about 30 minutes) the 15 cm finishing line prescratched horizontally), remove the TLC plates and air dry. Remove all traces of solvent and ammonia with a dryer (hair dryer) and then in a drying oven if necessary.

      Developing solvents:
      • (S-1: Davidow-Petri-Quame: *Tech Bull Reg Technol, 38:* 298, 1968.) Ethyl acetate:methanol:NH_4OH (85:10:5).
      • (S-2: Mule, S.J.: *Anal Chem, 36:*1907, 1964.)
        (a) NH_4OH:benzene:diaxane:ethanol (5:50:40:5)
        (b) Acetic acid:ethanol:H_2O (30:60:10)
      • (S-3: Steele, J.: *J Chrom, 19:*300, 1965.)
        (a) Ethanol:dioxane:benzene:ammonium hydroxide (5:40:50:5)

(b)	Chloroform:dioxane:ethyl acetate:ammonium hydroxide (25:60:10:5)

(c)	Ethanol:dioxane:chloroform:petroleum ether (30–60° C):benzene:ammonium hydroxide:ethyl acetate (5:50: 10:15:10:5:5)

(d)	Ethyl acetate:benzene:ammonium hydroxide (60:35: 5)

(e)	Methanol:$CHCl_3$:NH_4OH (200:18:2.5)

• Others

Chloroform:methanol (50:50) Rf 14 (Curry).

Chloroform:methanol (30:10) Rf 47 (Tudo de Lewis).

Methanol:ammonium hydroxide (100:1.5) Rf 45 (Sunshine).

b.	Detection by Rf:

Examine under UV light to identify quinine or any other drug that is sometimes used as diluent for heroin.

Iodoplatinate spray → dark blue.

Allow to dry and color intensifies; then spray with ammoniacal silver nitrate. The dark blue spot *disappears* completely. Put TLC plate in drying oven at 100°C and the reappearance of a dark chocolate-brown spot (within 10 minutes) confirms morphine. This is confirmatory for morphine because most other drugs do not fade; sensitive to about 0.2 μg/ml.

Reagents:

• Iodoplatinate: Ten (10) ml of 10% platinic chloride plus 250 ml of 4% potassium iodide are mixed and then diluted with H_2O to 500 ml. Store in dark bottle in refrigerator. Stable for about 2 weeks.

• Ammoniacal silver nitrate: Mix 20 ml of 5N ammonium hydroxide and 20 ml of 50% silver nitrate; prepare every 2 days.

• Dragendroff's reagent: 1.3 bismuth subnitrate in 60 ml of water plus 15 ml glacial acetic acid are mixed with 12 gm potassium iodide in 30 ml of water. To final mixture add 100 ml of water and 25 ml of glacial acetic acid.

This reagent may be sprayed on top of the dry iodopla-

TABLE XXXII

DRUG	Rf							
	S-1	S-2a	S-2b	S-3a	S-3b	S-3c	S-3d	S-3e
alvodine				97	98	98	93	
anileridine				95	95	93	77	
atropine	45							
caffeine	80							
cocaine	96			86	84	84	68	65
codeine	52	39	29	28	42	40	05	78
Dicodid				36	35	42	05	
dihydromorphine		10	21	09	16	17	01	
Dilaudid				18	19	21	02	
Dionin	63	46	25	40	46	47	05	
(ethyl morphine)								
heroin (pure)	80	76	35	74	67	73	19	56
hyoscine	84							
(Scopolamine)								
levo-dromorane				57	54	44	20	
meperidine	90	97	41	63	70	70	27	65
(Demerol)								
mescaline				21	23	27	04	
methadone	98	99	59	79	81	82	58	
metapon				28	30	34	03	
monoacetylmorphine		64	40	50	55	56	11	
morphine	40	11	27	18	20	23	02	50
narcotine				80	83	85	72	
nicotine	90							
Nisentil				83	79	87	25	
noscapine	99							
Numorphan				56	56	58	15	
papaverine				73	77	77	53	
peronin				53	51	52	09	
phenazocine				96	96	95	80	
procaine	97			67	69	68	41	
quinine	60			41	42	46	04	68
strychnine	60							
thebaine				65	73	74	23	
tetracaine				68	70	70	33	

For others see pages 109 to 117.

tinate spray (omitting the ammoniacal AgNO₃). Morphine will maintain its blue color, whereas interference by other drugs that show a distortion of similar colors will be minimized.

    c. To reconfirm TLC spot: Scrape spots of interest into individual screw-capped test tubes; add 1 ml of H_2O and 1 ml of buffer (pH 9); mix. Extract with 5 ml of chloroform: isopropanol (3:1). Allow layers to separate. Add 1 drop of 0.1N HCl to the solvent layer and gently evaporate to barely dryness on a water bath at about 80°C.

        Aliquot portions should be confirmed by using another developing solvent system (TLC as described above); precipitate or micro crystalline tests; Color tests, or fluorimetry.

2. Precipitate or microcrystal tests. See Alkaloids.

        Residue is dissolved in 3 drops of 2% acetic acid. Transfer 1 drop to a micro slide and add 1 drop of reagent barely to one side of sample.

    a. Wagner's reagent → red-brown precipitate (oil), which on standing → overlapping plates or rosette crystals

    b. Marme's reagent → gelatinous—colorless needles (single or in sheaths)

    c. sodium carbonate → small rod crystals often in rosettes

    d. Other crystalline precipitates are also formed with the following reagents: Mayer's; gold chloride; platinic chloride; phosphomolybdate; potassium iodide.

    e. morphine + Picric acid → nothing

    f. heroin   + Picric acid → precipitate

3. Color tests (see Alkaloids): Residue is dissolved in methanol; 1 drop is transferred and allowed to dry on a porcelain spot plate. Add 1 drop of reagent onto residue.

    a. sulfuric acid → colorless → purple (by heat)

    b. nitric acid → orange-red → red-yellow → green

    c. Frohde's → violet → green → gray

    d. Mandelin's → red → blue-violet → green

    e. Mecke's → blue-green → brown (by heat)

    f. Marquis → peach-red → violet → blue-violet

    g. $FeCl_3$ → blue in neutral solution (morphine) (acid or alcohol destroys color)

    h. $FeCl_3$ → blue (no change with codeine or heroin).

    i. iodic acid → liberates I_2, which is soluble in chloroform (I_2 is not liberated with codeine or heroin)

4. UV spectrophotometry, although not sufficiently sensitive for morphine in amounts found in urine or tissue, may be used on the residue found in the vial, syringe, or original container.

Dissolve in 5 ml of 0.5N sulfuric acid if residue is relatively dry and pure, or fix pH at 9 with buffer and extract with chloroform:isopropanol (3:1) as described in test 1.

Re-extract solvent with 5 ml of 0.5N sulfuric acid. Read (scan) acid extract in UV spectrophotometer:

Morphine: Maximum density, 285 nm; $E_{1cm}^{1\%}$ 55; minimum density, 260 nm; $E_{1cm}^{1\%}$ 17.

Heroin: Maximum density, 280 nm; $E_{1cm}^{1\%}$ 86; minimum density, 255 nm; $E_{1cm}^{1\%}$ 54.

Codein: Maximum density, 285 nm; $E_{1cm}^{1\%}$ 58; minimum density, 262 nm; $E_{1cm}^{1\%}$ 22.

5. Fluorimetry (Kupferberg, Burkhalter, and Way): UV technic is not sensitive enough to detect morphine in blood or urine. Conversion of morphine (which is weakly fluorescent) to pseudomorphine (which is very highly fluorescent) affords not only a very sensitive but also a highly specific means to determine morphine even in small traces (1 μg). Morphine is extracted by chloroform-butanol from tissue saturated with sodium bicarbonate; it is then re-extracted into an acid phase where it is oxidized to pseudomorphine by potassium ferri-ferrocyanide; this is then read in a spectrofluorometer.

a. Mix 1 to 3 ml of bile (plasma or urine) and 0.5 gm of sodium bicarbonate in a glass-stoppered test tube. Add 9 ml of 10% *n*-butanol in chloroform. Shake and extract for about 5 minutes; centrifuge at 2000 rpm. Carefully transfer 8 ml of the solvent to another glass-stoppered test tube containing 1.2 ml of 0.01M hydrochloric acid. Shake and extract for about 3 minutes, centrifuge, and convert the morphine to pseudomorphine.

One (1) ml of the 0.01M acid extract is carefully removed and is added to 1.0 ml of 0.1M pyrophosphate buffer (pH 8.5). To this is added 0.1 ml of potassium ferriferro-cyanide reagent and is thoroughly mixed. Allow to stand about 10 minutes; then transfer to a 1 cm quartz cuvette.

Emission at 440 nm resulting from excitation at 250 nm (wave length uncalibrated) is measured fluorometrically.

The excitation and emission of pseudomorphine in aqueous solution at pH 8.5 is sensitive and specific. When the emission wavelength is held constant at 440 nm, the excitation spectrum exhibits three peaks: at 250, 280, and 320 nm. When the excitation wavelength is held constant at 250 nm, the emission spectrum exhibits a single peak at 440 nm. Also at 250 nm, the tissue and reagent blanks show the minimal interference and can be quantitated.

Always do a tissue blank, which may sometimes be as high as a low positive unknown. This test may *only* be used, therefore, when it is confirmed.

Reagents: All reagents must be reagent-grade quality.

- Sodium pyrophosphate buffer (0.1H) and adjust to pH 8.5 with 1.0M hydrochloric acid. Should be made fresh each day.
- Potassium ferriferrocyanide stock solution: 57.7 mg of potassium ferricyanide and 4.9 mg of potassium ferrocyanide (trihydrate) is dissolved in 100 ml of water and stored in refrigerator. (Can be kept for 1 week.) Dilute tenfold prior to use.
- Standard morphine sulfate contains 0.1 μg to 10 μg per ml in distilled water calculated as free base. Keeps in refrigerator indefinitely.

b. To further confirm, TLC should be used. A small aliquot of the tissue extract is spotted onto a TLC silica gel G plate. Developed in a solvent system described above or with methanol:butanol:benzene:H_2O:NH_4OH (240:60:40:40:20).

Allow plates to dry and spray with potassium ferriferrocyanide and examine under UV light.

Normorphine, *n*-allyl normorphine, dihydromorphine, and 6-acetylmorphine also show fluorescence under similar conditions.

Heroin, codeine, apomorphine, meperidine, anileridine, and methadone do not show fluorescence, but heroin metabolizes to morphine in humans.

6. Immunoassay kits are available.
    a. Enzyme multiplied Immunoassay Technic (EMIT) (Syva).
    b. Radio immunoassay (RIA).
    c. Hemagglutination-inhibition (Baker).

Treatment

Immediate action is necessary to maintain all vital signs. Maintain respiration with a patent airway and artificial respiration (clear with suction if necessary to maintain a patent airway). Maintain blood pressure, body heat, water, and electrolyte balance. Support against shock and pulmonary edema.

Naloxone (Narcan) is the specific antagonist of choice. Nalline or Lorfan may also be used with caution but they may produce further depression if morphine or derivatives are absent.

These antagonists are very effective. They can reverse a fall in blood pressure; they can decrease pulse rate and cardiac arrhythmia when these are produced by morphine or derivatives. Loss of superficial and deep reflexes, corneal and gag reflexes, and pupillary constriction return to normal within 5 minutes. These dramatic changes may further confirm the presence of morphine or derivative, but *do not* remove the dangers of emergency. Most often treatment must be repeatedly given (as needed). Close observation is required for 24 hours. See package insert.

Since these antagonists inactivate action of morphine, they can also provoke withdrawal symptoms in those persons addicted to morphine (or its derivatives).

Symptoms and treatment for Demerol, methadone, heroin, codeine, Dilaudid, Dionin, pentazocine, and propoxyphene, generally are similar to morphine.

MOTHBALLS

Synonyms: Moth repellents, moth flakes, moth cakes.

Uses: Moth repellent, toilet deodorizers.

Properties: White crystalline, aromatic characteristic odor. Usually contain *p*-dichlorobenzene, naphthalene, or occasionally camphor.

MLD: For a 70 kg person: *p*-dichlorobenzene, approximately

15 gm; naphthalene, approximately 5 gm; camphor, approximately 2 gm.

Remarks: Since halogenation of aromatic compounds generally decreases toxicity, *p*-dichlorobenzene is the least toxic in this group. However, prolonged exposure to its vapors may cause liver damage and cataracts. Stimulates central nervous system.

Symptoms: Naphthalene: gastrointestinal irritation, abdominal cramps, nausea, vomiting, diarrhea, liver and kidney damage, painful urination, hemolytic anemia, cyanosis, hemoglobinuria (hemolysis), albuminuria, motor instability, jaundice, oliguria; wine-colored, black, or brown urine. Depression, convulsions, heavy breathing (sounds like snoring), coma, collapse.

Identification

Isolated by steam distillation. See Section I.

1. *p-Dichlorobenzene:* Mp 53°C (PDB).
   a. Test for organic halides.
   b. Characteristic odor.
   c. Extract steam distillate with ether and gently evaporate → white crystals (Mp 53°C).
   d. Extract steam distillate with *n*-heptane; UV spectrophotometry (maximum density, 265, 275 nm; minimum density, 270 nm). See Section I.

2. *Naphthalene:* Mp 80°C (Halowax).
   a. Extract steam distillate with ether and gently evaporate → white crystals (prismatic plates: Mp 80°C), characteristic odor.
   b. Extract steam distillate with *n*-heptane; UV spectrophotometry (maximum density, 265, 275, 285 nm; minimum density, 270, 280 nm).
   c. Penzoldt: 30 ml of urine is floated on 10 ml of sulfuric acid —green color is formed, which gradually spreads into acid phase.
   d. Partly eleminated in urine as β-naphthol. UV spectrophotometry. See Section I.

3. *Camphor:* Mp 176°C. (See tests, signs, and treatment listed under Camphor.

MUSCARINE (C₉H₂₀NO₂)

Synonyms: *Amanita muscaria,* toadstools, fly mushrooms, hydroxycholine, inedible mushroom.

Use: None

Properties: Basic, soluble in water; deliquescent crystals.

MLD: Approximately 50 mg/70 kg person.

Remarks: Alkaloidal properties. Symptoms come on within a few minutes to 2 hours after ingestion. Parasympathomimetic (similar to Parathion). *Not* to be confused with *A. phalloides* (delayed action).

Symptoms: Mainly respiratory difficulty, bronchial constriction and pulmonary edema. Parasympathomimetic (cholinergic) action, pin point pupils, nausea, vomiting, profuse sweating, lacrimation, thirst, diarrhea, and frequent urination, dehydration, hypotention, bradycardia, cardiac standstill or respiratory difficulties, terminal convulsions.

Identification

1. Yields typical crystals with alkaloidal precipitants. Refer to Alkaloids.
2. Determine blood cholinesterase activity; muscarine depresses cholinesterase activity. See Parathion.

Treatment

Poisoning* is similar for arecoline, mecholyl, acetylcholine, Doryl, physostigmine, pilocarpine, and organic phosphate esters of the parathion group. See under Parathion, for suggested treatment for the parasympathomimetic (cholinergic) symptoms.

Note: Mushroom poisoning of the *Amanita phalloides* or *A. virosa* or *A. verna* contain amatoxins (cyclopeptides) and are far more toxic, with a reported fatality of about 50 percent.

These poisonings have usually three phases: Severe abdominal cramps, watery diarrhea, nausea, and vomiting within 6–24 hours after ingestion; then a "transient" clinical improvement; then

---

*Poison toad known as the *Bufo-marinus* or *Bufo-giganticus* (native of Bermuda, southern United States, Mexico, Central and South America, and the Caribbean islands) produces similar symptoms.

hepatic and renal failure 2–5 days later.

Thiotic (α-lipoic) acid has been reported of some help. This can be obtained from the National Institute of Health at Maryland (telephone: 301-496-1518 or 301-656-4000) or at New York City (telephone: 212-244-5562).

Reference

Morbidity and Mortality Weekly Reports, Galerina Marginata or G. Autumnalis. Atlanta, C.D.C., 2/22/75.

NAPHTHOL

Symptoms: Phenollike symptoms, convulsions, coma, possible liver and kidney involvement; delayed action may produce anemia, retinal injury.

Identification

1. Extract urine or vomitus or residue with chloroform. Add 1 gm KOH to the CHCl₃ extract.
   a. α-naphthol → sky blue
   b. β-naphthol → blue → green
2. Alcoholic extract (several drops) is placed onto lignin (wood fibers) + several drops of HCl.
   a. α-naphthol → greenish
   b. thymol → green
   c. resorcinol → violet
   d. pyrrole → red
   e. pyrogallol → blue-green
   f. phenol → blue-green
   g. anisole → greenish yellow
   h. carbozole → cherry red
   i. indole → cherry red
   j. cresol → greenish

Treatment

Wash exposed areas with soap and water. If ingested, give activated charcoal and gastric lavage carefully. Sodium sulfate cathartics. Symptomatic and supportive as under Phenols.

NICOTINE ($C_{10}H_{14}N_2$)

Synonyms: Nicotia; Black Leaf 40; Barekil.

Uses: Insecticide; no therapeutic use.

Properties: Basic, liquid, water soluble; turns yellow-brown on standing. Bp 246°C. Volatile with steam. Soluble in ether or $CHCl_3$.

MLD: Approximately 60 mg (1 drop) /70 kg person.

Remarks: Alkaloid. Can be absorbed through skin. Death usually occurs within a matter of minutes. Tachyphylaxis. Mild poisoning may appear on overindulgence of tobacco. Absorbed through all portals.

Symptoms

Stimulation followed by depression of parasympathetic system, depending upon dose.

With toxic doses, paralysis of the central nervous system, including the respiratory center. Smaller quantities produce salivation, nausea, vomiting, purging, strong typical cigarette odor on breath and in blood, powerful gastrointestinal corrosion, burning sensation in mouth and throat. Blood is dark.

Toxic doses produce effects such as tachycardia, hypertension, curarelike effect on skeletal muscle, paralysis, abdominal pain, pupils first constricted, later dilated; disturbed vision, constriction of blood vessels, lowered temperature of limbs. Breathing is labored, pulse irregular, mental confusion, muscular weakness, giddiness, lack of coordination, partial or complete unconsciousness, clonic convulsions followed by collapse with muscular relaxation, slow and weak respiration that finally ceases although the heart may continue to beat for some time.

Identification

Isolated by alkaline-steam distillation or alkaline-chloroform extraction.

1. UV spectrophotometry (very sensitive) : See Section I. Maximum density, 259 nm; basic alkaloid.
2. GLC: See Section I.
3. Residue is dissolved in 1 ml of 1% acetic acid. Use 1-drop

aliquot portions for spot-test precipitate identification; examine for typical crystals.
   a. Wagner's reagent → brown precipitate
   b. Mayer's reagent → white precipitate
   c. picric acid → yellow precipitate (only in concentrated solution)
   d. gold chloride → yellow precipitate
   e. silicotungstic acid → white crystals
   Refer to Alkaloids.
4. Small aliquot portions of residue are transferred to spot plate and color reagents applied. See Alkaloids.
   a. sulfuric acid → colorless
   b. nitric acid → colorless
   c. sulfuric and nitric acid → colorless → yellow → red
   d. Fröhde's reagent → colorless → yellow → reddish white
   e. Mecke's reagent → bright yellow
   f. formaldehyde (1 drop) → stand 1 hour → add 1 drop of
   g. *p*-dimethylaminobenzaldehyde → violet zone
      nitric acid → pink to deep red
5. Nicotine has a strong characteristic odor, burning taste; blood is dark and has sharp odor like stale tobacco.

INTERPRETATION OF RESULTS: Smokers have 0.001 to 0.002 mg per 10 ml of blood and 0.001 to 0.010 mg per 10 ml of urine. A package of cigarettes (20) contains approximately 300 mg of nicotine. Much of this is burned off in smoking, and the remainder is absorbed. Ninety percent of the absorbed nicotine is rapidly metabolized and the remainder (10%) is distributed in the body fluids (50 liters). Above 0.5 mg/dl blood level may be lethal.

Treatment

Should be prompt; activated charcoal or proteins, then gastric lavage or potassium permanganate (1:10,000), emetics, demulcents.

Guard against respiratory and cardiac problems.

Valium, ether, or barbiturates for convulsions (with caution).

Supportive and symptomatic treatment. Symptoms and treatment are generally similar to that of coniine, lobeline, or gelsemium.

NITRATES (KNO$_3$; NaNO$_3$)

Derivatives: Potassium and sodium nitrates; saltpeter; Chile saltpeter.

Uses: Explosives, munitions, fertilizer.

Properties: White crystalline salt, soluble in water.

MLD: Approximately 8 gm/70 kg person.

Remarks: Usual poisoning by accident or mistaken identity. Some nitrates may convert to nitrites in the body by action of intestinal flora. Nitrites produce methemoglobin.

Symptoms: Gastrointestinal irritation, nausea, vomiting, diarrhea (bloody), abdominal pain, vertigo, muscular weakness, hematuria, albuminuria, oliguria, convulsions, collapse, coma, death.

Identification

Add some water to the vomitus or gastric lavage and then filter. Clear filtrate is tested.

1. several drops of filtrate + several drops of imipramine (2%) + several drops of H$_2$SO$_4$ → dark blue color (very sensitive)
2. diphenylamine test (very sensitive).
3. See tests under Nitric Acid. See below.

Normal urine may contain up to 0.4 percent nitrates (food products).

Treatment

Milk or water then gastric lavage, or emetics, and cathartics. Valium or short-acting barbiturates for convulsions. Support against kidney damage.

NITRIC ACID (HNO$_3$)

Synonyms: Aqua fortis; engraver's acid.

Uses: Industry, munitions, reagent.

Properties: Colorless liquid (or amber color). Sharp acrid penetrating odor; strong oxidizing agent; very corrosive.

MLD: Approximately 3 ml/70 kg person.

Remarks: Powerful oxidizing agent.

Symptoms: Acrid sour taste, yellow eschars on lips, mouth, and throat. Yellow-brown stains, corrosive on skin and tissue. Severe pain in mouth, throat, and stomach. Nausea, vomiting, diarrhea, thirst, difficult swallowing, acidemia, rapid weak pulse, slow shallow breathing, convulsions, collapse, shock, death.

Identification

In stomach contents:

1. Solution may be colorless or yellow; sharp odor; precipitates protein. Stains tissues, clothing, wood, paper, etc. yellow.
2. Turns litmus paper pink.
3. Drop in a piece of copper and, if acid is not too dilute, when heated will produce pungent dark brown heavy copious fumes (NO_2).
4. Add a pinch of diphenylamine and stratify over 2 ml of sulfuric acid; a deep blue band develops at interface (sensitive to 1:1,000,000).
5. First neutralize the acid; then add 2 ml of 10% ferrous sulfate and stratify over 2 ml of sulfuric acid. A deep brown band will develop at interface (specific).
6. Quantitative determination by comparing color intensity produced in tests 4 and 5 or by titration with standard sodium hydroxide solution.

Treatment

If tissue damage is extensive, avoid emetics and stomach tube. Avoid carbonate types of alkalizing agents (chalk, baking soda, sodium bicarbonate are contraindicated). Give milk or water to dilute acid. Neutralize with Amphogel or cremalin, limewater, soap suds, etc. Give demulcents such as cream, olive oil, raw eggs. Cracked ice to relieve thirst. Supportive.

Keep patient warm and quiet. If there are signs of asphyxia, tracheotomy may be necessary. If exposure was *external,* wash areas with water profusely and then apply a paste of baking soda.

Give morphine for pain, antibiotic if needed, corticosteroids for persistent shock. See Section I.

NITRITES (KNO$_2$, NaNO$_2$, C$_5$H$_{11}$NO$_2$)

Derivatives: Potassium, sodium, amyl nitrite; ethyl nitrite; nitroglycerin.

Uses: Medicinals (vascular drugs), antiseptics, to pickle and preserve smoked meat and fish.

Properties: White crystalline, water soluble, can produce methemoglobin, found in well water when surface water is allowed to seep in. Can be converted to nitrosamines (carcinogenic).

MLD: Approximately 5 gm./70 kg person.

Remarks: Symptoms may resemble cyanide. Death in $\frac{1}{2}$ to 3 hours. Is rapidly oxidized and thus can be only found in stomach contents as nitrites and nitrates. Nitrites are more toxic than nitrates. Nitrates may be converted in the body to nitrites.

Symptoms: Vomiting, colic, nausea, diarrhea, flushed face and neck, fullness and throbbing of head, dizziness, mental confusion, peripheral vasodilatation, *fall in blood pressure,* tachycardia, fainting, cyanosis, methemoglobinemia, anoxia, dilatation of pupils, peripheral circulatory failure, coma, death from cardiac or respiratory failure.

Identification

Stomach contents, vomitus, or drug is diluted with water and filtered. Divide into several aliquots and do the following tests for nitrites on the clear filtrate.

1. Mix a 10 ml portion plus 10 mg of diphenylamine sulfate and then layer with 5 ml of concentrated sulfuric acid. A blue ring forms at interface. This is also a good test for nitroglycerin.

2. Mix a 10 ml portion plus 10 mg of brucine sulfate and then layer with 5 ml of concentrated sulfuric acid. A red ring forms at interface.

3. Nitrites when treated with dilute H$_2$SO$_4$ $\rightarrow$ brownish red fumes (NO$_2$).

4. A few drops of potassium iodide solution (10%) and a few drops of dilute sulfuric acid added to a nitrite solution liberates iodine, which will turn a starch solution or starch paper a deep blue-black.

5. See imipramine test under nitrates.

6. Alcoholic solution of indole → orange → brown.

7. Test blood for methemoglobin. Methods described under Aniline.

Treatment

Emetics; or activated charcoal, and gastric lavage, cathartics; withdrawal of drug.

Do not give epinephrine! Use plasma expanders to maintain blood pressure!

Keep patient quiet, recumbent position; maintain body heat, fluid, and electrolyte balance. Artificial respiration and oxygen therapy, if needed. Exchange transfusion if cyanosis is severe.

Treat with 1% methylene blue IV when methemoglobinemia is severe or above 40 percent. Ascorbic acid is also effective but gives slower response. See under Aniline. Supportive.

NITROBENZENE ($C_6H_5NO_2$)

Synonym: Oil of mirbane.

Uses: Shoe polish, perfumes, dyes, soaps.

Properties: Yellow oily volatile liquid. Bp 207°C. Characteristic shoe polish odor.

MLD: Approximately 2 ml/70 kg person.

APPROXIMATE BLOOD LEVEL: Lethal, 0.05 mg/dl.

Remarks: Urine may have a characteristic shoe polish odor; will be brown due to *p*-aminophenol. Death after a few hours if untreated. Methemoglobin persistent for several days. Absorbed through all portals. Skin absorption is common.

Symptoms: Characteristic odor of bitter almonds (shoe polish), mental dullness, headache, nausea, vomiting, black tongue, diarrhea, ataxia, nystagmus, brown urine that has a characteristic odor, methemoglobinemia, severe cyanosis, weak respiration, irregular pupils, dyspnea, delirium, convulsions, coma, respiratory arrest, death. Toxic symptoms may sometimes be delayed 12 hours.

Identification

Separated by steam distillation.

1. Steam distill into chloroform; separate the chloroform and then evaporate → oily nitrobenzene (Bp 207°C).
2. To 2 ml of nitrobenzene, add 2 ml of sulfuric acid and 3 ml of fuming nitric acid → dinitrobenzene crystals (Mp 90°C).
3. To the dinitrobenzene (test 2) plus several drops of absolute alcohol (to dissolve), add 3 drops of sodium hydroxide (40%) and 1 ml of fructose (1%) → violet color → brown.
4. Test blood for methemoglobin, see Aniline.
5. UV spectrophotometry; See Section I.

Treatment

Charcoal with gastric lavage or emetic; saline cathartics. Avoid fats and oils. Maintain body heat, fluid, and electrolyte balance.

Artificial respiration, oxygen therapy as needed.

Ascorbic acid (oral) for methemoglobinemia or 1 mg per kilogram of 1% methylene blue (best). See Aniline.

Valium or short-acting barbiturates for convulsions. Symptomatic and supportive measures.

NOLUDAR ($C_{10}H_{17}O_2N$)

Synonyms: Methyprylon.

Properties: MW, 183. Mp 74°C.

MLD: Approximately 15 gm/70 kg person.

Approximate Blood Levels: Therapeutic, 1 mg/dl, lethal, 10 mg/dl.

Symptoms: Drowsiness, coma, respiratory depression, hypotension, reflexes hyperactive (early), reflexes hypoactive (late), slight bradycardia, convulsions (late), hyperactivity (late); pupils are usually normal or constricted; pyrexia or hypothermia.

Identification

1. Extract 2 ml of plasma, 1 ml of water, and 0.6 ml NaOH with 8 ml of ether for about 20 minutes. Centrifuge and transfer 7 ml of ether layer to a 15 ml centrifuge tube. Wash twice with 1 ml of 0.5N NaOH; centrifuge after each washing and remove washings by capillary pipette. Evaporate ether in a water bath at 60°C. Dissolve residue in 3 ml of water and add 1 ml of diluted (1:2.5) Folin-Ciocalteu phenol reagent and 1 ml of 0.8N NaOH and let stand for 10 minutes to develop full blue. Then add 2 ml CHCl$_3$ and shake vigorously for about 1 minute and centrifuge. Transfer the clean aqueous colored layer to another tube and read optical density at 600 nm. Run in parallel 2 ml of control plasma and 2 ml of control plasma plus 10 μg of Noludar standard (1 ml of standard replacing the 1 ml of water).

    A single oral dose in adults, about 19μg/ml at 2 hours. Half-life is about 4 hours. Urine eliminates less than 3 percent of dose. Test is sensitive to about 2 μg/ml in plasma.
    Reference: D'Aiconte of Hoffman-La Roche.

2. TLC: See Section I.
    * Benzene:acetone:NH$_4$OH (100:20:6) Rf = 55
    * Chloroform:ether (85:15) Rf = 52
    Spray
    * HgSO$_4$ and diphenyl carbazone
    * Iodoplatinate

Treatment

Charcoal and then gastric lavage; or emesis. Guard against convulsions. Support all vital signs. See general suggestions, under Barbiturates. Dialysis may be helpful. Symptomatic and supportive measures.

NONBARBITURATE HYPNOTICS

Synonyms: bromides; chloral hydrate (Triclos); ethchlorvynol (Placidyl); ethinamate (Valmid); flurazepam (Dalmane); glutethimide (Doriden); methaqualone (Quaalude); meparafynol (Darmison); methyprylon (Noludar); paraldehyde; and thalidomide.

Symptoms and Treatment: Generally similar to Barbiturates.

OPIUM

Synonym: Poppyseed (morphine group).

Uses: Drugs (paregoric, etc.), illicit smoking or chewing.

Properties: Basic. Contains morphine, codeine, thebaine, papaverine, narcotine, etc.

Remarks: Alkaloidal, parasympathomimetic.

Symptoms: Similar to morphine but milder in intensity. Refer to morphine for identification and treatment.

OXALATES ($H_2C_2O_4$)

Synonyms: Oxalic acid; sodium or potassium salts.

Uses: Bleaching, cleaning agents, ink eradicator, metal polish, rust remover, straw hat cleaner.

Properties: Colorless crystals, bitter taste; soluble in water or alcohol. Sparingly soluble in ether (1 gm/100 ml).

MLD: Approximately 5 gm/70 kg person.

APPROXIMATE BLOOD LEVELS: Normal, 0.2 mg/dl; lethal, 2 mg/dl.

Remarks: May be found in traces in some vegetables such as rhubarb or spinach. Strong reducing agent. Death may occur within 10 minutes. Strong corrosive.

Symptoms: Burning in mouth, stomach, and throat; swelling of tongue, extreme thirst; swallowing is difficult; nausea, vomiting, diarrhea, headache, cold cyanotic skin, dilated pupils, dyspnea, tremors. Shredded, bloody, and "coffee grounds" brown-black appearance of stomach contents; acidosis. Severe damage to kidneys; urine contains casts, and calcium oxalate crystals, Anuria, edema, convulsions, possible circulatory and respiratory failure, coma, death.

Identification

1. Acidify gastric contents, vomitus, or residue with hydrochloric acid; add large volume of alcohol to dissolve the oxalate and heat gently on steam bath to help precipitate extraneous proteins. Keep adding alcohol, heating, and filtering until no more proteins are precipitated. Finally heat until all the alco-

hol has been driven off. With minimal water, transfer this residue to a separatory funnel and extract with large volumes of ether. Oxalates are more soluble in alcohol or water than in ether; therefore, this may require several extractions. Finally, evaporate the ether and to several aqueous portions do the following:

a. To a 1 ml portion, add 1 drop of sulfuric acid; then add several drops of dilute potassium permanganate (1:2000). The pink color of the permanganate is decolorized.

b. To a 1 ml portion, add 1 ml of calcium chloride (10%) → typical crystalline precipitate (calcium oxalate). Insoluble in acetic but dissolves in hydrochloric acid.

c. To a 1 ml portion, add 1 ml of silver nitrate (10%) → typical crystalline precipitate (silver oxalate), which is soluble in nitric acid.

d. To a 1 ml portion, add 1 ml of lead nitrate (10%) → typical crystalline precipitate (lead oxalate), which is insoluble in acetic acid.

e. To a 1 ml portion, add 0.2 gm of resorcin and stratify with 3 ml of sulfuric acid. Blue ring at interface.

f. To a 1 ml portion, add 1 drop of sulfuric acid and 1 ml of indole solution by underlay. Then mix and place in water bath at 80–90°C → pink.
   Reagent: Indole solution: 10 mg in 10 ml of sulfuric acid, prepared fresh.

2. Grind 100 gm of kidney and steam distill with 100 ml of 2N sulfuric acid. Discard volatile distillate and filter the residue while hot. Extract the residue with several 25 ml portions of alcohol. The collected filtrate is evaporated on a steam bath to about 25 to 50 ml volume. Add another 100 ml of alcohol. Gently heat and quantitatively transfer and filter the residue. Extract the residue with several 25 ml portions of alcohol. Collected filtrates are evaporated to dryness on a steam bath.

   Transfer the residue to a sublimation tube with ether. Sublime with vacuum under 95°C. Dissolve and transfer sublimate with ether. Evaporate ether. Dissolve residue with 2 ml of 1N sulfuric acid; add 2 ml of indole reagent (prepared as in test 1). Place in water bath at 80–90°C for 45 minutes to develop pink color. Cool, read at 525 nm against reagent blank of 2 ml of indole and 2 ml of 1N sulfuric acid.

Milligrams of oxalic acid in 4 ml volume (100 gm of tissue) at 525 nm, 1 cm cuvette (Beckman):

0.2 mg — 80% T
0.4 mg — 64%
0.6 mg — 50%
0.8 mg — 40%
1.0 mg — 32%

Traces of oxalate crystals may normally be found in urine (20 to 50 mg per 24 hour output).

Treatment

Immediately give large amounts of calcium compounds such as milk or limewater. Avoid gastric lavage or emetics or cathartics if severe corrosive damage is evident. Give slaked limewater, milk, milk of magnesia, egg albumin, or aluminum or magnesium antacid gels as demulcents.

Calcium gluconate IV for hypocalcemia. Supportive and symptomatic : maintain airways, guard against edema of glottis and esophageal strictures. Maintain body heat; water and electrolyte balance. Guard against convulsions; kidney damage; aci-acidosis, and collapse. General supportive measures.

PARALDEHYDE ($C_6H_{12}O_3$)

Synonym: Tripolymer of acetaldehyde. Acetal and benzaldehyde are more toxic than paraldehyde.

Uses: In medicine as a hypnotic, anesthetic; for alcoholic withdrawal (DT) (*not to be used* if patient is still under the influence of alcohol).

Properties: Colorless liquid, pungent odor like fusel oil. Bp 120–125°C. Irritating, soluble in water.

MLD: Approximately 100 ml/70 kg person.

APPROXIMATE BLOOD LEVELS: Therapeutic, 5 mg/dl; lethal, 50 mg/dl; half-life, 6 hours.

Remarks

Synergistic with alcohol; metabolizes in part to acetaldehyde. Hypnotic action is rapid (sleep in 15 minutes). Less certain and less potent than chloral hydrate; not to be used intravenously.

Paraldehyde — unless stored in 4 ounce containers or smaller that are light-resistant, well-filled, tightly covered, and kept at temperatures below 30°C—may depolymerize to acetaldehyde, which then metabolizes to *acetic acid* within several months.

Oral administration of deteriorated paraldehyde may cause metabolic acidosis and death due to stomach and lung corrosion, while rectal administration can produce painful corrosive burns and late intestinal obstruction. The proof of this is confirmed by the presence of a new distinct odor of *glacial acetic acid,* which turns blue litmus to pink. The concentration and presence of this acid can be demonstrated by titration with standard sodium hydroxide.

Intravenous administration is extremely hazardous, with a narrow margin between minimum anesthetic and lethal doses. Intramuscular injection may cause skin sloughing, sterile abscesses, or sciatic nerve damage.

Symptoms: Disagreeable pungent odor on breath up to 24 hours (fusel-oil odor), irritation of mouth and throat, dizziness, faintness, hypotension, incoherence, muscular relaxation, rapid pulse, constricted pupils, no response to light, slow respiration, collapse, coma, deep narcosis, death due to respiratory failure. Death may be delayed 24 hours but, when given in large amounts to an acute alcoholic, death may occur within 2 hours (synergism).

Identification

Separated by steam distillation.
1. Urine gives a positive Fehling's test.
2. Blood and urine will have a characteristic odor of paraldehyde (even as low as 0.01%).
3. Paraldehyde in blood. One (1) ml of blood plus 7 ml of water; shake and let stand for 5 minutes. Then add 1 ml of 10% sodium tungstate and 1 cc of $\frac{2}{3}$N sulfuric acid. Shake well

until a brown coagulum develops. Place flask in an ice bath and chill for about 10 minutes; filter through Whatman filter #42 and catch filtrate in flask cooled in an ice bath.

Add 0.1 ml of filtrate to chilled 5 ml of 2% sodium bisulfite; mix. *Keep solution cool in ice bath during entire procedure.* Take 1 ml of this solution and add 1 drop of 5% copper sulfate plus 8 ml of sulfuric acid, and then 4 drops of *p*-hydroxydiphenyl reagent. Mix well and keep *cold* during mixing.

Let solution stand at room temperature for 1 hour and read color intensity in a spectrophotometer at 560 nm with a Beckman DU 1 cm cuvette.

Reagents:

• All solutions and dilutions must be made with redistilled water. Sulfuric acid must be of tested purity and must be added drop by drop from a burette with mixing and chilling in an ice bath.
• *p*-Hydroxydiphenyl: 1 gm in 25 ml of hot 2N sodium hydroxide; then add 75 ml of water. *Make fresh.*

4. Microdiffusion: See Section I.

5. GLC: See Section I.

Treatment: Remove exposure. Gastric lavage and/or emetics. Saline cathartics. External heat, maintain body heat, fluids, and electrolyte balance. Artificial respiration and oxygen therapy as needed. Supportive treatment for depression.

PARAQUAT ($C_{12}H_{14}Cl_2N_2$)

Synonyms: 1,1'-dimethyl-4,4,bipyridimium methyl sulfate; methyl viologen, Gramoxone-HCl.

HOMOLOGUES: Diaquat, difenzoquat.

Uses: Powerful herbicide, or plant desiccant.

Properties: H_2O soluble; quaternary NH_4 compound.

MLD: Approximately 75 mg/70 kg person.

Remarks: Eliminated in urine unchanged up to 3 (or more) days.

Symptoms

IMMEDIATE: GI irritation and burning sensation of mouth and throat; vomiting, corrosion of esophagus and stomach, which may produce ulceration or perforation. Persistent vomiting, restlessness, and hyperexcitability.

DELAYED: Lung involvement and death due to pulmonary changes have been reportd as long as 20 days after ingestion. Fever, tachycardia; liver involvement with jaundice; smoking marihuana contaminated with paraquat may sometimes produce severe lung hemorrhages.

INHALATION (MIST): May cause nasal bleeding, irritation and inflammation of mouth and upper respiratory tract; cough, chest pain, asthmatic attacks, frontal headache, vomiting.

SKIN CONTACT: Severe skin irritation and burning plus the same systemic symptoms as those seen following ingestion.

Identification

1. Five (5) drops of filtered vomitus or gastric lavage plus 5 drops of sodium dithionite → blue-green color. Read visually or in spectrophotometer.
   Reagent: Sodium dithionite (Na hydrosulfite; $Na_2S_2O_4$): 0.1 gm in 10 ml of 1N NaOH; prepare fresh and use within 1 hour.
2. Marihuana cigarette contaminated with paraquat is shaken and extracted vigorously with 5 ml H_2O for 15 minutes and is then filtered. The 5 ml clear filtrate (cigarette) or clear gastric lavage or vomitus is alkalinized with 0.1 gm $NaHCO_3$, then add 0.1 gm sodium dithionite; mix → blue color. Urine may require shaking with alumina to clear and then filter and dilute before testing. Read at 625 nm; 20 mcg/ml = absorbance 0.7.
3. UV spectrophotometer (0.5N H_2SO_4) See Section I. Maximum density: 257 nm $E_{1cm}^{1\%}$: 850
   Reference: Tomsett; Curry; and Clarke.

Treatment

Immediate ingestion of activated charcoal or milk followed by *careful* gastric lavage with 1% bentonite solution; 30% suspension of Fuller's earth or similar clay earth substances have been reported to help decompose paraquat. Saline cathartics to rush elimination. Hemodialysis as needed to support kidney. Maintain respiration and fluid and electrolyte balance; give demulcents (egg white). Cortisone has been reported to help survival. Symptomatic and supportive treatment for hyperexcitability, shock, respiratory difficulties. Keep patient at rest and under medical observation.

PARATHION ($C_{10}H_{14}NO_5PS$)

Derivatives

VERY TOXIC: Parathion (diethyl-*p*-nitrophenyl monothiophosphate); DFP (diisopropyl fluorophosphate); EPN (ethyl-*p*-nitrophenyl benzenethionophosphonate); HETP (hexaethyl tetraphosphate); TEPP (tetraethyl pyrophosphate); OMPA (octamethyl pyrophosphoramide); Bidrin; Co-ral; demeton (Systox); Di-Syston; fenthion (Baytex); Guthion; methyl parathion; Thimet; Trithion.

MODERATE TOXICITY: DDVP (dimethyl-dichlorovinyl phosphate); Diazinon; Dimethoate; Dicapthon; Phosphon; Dipterex; Proban; Karphos; Phosalone; Phosmet.

LOW TOXICITY: Malathion; Abate; Ronnel; Bromophos; Menazon; Baythion; tetrachlorvinphos; Betasan; Glyphosate; Phoxim.

Uses: Very powerful and effective insecticide; limited use in medicine (DFP for glaucoma and OMPA for myasthenia gravis). Potential in warfare as an extremely toxic nerve poison (breaks down activity of cholinesterase and allows acetylcholine to accumulate). Too dangerous to use or store at home. Used by fruit growers, tobacco farms, and greenhouses.

Properties: Parathion is a yellow-brown liquid. Organic phosphate ester. Insoluble in water, ether, or kerosene. Soluble in alcohol, hexane, petroleum ether, acetone, or xylene. Unstable in high (alkaline) pH (above 8); Bp 375°C. Onion-garlic odor.

MLD: *Very toxic:* approximately 30 mg/70 kg person (for parathion).

Remarks: Cholinergic; parasympathomimetic; "nerve poison," war gas; cholinesterase inhibitor; organic phosphate ester.

Symptoms

Produces approximately similar signs and symptoms and requires same treatment as other cholinesterase inhibitors or destroyers (muscarine, pilocarpine, physostigmine, etc.).

These agents may be absorbed through all portals of entry. Skin contact and inhalation can cause poisoning, as can ingestion.

Symptoms and signs usually appear rapidly, and this may be a diagnostic aid. Death usually occurs within $\frac{1}{2}$ to 4 hours but may occur within 10 minutes or may be delayed 24 hours or more.

ACUTE AND LARGE EXPOSURE: Rapid onset of gastrointestinal response: nausea, vomiting, and cramps. Later diarrhea and anorexia, increased peristalsis, epigastric and substernal tightness, heartburn.

The pupils are most usually pinpoint, but this sign is not always diagnostic or early. Rarely, pupils may be dilated due to excitement and nervousness (with low exposure).

Respiratory symptoms include tightness in the chest, wheezing, dyspnea, pain, cough, constricted bronchioles, and cyanosis.

Other symptoms are excessive sweating, salivation, lacrimation; nasal, bronchiolar, and gastrointestinal secretions, resulting in vomiting and diarrhea; pulmonary edema, and frothing at the nose and mouth. Muscular twitch, fasciculation, cramps and convulsions in conjunction with bradycardia, anxiety, tension, restlessness, and confusion, which is followed by stupor and coma.

Death is usually by respiratory failure from paralysis of respiratory muscles and/or depression of respiratory center following bronchiolar constriction, excessive respiratory tract secretions, and pulmonary edema.

MILD EXPOSURE: Headache, blurred vision, and mild muscarinic signs (may be delayed several hours after exposure).

Moderate doses increase intensity of glandular secretions; severe doses produce excessive secretions, convulsions, coma, loss of reflexes and sphincter control. Prognosis is poor, but vigorous treatment must be continued. Death may be rapid, even within 10 minutes.

If illness (onset of signs and symptoms) is delayed 12 hours or more, it is more likely due to something else.

CHRONIC EXPOSURE: Sometimes produces delayed paralysis that may persist for several weeks.

Identification

1. *Parathion has an onion-garlic odor* even in the breath, vomitus, or stomach contents.

2. *Parathion metabolizes easily to p-nitrophenol:* Steam distill 10 ml of vomitus, urine, stomach contents, or residue and collect about 10 ml of distillate. Add two pellets of sodium hydroxide then heat on water bath for about 10 minutes. The yellow color produced is positive for *p*-nitrophenol (metabolite). This can be reported as traces or moderate or large amounts as compared with standard parathion. This *p*-nitrophenol test is excellent to detect early exposures or chronic exposures to parathion because it is sensitive to very small amounts. EPN is another organic phosphate ester that contains this *p*-nitrophenol radical.

   Alternate: Extract with chloroform or ether or *n*-hexane or petroleum ether; then evaporate and pick up residue in ethanol. Add water and one pellet of sodium hydroxide to produce the yellow color with heat (water bath).

3. *Total organic phosphorus in stomach contents* (presumptive with a strong history and typical signs and symptoms). Caution: Rice in stomach may also give positive results.

   Extract with petroleum ether, separate and evaporate to dryness. To residue add 5 ml H_2O and 10 ml nitric acid. Gently heat in a water bath for about 30 minutes at 100°C. Filter and add ammonium molybdate reagent and a little HNO_3; gently heat. A canary-yellow precipitate is positive. Fiske-Sabarrow or any other test for the *phosphate* radical is equally good.

4. TLC. Extract stomach contents with *n*-hexane or petroleum ether and gently evaporate to dryness; reconstitute. Glass plates are coated with silica gel G (250 μ). Tissue extract is concentrated into a few drops of alcohol, which is spotted in usual manner on bottom of plate. Select proper solvent and ratio and suspend and contact for about 30 minutes. See section I.

a. *Solvent:* Benzene:ethyl acetate (9:1) (USPHS).
   Developer: Bromine vapors and fluorescein.

   Plate is removed from solvent tank and allowed to air dry. Plate is then put into another tank saturated with bromine vapors (an open bottle at bottom of tank) for about 3 minutes. Great caution with bromine should be exercised; it is *very toxic* to skin or on breathing. Remove plate and aerate free from bromine vapors; spray with fluorescein reagent (0.3% in ethanol).

   Yellow spots with background of pink indicate positive results. These spots will fluoresce a brilliant purple under UV light.

   If organic phosphates are negative, as above, then spray the plate (after fluorescein) with silver nitrate reagent (10%) and expose the plate to UV light. The presence of a chlorinated hydrocarbon would be shown by a dark gray spot. Compare with standards on the same plate.

b. *Solvent:* n-hexane:acetone (8:2).
   Developer: Bromine vapors and fluorescein.

	Rf
parathion	0.90
Diazinon	0.89
malathion	0.76

c. *Solvent:* n-hexane:acetone (9:1).
   Developer: Bromine vapors and fluorescein.

	Rf
parathion	0.68
Diazinon	0.81
malathion	0.52
Guthion	0.20

5. *Residue, vomitus, or gastric lavage is extracted with n-hexane or n-heptane* (spectral grade). Filter and scan in UV spectrophotometer with a reference blank of the solvent shaken with water and filtered. See Table XXXIII.

6. *Cholinesterase activity* (H. Michel): Blood is collected in heparinized tubes. *Do not use fluoride!* Separate red blood

TABLE XXXIII

UV Spectrophotometric Scan For Determination

Compound	Solvent	Max Den	$E \begin{smallmatrix} 1cm \\ 1\% \end{smallmatrix}$	Min Den
parathion	hexane	270	347	
	heptane	267	553	232
	ethanol	274	319	235
methyl parathion	hexane	270	377	235
	ethanol	272	319	235
diazinon	hexane	241	130	234
guthion	hexane	288	301	
	ethanol	285	268	261

cells as soon as possible and suspend in isotonic saline.

Centrifuge 5 ml of blood in a graduated tube at 2000 rpm for 15 minutes. Separate plasma. Mix red blood cells with two to three times volume with 0.9% NaCl and again centrifuge at 2000 for about 15 minutes. Discard supernatant fluid and repeat washing with 0.9% NaCl, freshly made. This time centrifuge at 2000 rpm for 20 minutes. Note volume of red blood cells (done in graduated tube). Remove sufficient supernatant fluid so that the exact remaining fluid is equal to the volume of red blood cells (total is about twice volume of red blood cells). Mix cells and fluid thoroughly. Remove 0.4 ml of cell suspension and hemolyze this with 9.6 ml of 0.01% saponin. One (1) ml of hemolyzed solution (RBC = 0.02 ml of original RBC) is added to 1 ml of buffer solution and is placed in a water bath at 25°C for 10 minutes to establish equilibrium. Determine the initial pH to the nearest 0.01 unit (pH_1). Add 0.2 ml of 0.11M acetylcholine solution with rapid mixing and record the exact time. Allow the enzymatic reaction to proceed for exactly $1\frac{1}{2}$ hours. Final pH (pH_2) is determined; record exact time at which pH was measured.

Calculate cholinesterase activity in Δ pH/per hour.

Calculations:

$$\Delta pH/hr = \frac{(pH_1 - pH_2 - b)}{t_2 - t_1} f$$

pH_1 = initial; pH_2 = final; t_1 mix with acetylcholine; t_2 time of pH_2; b = nonenzymatic correction for blank. f =

correction for variations both taken from table by Michel (XXXIV).

Sample

$pH_1 = 8.06; pH_2 = 7.82$

$t_1 = 913; t_2 = 10{:}27 \ (10{:}27 - 9{:}13) = 75 \text{ min} = 1.23 \text{ hr}$

$$\Delta pH/hr = \frac{(8.06 - 7.82) - 0.02}{1.23} \quad \Delta pH/hr = 0.170$$

Michel states the normal mean to be 0.703 Δ pH/hr. To express the Δ pH as % of normal:

$$\frac{0.170}{0.703} \times 100 = 22.6\%$$

However, normal values may have a wide range: 0.40 to 1.00 Δ pH/hr in humans.

TABLE XXXIV

CORRECTION FACTORS FOR USE IN SAMPLE EQUATION

pH_2	b	f
7.9	0.03	0.94
7.8	0.02	0.95
7.7	0.01	0.96
7.6	0.00	0.97
7.5	0.00	0.98
7.4	0.00	0.99
7.3	0.00	1.00
7.2	0.00	1.00
7.1	0.00	1.00
7.0	0.00	1.00
6.8	0.00	0.99
6.6	0.00	0.97
6.2	0.00	0.97
6.0	0.00	0.99

Reagents:

• *Buffer:* Dissolve 0.02M sodium barbital (4.1236 gm), 0.004 M potassium dihydrogen phosphate (0.5446 gm), and 0.60M potassium chloride (44.730 gm) in 900 ml of water. Add 28.0 ml of 0.1N hydrochloric acid while shaking. The volume is brought to exactly 1000 ml with water. pH is exactly 8.10 at

25°C. Add several drops of toluene and keep in refrigerator.

Check buffer before each use because *capacity* decreases after several weeks. If in doubt, discard and remake.

• 0.11M acetylcholine: 2.0 gm acetylcholine chloride in 100 ml water; add 2 drops toluene and keep in refrigerator.

• Acetylcholine perchlorate is perhaps better because it is not hygroscopic and will keep.

COMMENTS. A gradual low exposure to an organic phosphate ester may diminish the cholinesterase activity to a low level (0.2 Δ pH/hr) in man and yet may not produce severe symptoms or toxicity. A sudden large exposure, on the other hand, may also produce a low level (0.2 Δ pH/hr) but this time with severe symptoms and toxicity. Cholinesterase levels therefore must always be associated with symptoms and signs before an accurate evaluation can be made. (Death can occur at 0.10 △ pH/hr, and yet persons have survived with lower levels.)

PITFALLS TO BE AVOIDED IN CHOLINESTERASE DETERMINATION

1. Sample should not be contaminated with fumes or acids or alkali from the air.
2. To obtain good results, you must immediately separate plasma from red blood cells; put the cells in 0.9N saline solution.
3. Separated cells should be kept at 0–5°C because loss in enzyme activity can occur if the samples stay at room temperature for too long.
4. Plasma and the cells are stable for several weeks if kept at 0–5°C.
5. Plasma can be stored for several months in the frozen state.
6. Speed and duration of the centrifugation should be standardized.
7. Prevent overheating of the samples as might occur during centrifugation.
8. Concentration of substrate should be low.
9. Temperature of the reaction mixture during the incubation period should be controlled.

10. It is essential to control the pH of the reaction mixture within narrow limits, otherwise you get variables (check pH buffer before each determination) .
11. The most common source of error lies in the buffer solution. If in doubt, discard it and make fresh.
12. Before each use of the pH meter, the calomel electrodes should be checked to ensure free flow of the KCl.

7. Cholinesterase in blood: Blood drop is diluted in a leukocyte-counting pipette with acetylcholine chlorine. Incubate for 15 minutes at 23°C. Place 1 drop onto a 1.1.% agar gel containing bromthymol blue adjusted to an approximate pH of 8.

Shade of color from dark green to orange around the drop indicates approximate levels of activity.

Various kits are commercially available.

Reference: Davidson-Adie: *Anal Biochem, 12:*70, 1965.

8. *Plasma cholinesterase* (Curry) (paper color test) :
   • Bromthymol blue (0.04%) is made fresh in glass distilled H_2O. Acetyl choline bromide is added to this solution to make 100 mg/ml.
   • Whatman #1 paper is impregnated with this solution; allow to air dry at room temperature. Cut into strips and store in tightly sealed bottles in a dessicator; use within 1 month.
   • Place 2 drops of plasma onto a glass slide; place strip test paper onto this and then another glass slide is placed and pressed (gently) on top to eliminate air bubbles.
   • Record time required for aquamarine color $\rightarrow$ green $\rightarrow$ pale yellow.
   • Blank test paper is tested with 2 drops of pH buffer 5 to establish "normal" blank. This "normally" takes about 5 minutes for color changes at about 23°C.
   • Positive depression of plasma cholinesterase activity may prolong this color change to 30 minutes or more.
   • In testing, always parallel a "normal blank" for comparison.

9. Rapid field tests for cholinesterase:
   TLC plates are made with a cellulose slurry at pH 11.0.
   Development: Water:100% ethanol:$CHCl_3$ (56:42:2) .
   Detection: Human blood plasma for $\frac{1}{2}$ hour; then spray with

reagent. Intense blue spots.

Reagent: 1 part 0.6% bromthymol blue in 0.1N NaOH and 15 parts 1% acetylcholine–HCl in water.

Reference: Menn and Bain: *Nature, 209:*1351, 1966.

Treatment

If early, give activated charcoal and gastric lavage. Of utmost importance is to guard against respiratory difficulties; at all times maintain a patent airway and respiratory exchange. Artificial respiration (and suction) as needed to *clear cyanosis.* IV atropine, 2 mg (slowly), as soon as cyanosis is overcome. Repeat at 5–10 minutes intervals or as *needed;* or until signs of atropinization begins to appear (dry flushed skin, and tachycardia up to 140 per minute). When excessive secretions and symptoms again recur, repeat atropine at intervals as needed (up to about 40 mg/day).

Remove all clothing (use rubber gloves). Wash surfaces with soap and water as soon as supportive measures have been instituted.

Protopam, prolidoxime, or 2-pyridine aldoxime (PAM) 1000 mg IV and repeated several hours later may help to reactivate some cholinesterase. This is of assistance to the atropine but is not sufficient treatment without atropine. Together, they are remarkable.

Favorable response to atropine does not guarantee against sudden and fatal relapse. Mild degree of atropinization should be continued during entire crisis (24–48 hours if necessary). Glucose seems to augment the atropine antidotal action. For the first several hours full atropinization may be vital to counteract cholinergic effect. Carefully watch for cyanosis because of danger of it inducing ventricular fibrillation. Correct this before continuing with atropine.

Atropine dries secretions of the respiratory tract and reduces heart block. Maintain fluid balance (especially monitor fluid intake). Avoid morphine, aminophylline, theophylline, succinylcholine, or phenothiazine.

Symptomatic and supportive treatment.

Symptoms and treatment is generally similar for other parasympatomimetic (cholinergic) agents, except *do not* give PAM

(Protopam) for the *carbamate* group; it is contraindicated and *can be dangerous.*

PENTAZOCINE ($C_{19}H_{14}Cl_2N_2$)

Synonym: Talwin.

Uses: Potent analgesic.

MLD: 500 mg/70 kg person.

APPROXIMATE BLOOD LEVELS: Therapeutic, 0.02 mg/dl; lethal, 0.5 mg/dl (hydrolyzed: 5 mg/dl).

Symptoms: CNS depressant, nausea, vomiting, dizziness, light headedness, euphoria; visual hallucinations are possible; respiratory depression.

Identification

Soluble in water, ethanol, ether, or chloroform. Extract with alkaline-ether. An acid hydrolysis is necessary and can increase sensitivity ten times.

Blood or urine is first hydrolyzed with HCl for about 5–10 minutes in boiling water bath; then alkalinized with (concentrated) NaOH; then extracted with ether; and re-extracted with 0.5N H_2SO_4.

1. UV spectrophotometer (pure) :   See Section I.
    a. 0.5N H_2SO_4: Maximum density, 277 nm; $E_{1cm}^{1\%}$, 70; minimum density 245 nm.
       In an actual case, however, the minimum density is not 245 nm but has shifted to 263 with a different slope.
    b. O.5N NaOH: Maximum density, 298 nm; $E_{1cm}^{1\%}$, 110; minimum density, 278 nm.
2. TLC: See Section I.
    a. Methanol: NH_4OH (100:1.5)
    b. Ethyl acetate: methanol:NH_4OH:H_2O (85:13.5:0.5:1) Rf 81.
3. GLC: See Section I.

Treatment

Emesis or gastric lavage, maintain all vital signs and especially respiratory exchange and water balance. Oxygen as needed. Supportive and symptomatic treatment. Treatment generally similar as for morphine. Naloxone reported to be useful. Supportive!

PHENCYCLIDINE

Synonyms: Phenylcyclohexypiperidine (PCP); Sernylan; "PeaCe Pill"; "Angel dust"; HOG; "cyclone"; "superwood"; mintweed; elephant or horse tranquilizer; "rocket fuel"; "goon"; "surfer"; "scuffle."

Uses: Alleged as an analgesic or anesthetic but too risky because it may produce many toxic side effects. The therapeutic index (margin of safety) is very low; the risks are too great for the questionable benefit. It is smoked sprinkled on marihuana or parsley leaves in a "joint"; it is taken by mouth; it is snorted in doses of 5–100 mg each trip. Chronic users might take from 100 mg up to 1 gm in 24 hours.

MLD: Approximately 500 mg or more/70 kg person. Lethal blood level:0.05 mg/dl.

Symptoms

Acute intoxication is usually very unpleasant; time and distance is distorted; stagger as though drunk; feeling of extreme anxiety with fear of impending doom or death.

Effects are stronger than marihuana; more comparable with LSD but different. Great variability exists in effects. Some report distinct euphoria and others report marked depression. Symptoms in general may vary with dose and frequency or use, even in the same person.

At relatively low doses (5 mg leading to a serum level of about 25 ng/ml), patient may show agitation, excitement, incoordination, catatonic rigidity, catalepsy, inability to speak, horizontal or vertical nystagmus, no pain to pinprick, flushing, diaphoresis, bizarre behavior, hostility, disorientation, drowsiness, apathy (like drunk); later may be amnesic.

At moderate dose (10 mg leading to a serum level of 50–100 ng/ml), Aronow and Done describe coma or stupor with eyes open, nystagmus, vomiting, hypersalivation, muscle rigidity on stimulation, flushing, diaphoresis, fever, decreased peripheral sensations (pain, touch, and position), local anesthetic, delirium, hallucinations, paranoid delusions, schizophrenia.

At high doses (over 10 mg leading to serum levels over 100 ng/ml), Aronow and Done describe prolonged coma, eyes closed with variable pupil size but reactive, hypertension, decerebrate positioning, muscular rigidity, convulsions, absent peripheral sensations, decreased or absent gag and corneal reflexes, diaphoresis, hypersalivation, laryngeal spasm, flushing, fever, possible death.

If large amounts were ingested, PCP will be present in the urine for several days.

Identification

Alkaline-chloroform extraction. Urine is best specimen:

Urine (25 ml) is adjusted to alkaline with sodium carbonnate and then extracted four times with equal volume of chloroform. Combine, filter, and add 2 drops of hydrochloric acid and then evaporate the chloroform to dryness (with great care).

Parsley (.5 gm) is triturated with 0.1N HCl and extracted with 4 × 25 ml of chloroform. Evaporate, reconstitute with ethanol.

Tablets are weighed and then dissolved in methanol. Centrifuge, separate, evaporate solvent.

1. UV Spectrophotometry: See Section I. 0.5N H_2SO_4 maximum density, 251, 257, 262, 268, minimum density, 237, 245–247 (shoulder), 253, 260, 267.

    Curve in ethanol is the same and more sensitive. Curve in chloroform is approximately the same as in H_2SO_4.

2. TLC See Section I.
   * $CHCl_3$:ethanol:acetone:H_2O (40:36:20:4). Rf 85
   * Hexane:ethyl acetate:ethanol (70:25:5). Rf 80
   * Methanol:NH_4OH (100:1.5). Rf 60
   * Butyl ether:diethyl ether:diethylamine (45:45:10)
   Spray: Iodoplatinate

3. GLC: SE-30—3%; or 3% OV-1 on Chromosorb W. 4 feet by $\frac{1}{4}$ inch stainless steel; isothermal at 214°C, injection at 232°C, detector at 245°C.
   Also see Section I.

Treatment

Supportive and symptomatic. Maintain respiratory exchange and patent airway; guard against respiratory depression, convulsions, hypersecretions and coma. Acidification of urine (below pH 5) (with NH_4Cl) will hasten excretion of PCP. Guard against hypersecretions in the pharynx, hyperthermia, and hypertension. If it is *necessary* to administer tranquilizers, *do not use phenothiazines;* haloperidol (Haldol) have been reported of use (5 mg 1M) repeatedly hourly until under control.

Screen for the concomitant presence of other drugs and treat accordingly. Generally supportive.

References

Aronow, R. and Done, A.: Phenylcyclidine overdose. *J Am Coll Emer Phys, 7:*56, 1978.

Gupta, R.C., Lu, I., Lee Oei G., and Lundberg, G.D.: *Clin Tox, 8:*611, 1975.

Munch, J.C.: *Bull Narcotics, 26:*9, 1974.

Petersen, R.C. and Stillman, R.C.: Phenylcyclidine: A review, *Newsletter of the National Institute on Drug Abuse,* no date (1978).

PHENACETIN ($C_{10}H_{13}NO_2$)

Synonyms: Phenetids, *p*-acetophenetidin.

Uses: Antipyretic, analgesic.

Properties: Neutral, bitter, insoluble in water. White crystalline. Mp 135°C. Soluble in ether or $CHCl_3$.

MLD: Approximately 5 gm/70 kg person.

Remarks: Death may be sudden or delayed for several days. Cardiac patients seem to be especially susceptible. Frequent and continued use may cause serious blood disturbances. Rapidly metabolized in part to acetaminophen.

Symptoms: Skin eruptions and rashes; swelling of face, eyelids, forehead and upper parts of cheek. Bright yellow urine, cyanosis, methemoglobinemia, cold extremities, diaphoresis, anemia, muscular weakness, weak pulse, dyspnea, hypotension, lowered body temperature, jaundice, nephritis, collapse, shock.

Identification

Acid-ether extraction group.

1. Urine is intensely yellow. Reduces Fehling's solution.

2. To 10 ml of urine, add 1 ml of ferric chloride (10%) → brown-red color that changes to bluish green.
3. Positive indophenol test. Dissolve a small portion of residue in 1 ml of hot 10% hydrochloric acid; add 1 ml of saturated aqueous solution of phenol. A freshly prepared solution of calcium hypochlorite is added dropwise. A dirty red-violet color appears on shaking. Add ammonia and deep blue color is produced. This test is also positive for acetanilid.
4. Phosphomolybdic acid gives a yellow precipitate with both acetanilid and phenacetin. To differentiate, precipitate plus heat → dissolves acetanilid; Phenacetin is undissolved.
5. Small aliquot of acid-ether residue is boiled with 5 drops of hydrochloric acid for 5 minutes. Filter and dilute with equal amounts of water. To cold filtrate, add 5 drops of potassium dichromate (10%).
   phenacetin → ruby red color
   acetanilid → yellow color which turns green
6. Small aliquot of residue plus 1 ml of sulfuric acid plus 1 ml of ethyl alcohol and gently warm on steam bath → ethyl acetate, which has a characteristic odor.
7. When boiled with 10% nitric acid → mononitroacetophenetidin, which is fine-needle yellow crystals (mp 103°C) after repurification with hot and cold water.
8. Test for methemoglobin in blood; method described under Aniline.
9. UV Spectrophotometry: See Section I.
10. TLC: See Section I.
11. GLC: See Section I.

Treatment

Gastric lavage with charcoal. Emetics. Cathartics (sodium sulfate, 30 gm with large amounts of water).

Ascorbic acid and methylene blue for methemoglobinemia, if needed. See Aniline.

Artificial respiration and oxygen therapy for cyanosis. Keep patient quiet and warm. Combat shock or collapse. Blood exchange transfusion if indicated. Support against kidney and liver damage. See Aniline and Acetaminophen.

PHENOLS (C_6H_5OH)

Synonyms or Derivatives: Carbolic acid; cresols (*o, m, p*); thymol, catechol, menthol, resorcinol are quite toxic; naphthol, hexylresorcinol less toxic; tannic acid least toxic. Creosotes (wood tar or coal tar). Camphophenique (with camphor); "carnica."

Uses: Disinfectant, preservative, antiseptic, antipruritic, industry.

Properties: White, crystalline, hygroscopic, volatile, slightly soluble in water, corrosive to skin, mp 43°C, absorbed (rapidly) through all portals.

MLD: Approximately 8 gms/70 kg person.

Symptoms: Characteristic odor of phenol, severe gastrointestinal irritation and corrosion, nausea, vomiting, white burns, local anesthetic and edema on lips and mouth. Profuse sweating, thirst, abdominal pain, diarrhea, dizziness, headache, tinnitus. Weak irregular pulse, vaso motor depressor (VMD), hypotension, shallow respiration, cyanosis, fall in body temperature. Brown-purple urine (metabolite *p*-aminophenol), albuminuria, hematuria. Kidney and liver and bladder involvement, oliguria, acidosis, pulmonary edema, convulsions or excitement, depression, followed by coma. Death due to respiratory, circulatory, or cardiac failure.

Identification

Steam distill (with tartaric acid) or acid chloroform extraction. Cannot be tested with certainty 10 or more hours after exposure.

1. Typical carbolic acid odor. Color of urine:
   phenol, brown-purple;
   salol (phenyl salicylate) or creosote or resorcinol, dirty green; pyrogallol, brown-black.
2. To 10 ml of urine, add 1 ml of 10% ferric chloride → purple color. (Color persists with heat).
3. Boil 10 ml of urine with Millon's reagent → red color.

   Reagent: Millon's: Dissolve 10 gm of mercury in 20 ml of nitric acid. Dilute with an equal amount of distilled water. Allow to stand 2 hours. Decant.

4. Urine or blood (5 ml) made slightly acid with 1 drop of 10% HCl is extracted with 35 ml of chloroform. Separate and then re-extract with 5 ml of 0.5N NaOH and read in UV (very sensitive). See Section I.

    a. H_2O Maximum density, 270 nm; $E_{1cm}^{1\%}$, 147; minimum density 238 nm.

    b. NaOH, 0:5N: 1% maximum density, 234, 286, 370; $E_{1cm}^{1\%}$, 1100; minimum density, 260.

5. Isolate by Conway microdiffusion. Sodium hydroxide 10% is used as absorbent. React with Folin phenol reagent → blue. See Section I.

6. To differentiate between carbolic acid and other phenols, extract material with 25 ml of chloroform; add a little solid potassium hydroxide and warm:

    carbolic acid → red

    naphthols → blue

    thymol → dark red

7. Bromine water is added to distillate or an aqueous solution of the suspected residue until the fluid is permanently yellow. If phenol is present, small yellowish white crystalline stars or needles of tribromophenol separate out (mp 94°C).

8. Ammonium hydroxide is added to the distillate in the pro-portion 1:4 and 2 to 5 drops of freshly prepared solution of sodium hypochlorite, plus heat → blue color.

9. Phenol plus nitric acid → picric acid. Shake with ether and evaporate (mp 122.5°C).

10. Sulfuric acid plus potassium nitrite (KNO_2) → intense colors → brown → green → blue → red.

Treatment

Prompt action is necessary because response is rapid even when absorbed through skin. Carefully wash all exposed parts with water. If patient is conscious, give activated charcoal then care-fully remove by gastric lavage; olive or castor or vegetable oils have been used and egg white or milk as demulcent. Guard against acidosis, convulsions, and systemic action on heart and res-piration. Monitor all vital signs, including respiratory exchange, cardiovascular, blood pressure, heat; electrolyte, acid-base and water balance.

Guard against shock; morphine for pain; sodium sulfate as saline cathartic. Guard against kidney, liver, and bladder involvement. General supportive measures.

PHENOTHIAZINE DERIVATIVES
Members

	USUAL DOSE (oral)*	BLOOD LEVELS: Therapeutic (T) Lethal (L)
I. *Dimethyl* side chain chlorpromazine-HCl (Thorazine)	10–100 mg, t.i.d.	T, 0.05 mg% L, 0.5 mg%
promazine-HCl (Sparine)	50–100 mg, t.i.d.	L, 0.2 mg%
triflupromazine-HCl (Vesprin)	10 mg, t.i.d.	
II. *Piperazine* side chain prochlorperazine maleate (Compazine)	10–30 mg, t.i.d.	L, 0.2 mg%
perphenazine (Trilafon)	4–8 mg, t.i.d.	L, 0.1 mg%
fluphenazine-HCl (Prolixin) (Permitil)	0.5–3 mg, t.i.d.	
trifluoperazine-HCl (Stelazine)	2–5 mg, t.i.d.	
thiopropazate-HCl (Dartal)	10 mg, t.i.d.	
carphenazine maleate (Proketazine)	25–50 mg, t.i.d.	

*Physicians Desk Reference.

III. *Piperidine* side chain

thioridazine		T, 0.15 mg%
(Mellaril))	25–150 mg, t.i.d.	L, 2 mg%
mesoridazine		
(Serentil)	25–75 mg, t.i.d.	
mepazine-HCl		
(Pacatal)	25–50 mg, t.i.d.	

IV. *Antiemetics*
    (many of the above plus)

pipamazine	
(Mornidine)	5 mg, t.i.d.
thiethylperazine	
(Torecan)	20 mg, daily

V. *Antipruretics*
    (some of the above plus)

trimeprazine	
(Temaril)	2.5 mg, t.i.d.
methdilazine-HCl	
(Tocaryl)	8 mg, t.i.d.

MLD: Fatal (acute) dose varies widely with derivative. Approximately 15–150 mg/kg is suggested, although severe symptoms have developed with less.

Remarks

The phenothiazine group depresses the central nervous system. It enhances or potentiates the effect of (some) other central nervous system depressants and therefore should not be used in conjunction with morphine or other similar narcotics, barbiturates or other similar hypnotics, alcohol, or antihistaminics. Avoid preoperative use because severe hypotension has occurred during general anesthesia.

There is no apparent drug abuse or any accompanying "evil"

effects in spite of its great use. There is no "drug dependency" or withdrawal symptoms as such. However, abrupt withdrawal of drug following high dose therapy can produce discomfort and symptoms such as gastritis, nausea, vomiting, dizziness, and tremulousness. This can be avoided or minimized by a gradual withdrawal of drug, or by concomitant anti-Parkinsonism agents.

The phenothiazines are an excellent antipsychotic, but should not be given "indiscriminately" to the elderly (especially women).

Members of the piperazine group are generally more potent and toxic; they produce more extrapyramidal tract symptoms but less agranulocytosis, jaundice, and hepatitis than chlorpromazine. The aged (women) and children are more likely to show the dyskinesia effects.

The dimethyl group is generally less potent or toxic. There are fewer extrapyramidal effects but some danger of agranulocytosis and hepatitis. Chlorpromazine is the more widely used; triflupromazine is most potent of this group.

The piperidine group is generally least toxic, producing fewer side reactions. Thioridazine is perhaps the safest for the elderly; it produces relatively little extrapyramidal toxicity and there has been no reported jaundice or agranulocytosis; dermatitis is rare, but pigmentation of the retina has been reported by excessive use. Mesoridazine is more potent than thioridazine and is more' likely to produce hypotension. Mesazine may occasionally cause agranulocytosis and hepatitis.

In general, potency in position 2 is (from least to most) hydrogen, sulfur, chlorine, fluorine.

There has been an occasional report of "sudden death" with phenothiazines. In some cases, the cause appeared to be asphyxia due to failure of the cough reflex; in others, the cause was not clear.

PHARMACOKINETICS: Absorbed easily and quickly and is generally distributed widely. Rapidly becomes protein bound; partly destroyed in the liver and partly eliminated as the sulfoxide derivative in the urine. Fairly rapid onset of action, and it may still be detected in tissue even several weeks or more after high intake.

Symptoms

ACUTE: CNS depression, sedation, drowsiness, ataxia, apathy, nausea, fever, antiemetic, anticholinergic; dilated pupils, blurred vision, dry mouth, urinary retention, tachycardia. Chilliness, constipation, stuffy nose, hypotension, coma, edema, E.K.G. changes, ventricular arrhythmias, respiratory depression.

Stimulates the extrapyramidal system (Parkinsonism); depresses the hypothalamus; convulsions occur with very high doses.

Synergistic action with other CNS depressants such as alcohol, morphine, barbiturates, other hypnotics, analgesics, and general anesthesia.

GENERAL SIDE REACTION*

(1). Bone marrow depression with agranulocytosis: more frequent with the chlorpromazine group (but rare); less common with prochlorperazine group; no reported cases in the thioridazine group.

(2). Extrapyramidal tract symptoms: Withdraw drug, and control with anti-Parkinson drugs. Incidence is more common with the young and aged and also more usual with females.

Parkinsonism is more usually seen in the old and may be patient-related and dose-related and can occur at any time after conventional dosage. However, the larger the dose, the greater the incidence. The signs are similar to the classic illness, i.e. reduction in facial movement and arm movements followed by the typical shuffling gait and pill-rolling hand movements, tremulousness (spastic-jerky constant movements at rest). Reduction of dosage and/or anti-Parkinsonism drugs will help.

Acute dystonic reaction comes on suddenly and consists of bizarre muscle spasms that could be confused with tetany or hysteria. The muscles of the head and neck are mostly affected, producing an involuntary spasm of tongue and mouth muscles. These spasms may affect speech and swallowing; the mouth may be clamped shut with facial grimacing. There may also be spasm of the external ocular muscles with persistent painful upward gaze

*Task Force of FDA and the American College of Neuropharmacology: *N E J Med, 289*:20, 1973.

(for minutes to hours). The arms and leg muscles, although less frequently affected, can produce bizarre gait and difficulty in walking.

This acute reaction usually occurs 24 to 48 hours after starting medication. This can be dose-related and is noted to occur more often in the young and in males.

These reactions, although acute and violent in appearance, are easily treated by parenteral administration of antihistamines, barbiturates, and anti-Parkinsonism drugs. Response is usually dramatic.

Akathisia causes a desire to be in continuous motion with a restlessness, agitation, and an inability to sit or stand still. This may occur near the onset of treatment and therefore can easily be confused with a psychotic agitation, which could lead to continued or increased dosage. Anti-Parkinsonism agents may produce an immediate response.

Tardive dyskinesia can appear within a month or more of medication, but more usually it occurs after several years of treatment. It is more likely in the elderly and in women, and with patients with a history of some brain injury.

The most frequent signs are the "bucco-linguo-masticary triad," i.e. sucking and smacking movements of the lips, lateral jaw movements and puffing of the cheeks, with the tongue thrusting, rolling, or making fly-catching movements. This may be done with the mouth closed—the tongue hits the inside of the cheeks and a chewing-the-cud type of movement is seen.

Sometimes there is a ticlike movement of the lips and eyes; rocking, swaying, or restless limb movements may precede this. Symptoms of Parkinsonism also can coexist with tardive dyskinesia.

Tardive dyskinesia, which has a *very* late onset, should not be confused with acute dystonic reaction, which has a rapid onset. In many cases the tardive dyskinesia will be masked during dosage and thus will only be seen when the drug is stopped or dosage is markedly reduced. The reaction will be again masked when the drug dosage is resumed; it may get worse during emotional stress and disappear during sleep. Persistence of the symptoms after the drug is discontinued are characteristic manifestations.

(3). Hypotension may be more marked, especially when given parenterally or in patients who received general anesthesia following Chlorpromazine administration.

(4). Hepatitis: intrahepatic obstructive jaundice: chlorpromazine (Thorazine) group is more frequently involved; prochlorperazine (Compazine) group is less frequently involved; thioridazine (Mellaril) group is least frequently involved.

(5). Dermatitis is possible with exposure to sun (photosensitive).

Identification

Insoluble in chloroform. Blood is not as satisfactory as urine, bile, or liver; becomes protein bound and requires acid-hydrolysis to free the phenothiazine; requires NaOH ether extraction; should be extracted without delay. Chloroform is ineffective as solvent.

1. Simple, direct, color-screening tests
   a. To 1 ml of urine add 6 drops of sulfuric acid and 2 drops of 10% ferric chloride. A light pink to purple color indicates a positive reaction for a phenothiazine compound. Salicylates do not interfere.
   b. To 1 ml of urine add 1 ml of FPN. Read within 20 seconds. Phenylketonuria or impaired liver may give false positive reactions.
      (1) Chlorine derivatives → *pink*
         Compazine (prochlorperazine)
         Dartal (thiopropazate)
         Mornidine (pipamazine)
         Sparine (promazine) → pink-orange
         Tacaryl (methdilazine)
         Temaril (trimeprazine)
         Thorazine (chlorpromazine)
         Torecan (thiethylperazine)
         Trilafon (perphenazine)
      (2) Fluoride derivatives → *amber-flesh*
         Prolixin (fluphenazine)
         Permitil (fluphenazine)
         Stelazine (trifluoperazine)
         Vesprin (triflupramazine)

(3) Sulfur derivatives

Pacatal (mepazine) → pink

Mellaril (thioridazine) → blue (in large amounts)

(4) Tricylic antidepressants also give a positive FPN color. See under Tricyclic antidepressants.

Tofranil (imipramine) → green to blue

Norpramine (desipramine) → blue

Reagent: FPN.* 5 ml of 5% $FeCl_3$ + 45 ml of $HClO_4$ + 50 ml of 50% HNO_3.

2. Fifteen (15) ml of urine plus 15 ml HCl is gently hydrolyzed (with a watchglass lid) for 5 minutes on a water bath (boiling). Cool and then bring to *alkalinity* by carefully adding 50% NaOH, which was previously washed with ether. Cool and then extract with 2 × 50 ml of ether. Each portion is filtered to remove water droplets.

The combined ether extract is extracted with 5 ml of 0.5N H_2SO_4. This H_2SO_4 extract is transferred and examined by the following methods

Note: Extractions *cannot* be made with $CHCl_3$ alone, nor with $CHCl_3$ isopropanol because this gives false positive in UV curve; putrefaction also interferes (J.R. Rodriguez).

a. UV spectrophotometry (very sensitive) (See Section I): Urine, liver slurry, or blood is first hydrolyzed as described. Ether is the extracting solvent of choice.

Compare the maximum and minimum absorption spectra and quantitate by reference to standard curve ($E_{1cm}^{1\%}$) (Table XXXV). Range 350 to 220 nm. Solution is saved for further confirmation by following methods.

b. Thin Layer Chromatography (TLC): See Section I.

To the above 0.5N H_2SO_4 extract, add dropwise dilute NaOH to make it definitely alkaline. Extract with about 30 ml of ether. Separate and gently evaporate ether to dryness. Pick up residue with minimal amount of alcohol and spot it on a silica gel glass plate in the usual manner. On the same plate, spot several standards of possible suspected compounds. Allow to run until the solvent front reaches exactly

---

*Forrest and Forrest: *Clin Chem*, 6:11, 1960.

TABLE XXXV

	Minima	$E\,^{1\%}_{1cm}$	Maxima
Compazine	305		279
(prochlorperazine)	254	820	225
Dartal	305		278
(thiopropazate)	254	630	
Mellaril	310		285
(thioridazine)	263	1000	
Mornidine	304		278
(pipamazine)	254	800	225
Pacatal	301		
(mepazine)	253	930	275
Paraflex	290		264
(chlorzoxazone)	246	580	229
Phenergan	298		275
(promethazine)	249	980	
	265		263
Preludin	260		258
(phenmetrazine)	255	10	252
	249		228
Prolixin; Permitil	305		278
(fluphenazine)	255	660	
Sparine	300		227
(promazine)	252	820	278
Stelazine	304		278
(trifluoperazine)	255	680	
Thorazine	305		227
(chlorpromazine)	254	950	224
Tofranil	250	360	231
(imipramine)			
Trilafon	305		278
(perphenazine)	254	820	225
Vesprin	304		
(triflupromazine)	255	820	279

the 10 cm line (previously measured off). Examine and compare spots under UV light. Record colors and approximate Rf. Then spray with appropriate reagents: record resulting colors and exact Rf (Table XXXVI)

First view under UV light for color, location, and Rf. Then spray with 5% H_2SO_4, or FPN, or with iodoplatinic acid reagent.

TABLE XXXVI

	Solvents #								5% H_2SO_4	Colors When Sprayed with FPN	$PdCl_2$
	1	2	3	4	5	6	7	8			
chlorpromazine (Thorazine)	76	69	75	62	35	63	54	62	pink	pink	purple
prochlorperazine (Compazine)	40	34	51	45	20	63	40	63	pink	pink	purple
fluphenazine (Permitil)	18	84	6	68	48	80	70	75	flesh	flesh (fades)	flesh
	15	85			30						
(Proloxin)	100	85	67		60		52	50	flesh	flesh (fades)	flesh
imipramine (Tofranil)	76	65	86	60	45		70	56	white y-G border	white with blue border	light yellow
mepazine (Pacatal)		12	76			88		58	orange	orange	purple
perphenazine (Trilafon)	16			55	40	73	57		pink	pink	orange
pipamazine (Mornidine)	11	81	91	75	58	80	76	72	pink	pink	purple
promazine (Sparine)	75	51		52	30	47	50		orange	orange	purple
thioridazine (Mellaril)	68	74	65	60	35	62	62	56	turquoise	turquoise	purple
chlordiazepoxide (Librium)	60			85	75	79					
trifluperazine (Stelazine)	54	57	55	55	35	68	50		flesh	flesh	flesh
triflupromazine (Vesprin)	84	79	78	70	55	67	80	65	flesh	flesh	flesh
amitriptyline (Elavil)	82	69	87	58	35	58	55	52	white	flesh	yellow
desipramine (Norpramine)	24		36		40	34				blue	

Solvents, see Table XXXXVI.

1. • Benzene:acetone:NH_4OH (100:20:6). (Paulus.) Shake in a separatory funnel to saturate. Settle and discard excess NH_4OH.
2. • Pyridine:petroleum ether:chloroform (45:68:4.5). (Machata from Eberthardt.)
3. • Cyclohexane:diethylamine (90:10). (Sunshine.)
4. • Acetone:methanol:isopropylamine (170:30:2)
5. • Acetone:methanol:isopropanol (170:30:2).
6. • Methanol:NH_4OH:chloroform (400:5:36). (Steele.)
7. • Ethanol:water:acetic acid (20:20:1). (Clark-Cole.)
8. • Methanol:NH_4OH (100:1:5). (Sunshine.)

Other solvent developers
• Chloroform:diethylamine (9:1). (Sunshine.)
• Chloroform:ethanol (7:3). (Moza.)
• Methanol:acetone:triethanolamine (50:50:1.5). (Ganshirt in Stahl from Baumler and Rippstein.)
Spray: Iodoplatinate yields a purple spot in most cases.
c. Colors and crystals (see Alkaloids)
   (1) Marquis → purple color
   (2) Thorazine → positive with Wagners, Mayers, Picric acid
   (3) Compazine → negative with Wagners, Mayers, Picric acid
d. Gas liquid chromatography (GC): See Section I.

Treatment

Withdrawal of drug, gastric lavage, intestinal purge; try emetics, but they may not work due to antiemetic action of the phenothiazine. Keep patient in horizontal position to minimize postural hypotension. Maintain heat, water, electrolyte balance, and respiratory exchange.

Combat shock. Stimulants are to be avoided. Control convulsions or excitement carefully with Valium or short-acting barbiturates; avoid other depressants.

There is no specific treatment other than symptomatic and supportive. Physostigmine salicylates may help for anticholinergic symptoms.

Supportive measures for possible liver damage and agranulocytosis. Parkinsonlike symptoms may be relieved with Cogentin or Benadryl. Guard against arrhythmias (monitor).

Thorazine (and others) are strongly bound to blood proteins, and dialysis has been reported as not very effective.

Supportive measures.

PHOSPHORIC ACID (H_3PO_4)

Uses: Industry, tile cleaner, copper and metal polish, rust remover; Meracid.

Properties: Oily, heavy, colorless, liquid.

MLD: Approximately 8 ml/70 kg person.

Remarks: Powerful acid. Ortho, syrupy phosphoric (85%).

Symptoms: Burns on mouth and lips, sour acrid taste, severe gastrointestinal irritation, nausea, vomiting, bloody diarrhea, difficult swallowing, severe abdominal pains, thirst, acidemia, difficult breathing, convulsions, collapse, shock, death.

Identification

In stomach contents. (dilute & filter)
1. Neutralize specimen with ammonium hydroxide and then add 2 ml of dilute lead acetate (10%) → heavy white precipitate of lead phosphate.
2. Turns blue litmus paper pink.
3. Add 2 ml of silver nitrate (10%) → a yellow heavy precipitate, which is soluble often after adding 1 ml of nitric acid.
4. Add 2 ml of ammonium molybdate solution and 1 cc of nitric acid and gently heat for 1 minute. This will produce a canary yellow precipitate (specific test).

Treatment

Avoid stomach tube if strong acid or severe tissue damage is evident. *Avoid* alkalies such as bicarbonate or carbonate for internal use.

Neutralize with limewater, milk of magnesia, soap suds, Cremalin, or Amphogel. Demulcents such as cream, milk, white of egg, oils.

Keep patient warm and quiet. Cracked ice to relieve thirst.

If there are signs of asphyxia, tracheotomy may be necessary.
If burns are external, wash with large amounts of water and
then apply sodium bicarbonate to make a paste.

Morphine for pain; combat shock; guard against secondary
infection. Symptomatic and supportive measures.

PHOSPHORUS

Synonym: Yellow phosphorus.

Uses: Rat or roach paste, "Pasta electrica," J-O, electric paste,
matches, fireworks.

Properties: Volatile; garlic odor; flammable. Gives off fumes;
luminescent in the dark.

MLD: Approximately 0.1 gm/70 kg person.

Remarks: Yellow phosphorus is very toxic; red phosphorus is
relatively nontoxic. Zinc phosphide is very toxic.

Symptoms: Gastric symptoms may be immediate or delayed
several hours. Nausea, vomiting, bloody diarrhea (strong corrosive). Possible death from severe shock within several hours.
Jaundice, nausea, and vomiting increases, hypoprothrombinemia,
hematuria, tender enlarged liver, skin eruptions, great prostration, greatly reduced blood pressure, dyspnea, albuminuria, increased blood coagulation time, petechial hemorrhages, nephritis,
renal and hepatic insufficiency, or acute yellow atrophy of liver
may develop after 24 to 60 hours. Convulsions, depression, delirium, coma, collapse, death (may be delayed several days).

Chronic symptoms are similar to above but less severe; necrosis of lower jaw (glass jaw), poor dental hygiene, brittle bones.

Identification

A garlic odor with white fumes coming off.

1. Ground liver or stomach contents (5 gm) is placed in an
   Erlenmeyer flask with 10 ml of water. Two strips of filter
   paper are impregnated: one with silver nitrate (10%) and the
   other with lead acetate (10%). These both are suspended and
   supported with a cork in the flask. Gently heat at about 50°C
   for 5–10 minutes. The presence of yellow phosphorus, even in
   traces, would darken the silver nitrate paper. Hydrogen sulfide

or formaldehyde or other volatile organic compounds if present will also give a positive test. The hydrogen sulfide can be detected by odor and the darkening of the lead acetate paper. The formaldehyde can be detected by odor and by the chromotropic acid test.

2. Ground liver or stomach contents (25 gm), plus 25 ml of water, acidified with tartaric acid, is steam distilled into 5 ml of 0.1N silver nitrate. Continue to distill until no more brownblack clumpy silver phosphide precipitate is formed.

During this distillation, darken the room and notice the very pretty green phosphorescence flickering up and down the condenser.

When the distillation is stopped, allow the Ag_3P to clump; then gently decant off the liquid and excess silver nitrate. Rinse once with minimal (1–2 ml) water and again carefully decant to remove excess $AgNO_3$.

Transfer the clumpy silver phosphide to a Gutzeit apparatus as described under Arsenic. Impregnate a paper disc with mercuric bromide and connect with flanges. Connect a cotton trap impregnated with saturated lead acetate. To the Ag_3P, add a few small pieces of pure mossy zinc and 10 ml of 15% sulfuric acid. Attach all parts and allow phosphine to generate (usually about 30 minutes is sufficient). A canary yellow disc confirms the presence of yellow phosphorus. The intensity of this yellow disc may be compared with standards similarly prepared. This is sensitive to about 20 μg of phosphorus. All reagents must be reagent-grade, and a reagent blank must be established first.

The formation of H_2 (action of H_2SO_4 on Zn) must proceed slowly. If too rapid, dip the apparatus into an ice bath to slow it down. If the blank shows that H_2S in excess is getting through, then lead acetate solution in a small bubbling trap is necessary. See Arsenic.

3. The above test can be performed directly on 5 to 10 gm of ground liver using nitrogen as the carrier gas (Schwartz). Phosphine or zinc phosphide is easily liberated; yellow phosphorus may require gentle heat (Curry).

Treatment

Physician should use rubber gloves. Gastric lavage with 250 mg of copper sulfate (several small portions with caution). or emetics; mineral oil followed by sodium sulfate (in water) with caution. Wash external surfaces with plenty of water and treat burns. Do not use oil demulcents. Calcium gluconate (4–10 ml of 10% IV). Support against possible liver damage with low-fat and high-carbohydrate intake. Avoid fats or oils. Calcium salts and B complex vitamins, vitamins K and C may be helpful. Morphine for pain.

Keep airways open. Maintain body heat, fluids, and electrolyte balance; prevent and support against shock. Sodium bicarbonate for acidosis; antibiotics for secondary infection. Supportive and symptomatic treatment.

Recovery may be slow; especially support against shock and liver involvement. Guarded prognosis for several weeks.

PHYSOSTIGMINE ($C_{15}H_{21}N_3O_2$)

Synonyms: Eserine, generally as the sulfate or *salicylate*. Calabar beans of *Physostigma venenosum*. Neostigmine is similar in action.

Uses: Treatment of myasthenia gravis; and curare, atropine-like drugs, phenothiazines, tricyclic antidepressant, and antihistamine poisoning. Diagnostic agent for some neurological disorders, and for anticholinergic action.

Properties: Basic, can be crystallized from benzene. Mp 105° C. Soluble in ether or ethanol. Strong alkali destroys it.

MLD: Approximately 60 mg/70 kg person.

Remarks: Parasympathomimetic (cholinergic), see Parathion.

Symptoms: Parasympathomimetic stimulation, constriction of pupils, dizziness, vertigo, weakness, vomiting, violent purging, cramps, nystagmus, sweating, salivation, lacrimation, bradycardia, pulmonary edema, fall in blood pressure, muscular twitching, bronchoconstriction, dyspnea, collapse, death due to respiratory failure or cardiac paralysis. See Muscarine.

Identification

Use sodium bicarbonate (avoid sodium hydroxide) in chloroform extraction. Ether extract yields a gum rather than crystals.

1. To 5 mg of residue or solution, add 2 drops of ammonia. Evaporate on steam bath → blue residue. When dissolved in alcohol → red fluorescent solution upon addition of 1 ml of acetic acid.
2. To 5 ml of saturated solution of physostigmine salicylate, add 2 drops of sodium hydroxide (10%) → pink color appears immediately.
3. Physostigmine solution plus 10 drops of ferric chloride (10%) → deep violet color.
4. a. Wagner's reagent → brown precipitate
   b. Mayer's reagent → white precipitate (Mp 70°C)
   c. picric acid → yellow precipitate (only in concentrated solution), Mp 114°C
   d. benzoic acid → benzoate (Mp 115°C). Examine for characteristic crystals.
   Refer to Alkaloids.
5. Color reactions. See Alkaloids.
   a. nitric acid → yellow → olive green → red
   b. nitric acid plus sulfuric acid → yellow → red
   c. Mandelin's reagent → green-yellow → yellow-brown (by heat)
   d. Mecke's reagent → brown-yellow → light red (by heat)
6. Physiologic test: 1 drop in cat's eye → constricted pupils. Very sensitive (0.001 mg).
7. UV spectrophometry; TLC; see Section I.

Treatment

Keep patient fully atropinized during entire crisis (give intravenously). This especially is for control of respiratory symptoms (pulmonary edema and bronchial constriction). Glucose when given with atropine appears to augment antidotal action. *Avoid morphine, aminophylline,* or *theophylline!* Use gloves when giving treatment. Remove all of patient's clothing; wash skin with soap and water (or water and sodium bicarbonate) if there has been skin contact.

Induce vomiting, perform gastric lavage if stomach is distended, use Levine tube) , if early and in absence of convulsions.

Oxygen therapy and artificial respiration as needed. Keep patient quiet and comfortable. Watch patient constantly; need of artificial respiration may develop suddenly. Acute emergency may last 24 to 48 hours.

Favorable response to one dose of atropine does not guarantee against sudden and fatal relapse. Atropine must be continued during entire emergency, in absence of cyanosis.

PAM plus the atropine therapy has been used as a means of treatment in man. These agents reverse the cholinesterase inhibition and neuromuscular block caused by the organic phosphate ester. See under Parathion.

PICROTOXIN ($C_{30}H_{34}O_{13}$)

Synonyms: Cocculin. Fish-berry (cocculus) and coriamyrtin are chemically and symptomatically related.

Uses: Central nervous system stimulant.

Properties: Shining prismatic crystals, very bitter, neutral. Mp 199–203 °C.

MLD: Approximately 30 mg/70 kg person.

Remarks: Deaths have occurred from antidotal use in suspected barbiturate poisoning when barbiturates were not present. Also its antidotal effects may set in late and persist and may be dangerous.

Symptoms: Mental confusion, restlessness and apprehension, respiratory center stimulation, excitement, dyspnea, muscular rigidity, dilated pupils, vomiting, palpitation. Bulbar convulsant (clonic) , asymmetrical, irregular convulsive seizures. Respiratory failure, stupor, and unconsciousness followed again by the convulsions.

Identification

Acid-chloroform extraction group.
1. residue made ammoniacal; add lead acetate solution (5%) → precipitate → yellow → yellow-red → violet-red when treated with sulfuric acid

2. residue plus concentrated sulfuric acid → golden yellow solution → changes gradually to reddish brown

3. Mix about 0.2 gm of potassium nitrate with 4 drops of sulfuric acid in small evaporating dish. Sprinkle several crystals of picrotoxin on this mixture and add sodium hydroxide (20%) dropwise until alkaline → crystals of picrotoxin acquire a red color, which gradually fades.

4. sodium hydroxide (40%) several drops → peppermint odor

5. sulfuric acid plus a trace of potassium dichromate → violet → brown

6. sulfuric acid plus vanillin → yellow → deep brown (with heat)

7. fuming nitric acid → blue-green (fades with excess)

Treatment

Valium or sodium pentobarbital intravenously to relieve convulsions. This is to be done first before further treatment. Keep patient quiet and warm. Avoid morphine or long-acting barbiturates. Gastric lavage with potassium permanganate (1:10,000), if taken orally. Artificial respiration and oxygen therapy as needed. and oxygen therapy as needed.

Symptoms and treatment are similar for Absinthe, cicutoxin, and coriamyrtin. Supportive measures.

PILOCARPINE ($C_{11}H_{16}N_2O_2$)

Synonyms: Pilosine, jaborandi.

Properties: Mp 128°C.

MLD: About 100 mg/70 kg person.

Symptoms: Generally similar to physostigmine.

Identification

1. Crystal tests see Alkaloids
   a. Mayers → derivative mp 70°C
   b. Picric acid → derivative mp 114°C
   c. Benzoic acid → benzoate mp 115°C

2. Color tests see Alkaloids
   a. Sulfuric acid → blue color

   b. Nitric acid → yellow → green → red

   c. Mandelin's → green → yellow → yellow brown (heat)

   d. Mecke's → brown yellow → light red (heat)

3. Physiologic test: 1 drop in cat's eye — constricted pupils. Very sensitive (0.001 mg)

4. UV: See section I

5. TLC: See section I

6. GLC: See section I

Treatment

Generally similar to physostigmine.

POISONOUS PLANTS

MLD: Varies with species, parts of plant eaten.

Identification

Botanically, and by signs and symptoms.

Symptoms and Treatment

ABSINTHE (thujone). Gastrointestinal irritant, convulsant. Symptoms and treatment generally similar to camphor.

AKEE. The unripened fruit is highly toxic and contains saponins. This is especially prevalent in Florida, Cuba, and Jamaica.

Acts as a severe gastrointestinal irritant, with apparent recovery within several hours. However, this recovery may be short and symptoms may recur followed by convulsions, coma, and hypotension. Liver and kidney damage, congestion of lung and brain may also develop.

AMYGDALIN GLUCOSIDE. Forms hydrocyanic acid on hydrolysis. See under Cyanide. Nausea, vomiting, abdominal pain, fever, semicomatose state; *4 plus glucosuria* and acetonuria, but no albuminuria; acidosis, convulsions.

ARNICA. Excess local application may produce skin irritation, ulcer, even gangrene. Ingestion produces nausea, vomiting, abdominal pain, diarrhea, pallor, dry skin, drowsiness, coma, oliguria, pinpoint pupils, respiratory difficulty.

Symptomatic treatment.

BELLADONNA GROUP (belladonna; Jimson weed, Jamestown weed, thorn apple, stinkweed, *Datura stramonium*). Contain atropine, stramonium, scopolamine, hyoscyamine. While all parts of these plants are poisonous, the seeds are especially toxic. See under Atropine for symptoms and treatment.

BERBERINE (alkaloid). Gastrointestinal upset, convulsant. Not very toxic.

CICUTOXIN (fleshy roots of water hemlock; looks like parsnip or artichoke). Stems and roots are very toxic. Yellow oil with odor. Nausea, vomiting, abdominal pain, diarrhea, dilated pupils, excitement, respiratory difficulty, *convulsions*. Can kill in 15 minutes. Symptoms and treatment similar to picrotoxin.

CONIINE (is found in poison hemlock or fool's parsley; *not* to be confused with water hemlock, which contains cicutoxin). Very toxic. MLD, 60 mg (1 drop). Symptoms and treatment generally similar to both nicotine and curare poisoning.

DOGBANE FAMILY. Soreness of mouth, gastrointestinal irritation, dilatation of pupils, sweating, anorexia, elevated temperature and pulse, respiratory difficulty.

GELSEMIUM. Frontal headaches, visual disturbance, muscular weakness, perspiration, dry mouth, thirst, vertigo, dilated pupils, slow respiration, lowered body temperature, respiratory difficulty, possible convulsions prior to death.

LABURNUM (cytisine). Severe nausea, vomiting, diarrhea, burns in mouth and throat, gastrointestinal pain, thirst, irregular pulse and respiration, delirium, twitchy coma, renal damage.

Give morphine for severe pain and symptomatic treatment.

LOBELINE (alkaloid). Liquid. Very toxic; MLD, 60 mg (1 drop). Symptoms and treatment generally similar to nicotine poisoning.

LYCORINE (alkaloid). Usually found in the bulb of many of the lily family and other bulb-type plants. The leaves and stems may also contain some lycorine. Fatalities are usually unlikely because of the prompt irritation and emetic action following nausea, vomiting, and gastroenteritis.

MESCALINE (mescal buttons or peyote) is derived from the dried tops of a species of cactus, *Lophophora williamsii*. These buttons contain mescaline, which is readily absorbed when chewed. Generalized muscular relaxation similar to marihuana. Visual disturbance (vivid beautiful colors), dilatation of pupils, hallucinations, slow pulse, shallow breathing, nausea, vomiting, drowsiness, depression, respiratory failure. Treatment similar to marihuana poisoning.

MILKWEED FAMILY. Gastrointestinal irritant, loss of muscular control, fever, respiratory difficulty.

TREMETOL. *Milk sickness* is produced by tremetol, which is found in leaves and stems of white snakeroot. It is soluble in milk and may be transmitted from cow to human. In animals, it is called "trembles"; in humans, milk sickness. Weakness, nausea, vomiting, diarrhea, loss of appetite, dry skin, constipation, slow respiration, subnormal temperature, collapse.

MUSHROOMS *(inedible)* and TOADSTOOLS. Most common are *Amanita muscaria* and *A. phalloides (A. brunnescens* and *A. verna).* *A. muscaria* contains muscarine and usually produces typical symptoms within 2 hours, which are characteristic of muscarine: salivation, sweating, lacrimation, constricted pupils, bradycardia, hypotension, gut motility and spasm, diarrhea, abdominal pain, difficult breathing, pulmonary edema and constricted bronchioles, delirium, convulsions, collapse, coma, and finally respiratory arrest.

Although these mushrooms have striking colors of orange-red, or scarlet to yellow, they are often confused with the edible species.

Immediate gastric lavage and saline cathartic are essential. *Keep patient fully atropinized,* which is essential to correct respiratory difficulties. For details, see under Muscarine.

A. phalloides is a very toxic fungus. (*A. brunnescens* and *A. verna* are closely related.) Symptoms usually are delayed 5 to 15 hours and are severe. Rapid removal is essential. Gastric lavage and saline cathartics should still be attempted even hours later to remove any possible unabsorbed fungi.

The severe gastrointestinal upset is treated with demulcents; opiates for pain. Valium or fast-acting barbiturates (with caution) for excitement. Keep patient warm and quiet; fluids or whole blood as indicated for thirst, dehydration, agglutination of red blood cells, or collapse. Recovery is slow and uncertain. Beware of temporary improvement; this may be followed by cyanosis, hypoglycemia, and collapse. Oxygen therapy; intravenous glucose. Liver, kidney, and myocardium damage usually occurs; these are treated with supportive therapy and diet. Maintain water, heat, and electrolyte balance. Atropine appears of little value.

No specific antidote is available. However thiotic (a-lipoic) acid has been reported of some help. If available, it is worth trying because of the poor prognosis with this poison. It may be available at the N.I.H. (Maryland) or in N.Y.C. See page 418.

POISON IVY, poison oak, sumac, elder, ash, and dogwood may grow as shrubs, vines or bushes. Powerful skin irritant, rash or vesicant blisters; if internal, may produce nausea, vomiting, corrosion, bloody diarrhea, hematuria, kidney and liver damage, possible convulsions, and collapse.

Treat skin irritation topically with water and sodium bicarbonate paste. If internal: gastric lavage with caution, demulcents and morphine for pain, fluids and catheterize to maintain urinary flow. High carbohydrate, and low-fat diet; other supportive measures.

Severe dermatosis; inflammatory reactions may be treated with corticosteroids and/or antihistamines.

POKEROOT (contains Saponins). Berries, root, and bark are toxic especially for children. Powerful emetic but action may be delayed several hours.

Symptoms are burning sensation in mouth, stomach cramps, severe vomiting, diarrhea, weakness, dizziness, visual disturbances, excessive salivation, and perspiration with recovery — usually in 24 hours.

Large amounts may produce convulsions, coma, and respiratory paralysis. Treat by giving milk, water, activated charcoal; gastric lavage or induce emesis unless convulsions. Maintain respiration, supportive and symptomatic measures.

PYRACANTHA (fire thorn, fire bush) (rose). Thorny evergreen shrub (6–20 ft); white flowers and brilliant orange-red berries. Common in landscaped gardens. Symptoms similar to belladonna: vomiting, nausea, abdominal cramps, stupor, coma, dilatation of pupils, convulsions, dry skin, and mouth, tachycardia, headache. Treatment same as for belladonna: emesis, gastric lavage, short-acting barbiturates for excitement or convulsions. Usually *not very toxic* (low toxicity) ; if symptoms are mild, vigorous treatment not necessary.

SELENIFEROUS WHEAT. Soil in the Midwest of the United States is rich in selenium. Plants, especially wheat, pick up selenium and incorporate it into the protein molecule. It replaces in part the sulfur molecule. This wheat or forage is especially toxic for stock animals (alkali disease) . Selenium is cumulative; eliminated in urine.

Symptoms generally resemble those of arsenic: nausea, vomiting, abdominal pain, diarrhea, restlessness, somnolence, fall in blood pressure, cough, dyspnea, convulsions, respiratory failure. Chronic: garlic odor to breath is strong; loss in weight, marked pallor, depression. Red staining of fingers, teeth, and hair. Dermatitis, marked debility, gastrointestinal disturbances, and possible liver involvement.

Treat with change of diet, gastric lavage, emetics, cathartics, demulcents, high-carbohydrate and low fat, other supportive measures for possible liver involvement. Short-acting barbiturates for convulsions. Oxygen therapy and artificial respiration as needed. General treatment similar for Selsun (selenium sulfide).

TAXINE (Yew) . Gastroenteritis, dyspnea, mydriasis, dizziness, epileptiform convulsions, coma, cardiovascular and respiratory depression, shock.

Treatment: activated charcoal, then gastric lavage; maintain a respiratory exchange and all vital signs; Valium for convulsions.

VERATRUM. Gastrointestinal irritation, sneezing, burning sensation of mouth, skin, and eyes. Nausea, vomiting, abdominal pain, diarrhea, muscular weakness, sweating, salivation, unresponsive thirst, paralysis, tremors and spasms, occasional convulsions, numbness and tingling in fingers and mouth; feeling of warmth in head, neck, and shoulders; cardiac arrhythmias, bradycardia. Bronchiolar constriction corrected by atropine therapy. Hypotension treated with plasma expanders. Shallow respiration, coma, respiratory depression, collapse.

Plant Sources of Poisons and Irritants

Some of the more common poisonous plants (wild and cultivated) are listed below with the particular toxic agent or cardinal signs and symptoms.

Treatment in general is symptomatic and supportive, after stomach is evacuated by gastric lavage.

Gastrointestinal (GI) irritants or corrosives may produce edema of lips, tongue, and throat; fever, delirium, tremors, or convulsions. Kidney involvement is always a possibility. Nausea, vomiting, abdominal pain, diarrhea (sometimes bloody) usually come on early.

abrin	toxalbumin
Abrus precatorius	toxalbumin
Absinthe	essential oil and powerful convulsant
Acacia (Arabic) gum	low toxicity
Acckanthera venenata	ouabain
almond	amygdalin (cyanide)
aloe	GI irritant
American false hellebore	veratrum
American hemp	dogbane family
angel's trumpet	atropinelike
appleseed	traces of amygdalin
arborvitae	thujone (Absinthe)
Arnica montana	arnica (essential oillike)
arrow grass	amygdalin (cyanide)
asthma weed	lobeline
autumn crocus	colchicine
azalea	curarelike
baneberry	purgative irritant and heart depressant
barberry	berberinelike
Bedstraw milkweed	milkweed family
belladonna	atropine
betel nut	physostigminelike
Betula	methyl salicylate
bird of paradise (green seed)	severe GI irritant

bitter almond	amygdalin (cyanide)
bittersweet unripe berries	solanine
bitter apple	colocynth
bitter cucumber	colocynth
bitter gourd	colocynth
black locust (robin)	toxalbumin
black laurel	veratrumlike
black nightshade	solanine
bloodroot (red juice)	GI irritant, digitalislike
blue nightshade	solanine
blue rocket	aconite
box (boxtree)	buxine irritant and convulsant
boxwood	berberine
broom tops	sparteine
bryonia	powerful purgative
bryony	GI irritant
buckthorn family	GI irritant
buffalo bur	solanine
bufotenine (seeds)	DMT (dimethyl tryptamine)
bull nettle	solanine
burning bush	convulsant
buttercup	aconitine
Buxus (box)	severe irritant
calabar bean	physostigmine
caladium	calcium oxalate
California poppy	berberine
calla lily	GI upset
camellia	digitalislike
cassava	amygdalin (cyanide)
castor bean (ricin)	toxalbumin
ceriman	GI upset
cervadilla	severe GI irritant
cherry laurel	traces of amygdalin
cherry seeds and plant	amygdalin (cyanide)
chinaberry	Absinthe (thujone)
chokecherry seed	amygdalin (cyanide)
Chinese forget-me-not	curarelike
Christ thorn	GI and skin irritant

Christmas berry	amygdalin (cyanide)
Christmas rose	GI upset and convulsant
cicuta	cicutoxin
cinchona bark	cinchonine (quininelike)
cinnamon	saponin
clematis	GI irritant
climbing lily	colchicine
Colchicum autumnale (autumn crocus)	colchicine
Colorado bur	solanine
colored elephant ear	GI irritant
columbine	GI irritant
colocynth	powerful cathartic
Coniumn maculatum	coniine
corn cockle	saponin
cowbane	cicutoxin
cow cockle	saponin
croton oil	toxalbumin
crowfoot family	aconitine
crown imperial	veratrumlike
cry baby tree	curarelike
cubeb	GI irritant; excitant
curcin	toxalbumin
cyclamin	saponin
cytisine	severe GI irritant; excitant
daffodil	lycorine, severe irritant
daphne berry (red)	corrosive and convulsant
datura	atropinelike
Datura stramonium	atropinelike
deadly nightshade	atropine
death camus	veratrum
devils dung	asafetida
deer wort	milk sickness (tremetol)
dogbane	digitalislike
dog parsley	GI irritant; convulsant
dumb cane (dieffenbachia)	oxalates
dumbeane	severe irritant
dumb plant	GI irritant

elderberry (black elder)	cyanide
elephant ear	GI irritant (calcium oxalate)
European bittersweet	solanine
evergreen trees	taxine
eyebright	lobeline
fava bean	very toxic, severe corrosive
finger cherry	optic nerve damage
firethorn (fire bush or pyracantha)	low toxicity
flag lily	GI and skin irritant
flax	amygdalin (cyanide)
food of the gods	asafetida sedative
fool's parsley	coniinelike
four o'clock	GI irritant and narcosis
foxglove	digitalis
gamboge gum	powerful cathartic
garget	pokeroot
Gelsemium sempervirens (jessamine)	strychninelike
Gloriosa superba (glory or climbing lily)	colchicine
goldenrod (rayless)	milk sickness (tremetol)
golden seal	berberine
goosefoot family	oxalate
grape hyacinth	lycorine
grape (wild)	respiratory depressant
greasewood	oxalate
heather	curarelike
hedeoma	oil of pennyroyal
hellebore	veratrum
hemlock	coniine
henbane	atropinelike
holly berries	GI irritant
horse nettle	solanine
horsetail milkweed	milkweed family
hyacinth (bulb)	severe GI irritant
Hyascyamus niger	atropinelike
Indian hemp	dogbane family

Indian physic	dogbane family
Indian tobacco	lobeline
inkberry	pokeroot
iris	severe GI irritant
Irish potato	solanine
ivy	saponin
jaborandi	pilocarpine
Jamestown weed	atropinelike
jasmine	gelsemium
Japanese plum	trace of amygdalin
Japanese yew	taxine
Jatropha curcas	toxalbumin
jequirity (abrin)	toxalbumin
Jerusalem cherry	solanine
jessamine	gelsemium, strychninelike
jet bead berry	amygdalin (cyanide)
jet berry bush	amygdalin (cyanide)
Jimmy weed	milk sickness
Jimson weed (Jamestown)	atropinelike
Johnson grass	amygdalin (cyanide)
jonquil	lycorine, severe irritant
kif	marihuana
laburnum	cytisine
Latana camara	severe irritant
latana berries	severe irritant
larkspur	aconitine (very toxic)
lemon grass	essential oil
leopard's bane	arnica
lily of the valley	digitalislike
lobelia	lobeline
love-in-a-mist	curarelike
Lupin	convulsant
Mahonia	berberine
machineel (sap and fruit)	severe irritant
may apple	potent cathartic
meadow saffron	colchicum
melilotus	irritant and liver damage
menthol	essential oil

milk ipecac	similar to dogbane
milkweed	GI and skin irritant
mimosa	saponin
mission bells	veratrumlike
mistletoe berries	digitalislike
mock orange	saponin
monkshood	aconitine
morning glory (seeds)	LSD-like; irritant
mountain laurel	veratrumlike (curarelike)
mountain mahogany	amygdalin (cyanide)
mountain tobacco	arnica
Myristica fragrans	nutmeg (essential oil)
narcissus (bulb)	lycorine, severe irritant
natal cherry	solanine
nels	aconitine
nerium oleander	digitalislike
night-blooming cereus	digitalislike
nutmeg	essential oils
nux vomica	strychnine
oleander (yellow)	digitalislike
oriental poppy	berberinelike
pansies	GI irritant and narcosis
parsley family	coniine or cicutoxin
peach seed	trace of amygdalin (cyanide)
pear seed	amygdalin (cyanide)
peony	taxine
periwinkle	saponin
peyote (cactus)	mescaline
pheasant's eye	digitalislike
philodendron	oxalates
pie plant	oxalic acid
pilocarpine	parathionlike
pilosine	pilocarpine
pimpernel	saponin
pin cherry	amygdalin (cyanide)
pink family	saponin
plum seed	amygdalin (cyanide)
podophyllum	potent cathartic

poincianna (pods)	severe irritant
poinsettia	GI and skin irritant (severe)
poison dogwood	vesicant; poison ivy-like
poison elder	vesicant; poison ivy-like
poison hemlock	coniine
poison ivy	vesicant
poison oak	vesicant; poison ivy-like
poison parsley	coniine
poison sumac	vesicant; poison ivy-like
poke	pokeroot, pokeberry
pokeberry	GI irritant and narcosis (saponins)
pokeweed (inkberry)	pokeroot (saponins)
poke root	saponins
pool wort	milk sickness (tremetol)
poppy family	opium
prickly poppy	berberine
primrose	vesicant
privet	GI irritant; nervous symptoms
purple cockle	saponin
quince seed	traces of amygdalin
ragwort groundsel	liver damage
rain lily	lycorine
rain tree	saponin
rattlebox	liver damage
Rauwolfia serpentina	depressant (mild)
rayless goldenrod	milk sickness (tremetol)
rhododendron	veratrumlike; curarelike
rhubarb	oxalate; leaf is severe irritant
richweed	milk sickness (tremetol)
ricin	toxalbumin
Ricinus communis	toxalbumin
robin	GI irritant and heart depressant
rue	essential oil
sabadilla	GI irritant (severe)
sage	Absinthelike
sago palm	GI irritant
sandbur	solanine
Scotch broom	nicotine

sedum	GI irritant
skunk cabbage	oxalate (irritant)
shirley poppy	berberine
snowdrop	lycerine
snow-on-the-mountain	GI and skin irritant
soapberry family	saponin
solanum	solanine
sorghum	amygdalin (cyanide)
Spanish bayonet	saponin
Spanish broom	quinidinelike
spreading dogbane	dogbane family
spider lily	lycorine
spinach	oxalate
spindle tree	GI irritant and convulsant
squaw weed	milk sickness (tremetol)
squaw mint	oil of pennyroyal
St. Joseph's lily	lycorine
staggerbrush	veratrumlike
staggerbush	curarelike
star-of-Bethlehem	GI irritant and narcosis (digitalislike)
stinkweed	atropinelike
strawberry bush	digitalislike
strophanthin	digitalislike
Strophanthus sermentosus	strophonthin
suckleya	trace of amygdalin
Sudan grass	amygdalin (cyanide)
sweet cloves	liver damage
sweet pea (pod)	paralysis
sweet shrub	thujone (Absinthe)
tansy	essential oil
tartago	strong cathartic; irritant
Taxus baccata	taxine
Texas thistle	solanine
tobacco	nicotine
thorn apple	atropinelike
tomato	trace of solanine
trompillo	solanine
tulip	veratrumlike

tung nut	toxalbumin
velvet grass	amygdalin (cyanide)
violet	GI irritant and narcosis
wandering milkweed	similar to dogbane
water hemlock	cicutoxin
white cedar	Absinthelike (convulsant)
white horse nettle	solanine
white sanicle	milk sickness (tremetol)
white snakeroot	milk sickness (tremetol)
whorled milkweed	milkweed family
wild black cherry	amygdalin (cyanide)
wild tomato	solanine
wisteria (pod)	severe GI irritant
woody nightshade	solanine
yellow jasmine	nicotine
yellow jessamine	gelsemium
yerba-de-pasmo	milk sickness
yew family	taxine

POTASSIUM PERMANGANATE (KMnO₄)

Uses: Fungicide, oxidizing agent, in industry.

Properties: Purple-black crystals; soluble in water; wine color.

MLD: Approximately 5 gm/70 kg person.

Remarks: Powerful oxidizing agent.

Symptoms: Severe gastrointestinal irritation, pink-purple coloring of skin, lips and mouth. Nausea, vomiting, diarrhea, abdominal pain, edema of glottis, renal damage, paresthesia, shock, death.

Identification

1. Stomach contents: vomitus is pink to purple.
2. Permanganate pink color is decolorized with addition of oxalic acid plus trace of sulfuric acid.
3. Color is decolorized with sodium bisulfite.
4. Color is decolorized with hydrogen peroxide.
5. Atomic absorption for manganese.

Treatment

Induce vomiting with emetics; or gastric lavage with dilute hydrogen peroxide if corrosion is not too severe (10 ml of 3% hydrogen peroxide plus 100 ml water) or with milk.

Demulcents such as egg white, egg albumin, oils. Combat corrosion, collapse, and shock. Keep air passages open; maintain respiration. Symptomatic and supportive measures.

PROCAINE ($C_{13}H_{20}N_2O_2$)

Synonyms: Diethylaminoethyl *p*-aminobenzoate. Procaine hydrochloride: Novocaine, Neocaine, Ethocaine.

Uses: Local anesthetic, nerve block; by injection or by mucous membranes.

Properties: Alkaloid, white crystals. Base mp 51°C; procaine HCl mp 153–156°C. Hygroscopic, soluble in alkaline ether or chloroform.

MLD: About 1/20 as toxic as cocaine.

Remarks: About 90 percent rapidly metabolyzes to *p*-aminobenzoic acid (Clarke). Allergy and hypersensitivity is not uncommon and is severe.

Symptoms

MILD CASES: Dizziness, confusion, loquacity, excitement, rapid heart rate, irregular respiration, anxiety.

SEVERE CASES: Extreme pallor, rise in temperature, sweating, dilated pupils, nausea, vomiting, loss of sensation, delirium, difficult breathing, cyanosis, fall in blood pressure, muscular tremors, convulsions, Cheyne-Stokes type respiration, coma, relaxation of sphincters, respiratory failure, and cardiovascular collapse.

Identification

Alkaline-chloroform or ether extraction.

1. Crystal tests: See Alkaloids.
    a. Wagners → brown oily precipitate
    b. Mayers → white precipitate, which is oily at first
    c. picric acid → yellow precipitate (mp 153°C)

d. gold chloride → yellow precipitate
e. mercury chloride → best crystals; plus 5 drops dilute H_2SO_4 (1:50) → procaine dissolves; cocaine will not.

2. Color tests; See Alkaloids.

To differentiate from cocaine:

a. procaine + sodium hypochlorite solution (fresh) → red-yellow precipitate, which is soluble in ethanol or chloroform or acetone

b. plus *p*-dimethylaminobenzaldehyde in ethanol + $\frac{1}{2}$ drop H_2SO_4 → red orange color

c. plus furfural (1% in ethanol + 2 drops of H_2SO_4 → rose-red

d. Sanchez (aqueous furfural saturated) + 2 drops acetic acid → deep red

e. Trace of alkaloid is dissolved in 0.5 ml of 2% furfural in H_2O and is floated (carefully) on top of 1 ml of H_2SO_4 color ring formation at interface:

procaine → rose-red
morphine → rose to violet
codeine → red to violet; blue on adding H_2O
veratrine → red—below a blue green
quinine → brown with yellow edge
cinchonine → brown border on cherry red

f. Chromic acid test → negative; see Cocaine.

g. Cobalt thiocyanate test → negative; see Cocaine.

h. Plus few drops $KMnO_4$ (5%) + gentle heat for few seconds → brown MnO_2 and odor of acetaldehyde. Cocaine does not react.

i. Doper's → flaky chocolate brown. (See Alkaloids).

3. Physiologic tests

a. E.C.G. may show atrioventricular block.

b. Trace to tip of tongue → numb sensation.

4. UV spectrophotometry: See Section I.

Maximum density: 227, 272 nm in 0.5N H_2SO_4

5. Thin layer chromatography: See Section I.

6. Gas liquid chromatography: See Section I.

Treatment

Immediately correct fall in blood pressure and convulsions. Remove from mucous membranes by washing it out; limit absorption from injection, by tourniquet and ice packs. Supportive.

Succinylcholine chloride or Valium to minimize convulsions. Artificial respiration and oxygen until blood pressure and pulse rate return to normal.

Placing patient in a head down position and IV saline or plasma expanders may help to restore blood pressure. Guard against peripheral circulatory collapse. Do not give epinephrine nor other vasopressors.

PROPOXYPHENE ($C_{22}H_{29}NO$)

Synonyms: Dextropropoxyphene; Doloxene; Darvon and Darvon compound; 32 and 65 mg capsules with and without aspirin, phenacetin, and caffeine. APC intensifies analgesic action.

Uses: Relief from mild to moderate pain; up to 65 mg $\times$ 6 daily.

Properties: Odorless, white, crystalline powder with a bitter taste; very soluble in chloroform or water; moderately soluble in ether; mp 170–171°C.

MLD: Approximately 1 gm/70 kg person.

Approximate Levels: Therapeutic blood level, 0.02 mg/dl; half-life 8 hours. Lethal level: blood, 3 mg/dl; liver, 8 mg/dl; urine, 5 mg/dl.

Remarks: Generally similar in structure to methadone. Some cross tolerance with some other CNS depressants. Analgesic somewhat less potent than codeine. Although it is unlikely to be used as an addicting agent, some drug dependency (rare and mild) has been reported (PDR) that includes tolerance and psychological and physical dependency. In degree, this is probably qualitatively similar to codeine but definitely quantitatively less. It will not support morphine dependency. The compound combination with aspirin may confuse the clinical picture.

Symptoms: *Rapid* onset of action, nausea, vomiting, lethargy, CNS depressant, fixed miosis, deep coma; respiratory depression and cardiovascular collapse may occur within 1 hour or may be delayed. Marked congestion of lungs, liver, spleen, and pancreas. Action generally similar to narcotic overdose but persistent *convulsions* also occur. Prolonged deep coma may be further complicated with hypoxia and brain damage and bronchial pneumonia.

Identification

Rapidly cleared from blood; rapidly metabolyzed; may possibly concentrate in body fat.

Soluble in water, butyl chloride, chloroform, or ether. Can be extracted from weakly alkaline solutions.

Distills from pH 8 after refluxing with HCl for 15 minutes. (Fiorese).

1. *Extract:* Ten (10) ml sample plus 10 ml water plus 15 ml hydrochloric acid in an Erlenmeyer flask with a watch glass cover is placed on a boiling bath for 20 minutes. Cool and transfer to a 500 ml Erlenmeyer flask and add 15 ml 50% sodium hydroxide. Cool and vigorously extract with 150 ml of ether. Separate and filter the ether through Whatman #1 filter paper. Wash ether with water and again filter the ether (McBay-Turk-Corbett-Hudson).

    a. UV: Extract the ether from above with 5 ml 0.2N H_2SO_4 with vigorous shaking. Filter the HCl extract through water-washed Whatman #5; then determine absorbance. Maximum was at 255 nm, $E_{1cm}^{1\%}$ 210, with a broad peak. See Section I.

    b. To increase sensitivity and specificity, simultaneously irradiate each cuvette (unknown and HCl reference blank) for 5 minutes place a few mm from a 257.3 nm UV light. Determine absorbance. Maximum is at 255 nm, $E_{1cm}^{1\%}$ 480, with a very sharp and distinct peak; with a shoulder at 247 nm.

2. Thin layer chromatography (TLC) : See Section I.
    Developer:
    • ethyl acetate:methanol:NH_4OH (85:10:5)
    Darvon Rf 0.90
    methadone Rf 0.91
    • ethyl acetate:methanol:NH_4OH:H_2O
    (85:13.5:0.5:1) (modified Davidow)

Darvon Rf 0.95

methadone Rf 0.77

Can now differentiate.

• Methanol:NH₄OH (100:1.5) Rf 0.66

(Sunshine in Clarke) .

• Acetic acid:ethanol:H₂O (30:60:10)

Rf 0.82 (Fiorese)

Spray:

• Iodoplatinate

• Ninhydrin then iodoplatinate

3. Color reactions: See Alkaloids.

   a. Marquis (H₂SO₄:formaldehyde—20:1) → dark purple → dull green (0.5 μg)

   b. Froede (ammonium molybdate 0.1% in H₂SO₄) → black → green (0.5 μg)

   c. Mecke (selenic acid 0.5% in H₂SO₄) → faint brown (0.5 μg)

   d. Mandelin (1% ammonium vanadate in H₂SO₄) → gray (0.5 μg)

   e. chloriodoplatinic acid → blue (0.5 μg)

4. Crystals

KI-triiodide (2 gms I₂ + 4 gms KI in 100 ml H₂O) → small plates

5. Gas chromatography (GLC) (Manno-Jain-Forney) . OV-1 on Chromosorb W and dimethyldichlorosilane. Column temperature 195°C; flame ionization detector. 5 ml plasma + 2 × 5 ml butyl chloride; shake; centrifuge; extract solvent with 0.2N HCl; centrifuge; remove and discard solvent by aspiration. The aqueous is flash evaporated to dryness under vacuum. Extract with 3 × 0.25 ml chromatographically pure chloroform. Dry with stream of N₂ gas. Pick up residue in 20 μl of chloroform containing 0.125/ml cocaine as internal standard. Keep column temperature at 195°C (at 210°C, 50% is destroyed; 180°C is too low) . With butyl chloride, can extract at pH 6 to 11.

Treatment

Maintain all vital signs including respiration, blood pressure, water and electrolyte and body heat balance. Do not use any analeptics; this can precipitate a fatal convulsion. If not in deep coma, gastric lavage may be useful within a few hours of ingestion but this must be weighted with the possible dangers of aspiration or triggering a convulsion.

Support (if possible) against shock, hypoxia, cerebral edema, atelectasis, and bronchial pneumonia. Apparently hemodialysis or peritoneal dialysis, is not much help, except for the complication of aspirin if present. Guarded prognosis is essential. Death can occur a month later with bilateral cortical atrophy, atelectasis, and bronchial pneumonia. Supportive. See Morphine

The narcotic antagonists such as Naloxone or Nalorphine may antagonize the respiratory depression, but not the convulsions.

PYRETHRUM ($C_{21}H_{28}O_3$)

Synonyms: Chrysanthemum extract, pyrethrin I and II.
Uses: Insecticide.
Properties: Viscous liquid. Soluble in alcohol, ether, or kerosene; insoluble in water.
MLD: Relatively low toxicity.
Remarks: Usually the vehicle kerosene is the more toxic agent.
Symptoms: Gastrointestinal irritation, nausea, vomiting, diarrhea, sternutatory effect, acrid bitter taste, numbness of tongue and lips, syncope, hyperexcitability, incoordination, tinnitus, convulsions, muscular paralysis, prostration, collapse. Death due to respiratory failure.

Treatment

If kerosene is the insecticide base, treat for kerosene poisoning.

Treat symptomatically. Gastric lavage, emetics, cathartics, demulcents, artificial respiration. Valium or short-acting barbiturates for convulsions. Supportive.

QUATERNARY AMMONIUM COMPOUNDS

Members: Zephiran chloride (alkyldimethylbenzylammonium chloride); Triton K-12 (cetyldimethylbenzylammonium chloride);

Triton K-60 (lauryldimethylbenzylammonium chloride) ; Retander LA (stearyltrimethylammonium bromide) ; Hyamine 2389 (methyldodecylbenzyltrimethylammonium chloride) .

Derivatives: Benzalkonium chloride (alkyl C_3H_{17} to $C_{18}H_{37}$); benzethonium chloride; cetylpyridinium chloride; methyl benzethonium chloride.

Uses: Antiseptics, detergents, bacteriocides, disinfectants, fungicides, sanitizers, and deodorants.

Properties: Viscous liquids; astringent taste; detergent; precipitate proteins; concentrated solutions are caustic.

MLD: Approximately 25 ml of 10% methyldodecylbenzyltrimethyl NH_4Cl in ethanol for adult. In general, it appears that quaternary ammonium compounds with two long-chain alkyl group (i.e. dimethyl distearyl ammonium chloride) are much less toxic than those with a single such substitution.

Symptoms: Local gastrointestinal irritation, nausea, vomiting, restlessness, confusion, chills, shortness of breath, apprehension, hypotension; convulsions may occur; skeletal muscle weakness or paralysis, severe laryngeal edema, respiratory difficulty, cyanosis, tachycardia, arrhythmias, oliguria, circulatory shock, death (death may be due to asphyxia with or without convulsions, usually within three hours) .

Treatment

Give milk, egg white, gelatin, or weak soapy water (not detergent). If mucosa is not damaged, gastric lavage or induce emesis. Support all vital functions; maintain respiratory exchange and blood pressure; oxygen or artificial respiration if needed. Treat convulsions with Valium or short-acting barbiturates. Guard against hypotension and circulatory shock, and stricture of the esophagus.

Corticosteroid therapy may be helpful to minimize severe laryngeal edema and to minimize possible esophageal stricture.

QUININE ($C_{20}H_{24}N_2O_2$)

Uses: Antipyretic, antimalarial; for colds; analgesic.

Properties: White crystalline, bitter taste. Mp 175°C. Soluble in $CHCl_3$. Chemically similar to quinidine.

MLD: Approximately 20 gm/70 kg person.

Approximate Blood Levels: For quinine: therapeutic, 0.2 mg/dl; lethal, 2 mg/dl; half-life, 15 hours. For quinidine: therapeutic, 0.5 mg/dl; lethal, 4 mg/dl.

Symptoms: Bitter taste, tinnitus, visual impairment, headache, flushing of skin, skin rash, mental confusion, low prothrombin blood level, diarrhea, decrease in body temperature, bradycardia, delirium, convulsions, unconsciousness, coma, collapse, circulatory failure, heart is depressed and blood pressure falls, renal damage. Death usually brought about by respiratory paralysis and/or paralysis of the heart.

Identification

$NaHCO_3$-chloroform or ether extraction group.

1. Use 10 ml of urine + 1 ml of quinine reagent → white precipitate.

    Sensitivity is 0.010 mg per 10 ml urine.

    Other alkaloids and albumin in large amounts will also give positive results. Other alkaloids are unlikely to be present in such large amounts. The interference of albumin may be ruled out by heating the solution gently. The precipitate, if due to quinine, will dissolve when heated and will reappear on cooling. Albumin precipitate will intensify and persist during heating.

    Reagent: Quinine: 3 gm of red mercuric iodide, 2 gm of potassium iodide, 20 ml of glacial acetic acid, and water of sufficient quantity to make 60 ml.

2. Neutralize 10 ml of urine with ammonium hydroxide. Add 3 drops of fresh chlorinated lime solution. Shake and make slightly alkaline with ammonium hydroxide → greenish precipitate.

3. To a tablet, powder, or residue (after extraction with alkaline chloroform), do following color tests:

    a. sulfuric acid → colorless to light yellow → changing to brown with heat

    b. Mecke's reagent → colorless → light brown with heat

c. *p*-dimethyl aminobenzaldehyde → red
For details, see under Alkaloids.

4. Dissolve a portion of the tablet powder, or residue from the alkaline-chloroform extract, with 1 ml of acetic acid (2%). Use 1 drop of this to perform the following alkaloidal precipitate tests. Examine for typical crystals. (See under Alkaloids.)
   a. Wagner's reagent → brown precipitate
   b. Mayer's reagent → white precipitate
   c. picric acid → amorphous yellow precipitate
   d. bromide water + ammonium hydroxide → green
   e. potassium dichromate (10%) → yellow precipitate

5. One drop of half-saturated bromine water + 1 drop of potassium ferricyanide (10%) + 1 drop of ammonium hydroxide (10%) is added to quinine solution that has been acidulated with acetic acid. Shake → gradually turns red. Shake with chloroform. The chloroform layer will pick the brilliant red-violet color.

6. Quinine solutions give a good fluorescence with UV light after addition of dilute sulfuric acid.

7. UV spectrophotometry. Maximum density, 250 nm. See Section I.

8. TLC to differentiate quinine from quinidine:

Developing Solvent	Rf Quinine	Rf Quinidine
• benzene:ether:diethylamine (20:15:5)	0.53	0.73
• cyclohexane:chloroform:diethylamine (50:40:10)	0.37	0.56
• chloroform:acetone:diethylamine (50:40:10)	0.73	0.89
• chloroform:diethylamine (90:10)	0.61	0.82

View under UV light before spraying (fluoresces) ; Ninhydrin then iodoplatinate spray; see Section I.

9. Spectrofluorimetry: Very sensitive (if available).

Treatment

Withdrawal of drug. Give activated charcoal or proteins. Gastric lavage with potassium permanganate (1:10,000). Emetics, cathartics. Keep patient warm and quiet.

Symptomatic treatment, especially for cardiovascular and respiratory symptoms. Artificial respiration and oxygen therapy if needed.

REPTILE BITE

Remarks: Poisonous reptiles in the United States include rattlesnake, copperhead, water moccasin (hemotoxic) ; coral snake (neurotoxic) ; gila monster (neurotoxic).

Symptoms: Sharp burning pain, bitten area swells, rapid fall in blood pressure, syncope, anaphylactoid type of reaction, nausea, vomiting, malaise, prostration, numbness of extremities, respiratory difficulty, possible convulsions, coma, respiratory failure and/ or cardiovascular collapse.

Identification

By common recognition, or by a zoologist or zoo curator.

Treatment

Apply tourniquet above the bite; use no alcoholic drinks. Local incision to promote drainage of venom; apply suction to help drainage. Disinfect wound, prevent secondary infection.

Specific antivenin therapy is recommended, especially if available. Morphine for pain and Valium for apprehension. Transfusion of whole blood if indicated.

Symptomatic treatment and supportive measures especially in maintaining normal respiration and circulation.

Antivenin Index Center, Oklahoma City, is a 24-hour-a-day, 7-day-a-week information retrieval service; telephone: (405) 271-5454. Special antivenin and expert advice may be available at an area zoo or visiting circus. Also, serum may be available at Wyeth Laboratories for some reptiles.

ROTENONE ($C_{23}H_{22}O_6$)

Synonyms: Derris root extract.

Uses: Insecticide.

Properties: White neutral powder. Mp 163°C Soluble in alcohol, ether, and chloroform, insoluble in water.

MLD: Relative low toxicity.

Remarks: Not absorbed through skin; may cause a mild irritation; fat and oil-soluble.

Symptoms: Gastric irritation, nausea, vomiting, diarrhea, hypoglycemia. Respiration is first stimulated and then depressed. Stupor, frequent convulsive seizures. Liver damage. Death due to respiratory failure. Cardiovascular system not especially affected. Symptoms may appear within a few minutes to a few hours. Death can occur as early as 5 hours after ingestion and can be delayed 10 days.

Identification

Low blood sugar may be suggestive. UV spectrophotometry in Ethanol. See Section I.

Treatment

Acts as a gastric irritant and also stimulates the emetic center. Much may be removed automatically by these two mechanisms. Gastric lavage as an additional measure. No specific antidote known. Keep patient warm and quiet. Artificial respiration. Valium or short-acting barbiturates for convulsions. Saline cathartics (30 gm of sodium sulfate). Avoid fats and oils. Oxygen, artificial respiration. Intravenous glucose to correct hypoglycemia. Symptomatic and supportive measures.

SANTONIN ($C_{15}H_{18}O_3$)

Synonyms: None; extracted from dried flowers of artemisia.

Uses: Antihelmintic.

Properties: White crystals, four-sided flat prisms. Mp 170°C. Sparingly soluble in chloroform, ether, or ethanol.

MLD: Approximately 1 gm/70 kg person.

Remarks: Urine is yellow-green color when acid; red when alkaline. These same colors are given by rhubarb, senna, or emodin.

Symptoms: Gastrointestinal irritation, nausea, vomiting, abdominal pain, diarrhea. Yellow vision, disturbed vision, which may last a week, Hematuria, dysuria, headache, later delirium, convulsions, collapse, coma, feeble heart, disturbed respiration, prostration, death.

Identification

Isolated by acid-chloroform extraction.

1. Acidify 5 ml of urine with 1 ml of hydrochloric acid → bright yellow color.

2. Alkalinize 5 ml of urine with 1 ml of 10% sodium hydroxide → pink to scarlet color, which is soluble in chloroform.

3. Add 10 ml of calcium hydroxide (saturated) to 25 ml of urine → carmine red color.

4. Extract 30 ml of urine with 30 ml of chloroform; separate and evaporate chloroform. Add 2 drops H_2SO_4 to residue → violet color.

5. KCN plus heat → red residue.

6. H_2SO_4 (1:1) plus heat → yellow → add drop of $FeCl_3$ (10%) → red → purple.

7. UV Spectrophotometry in ethanol. Maximum density, 245 nm (very sensitive). See Section I.

Treatment

Gastric lavage or emetics. Saline cathartics (sodium sulfate, 30 gm). Valium or short-acting barbiturates for convulsions. Supportive.

SEA NETTLES

Remarks: Portuguese man-of-war, agua viva, and jellyfish are generally included under this classification.

Symptoms: Immediate sensation of sharp sting when tentacles strike. Tentacle releases a sticky vesicant fluid that produces urticaria within 2 minutes. Pain increases in intensity up to about 1 or 2 hours. Nausea, vomiting, severe abdominal pain, syncope, drop in blood pressure, respiratory difficulty, collapse.

Identification

Vivid color, sac, and long tentacles.

Treatment

Antihistaminics; transfusion of fluids or whole blood. Calcium gluconate (1–2 gm IV) ; repeat as necessary.

Symptomatic treatment especially for cardiovascular and/or respiratory difficulties. Support against shock.

Sponge with alcohol or dilute vinegar; then cover with sand. After 1 minute, scrape free with a knife. (Do not *rub* or spread.)

SILICA

Identification

(Gettler-Umberger method) :

Dry 10 gm of lung in a nickel crucible and ash and fuse for several hours at 800–900°C with 2.5 gm of fusion mixture.

Cool the *fused salts* and dissolve by boiling with three successive 20 ml portions of distilled water. Bring each to boil and heat for an additional 5 minutes; then filter and wash the residue.

Collect all filtrates into a 600-ml Erlenmeyer flask with a pencil mark to indicate the 500-ml level.

Neutralize with acetic acid and add 15 ml of acetic acid in excess. Heat on a hot plate for about 15 minutes to expel all of the carbon dioxide. Allow to cool to room temperature; add 20 ml of 13% ammonium molybdate and allow to stand for 20 minutes. Add 20 ml of 10% oxalic acid and allow to stand for 10 minutes.

Then add 10 ml of hydroquinone sulfite solution and gently heat the solution on a hot plate for 30 minutes to develop the blue color fully.

Cool and dilute with water to the 500 ml mark. Read at 570 nm. *Normal lung:* 2–4 mg per 10 gm of wet lung. *Silicotic lungs:* 10–40 mg or more per 10 gm of wet lung.

If the color is too dark, dilute with water and reread. Make certain that the lung and silicon dioxide are fused at 900°C for several hours.

A normal lung blank and a standard silicon dioxide with a lung control should be run in parallel.

Reagents

• Fusion mixture: Sodium carbonate plus potassium carbonate (1:1).

• Hydroquinone sulfite: 0.75 gm of hydroquinone + 10 gm of sulfite + 100 ml of water.

SILVER

Derivatives: Argentum; Argyrol; silver proteins. Most common member is silver nitrate.

Uses: Antiseptic, photography, chemical reagent, indelible ink.

Properties: White crystalline. Water-soluble salt. Acid reaction. Corrosive.

MLD: Approximately 2 gm/70 kg person (silver nitrate).

Remarks: Relatively nontoxic, cumulative. Silver nitrate is toxic and corrosive. Blue coloring of skin (argyria) is irreversible.

Symptoms: (Silver nitrate, most toxic member.) Metallic taste, severe gastrointestinal irritation, nausea, vomiting, diarrhea, vomitus of white and brown masses that turn darker on exposure to light; yellow burns on mouth, skin, and mucosa; dizziness, paresis, coma may occur. Fingernails and gums may become colored, paralysis, permanent bluish pigmentation of skin may occur after long exposure.

Identification

1. Water-soluble salt; acid reaction to litmus (silver nitrate); corrosive to skin; discolors skin a dark gray to black color; solution turns dark in sunlight; silver precipitates out.
2. To solution, add 1 ml of dilute hydrochloric acid (10%) → a white curdy precipitate silver chloride, which is insoluble in concentrated nitric acid.
3. Deposits on copper spiral with dilute hydrochloric acid → gray deposit. See Section I. Quantitate with atomic absorption.

Treatment

Gastric lavage with sodium chloride; or emetics if corrosion is not too extensive. Wash externally with plenty of water. Use demulcents, milk. Morphine for pain or Valium for irritability. Support against shock.

SOLANINE ($C_{45}H_{73}NO_{15}$)

Synonyms: Immature, rotten, or sprouting potatoes (large amounts). Solatunine: only tuber is edible; shoots, leaves, and stem are toxic.

Uses: None.

Properties: Glycosidal alkaloid. Insoluble in water, ether, and chloroform; soluble in hot ethyl alcohol and in amyl alcohol. Mp 250–260°C.

MLD: Approximately 0.2 gm/70 kg person.

Remarks: Symptoms appear within a few hours.

Symptoms: Nausea, vomiting, abdominal pain, diarrhea, headache, mydriasis, blurred vision, vertigo, depression, constriction of the throat, mental confusion, cardiac depression, prostration and sometimes jaundice, collapse. These symptoms are rarely severe. Usually, patients recover.

Identification

Separated with amyl alcohol or alkaline-ether. *Urine:* Alkaline-ether extraction. Evaporate ether. Residue + 1 drop of acetic acid + 2 drops of sulfuric acid + 1 drop of formaldehyde or hydrogen peroxide (5%) → purple-red color. Morphine interferes with formaldehyde but not with peroxide.

Treatment

Activated charcoal with warm water and then gastric lavage or emetics. Ice bag to head. For excitement or delirium, use Valium or *short-acting* barbiturates. Maintain body heat and fluid balance. Artificial respiration if needed. Symptomatic and supportive.

SPIDER BITE

Remarks: Black widow spider has neurotoxic venom. Bite is very toxic for infants.

Symptoms: Slight swelling at site of bite, with pain that increases in intensity. After several hours, pain spreads to extremities. Stomach muscles become rigid. Abdominal pain, nausea and vomiting, rapid feeble pulse rate, fever, urticaria, increased blood pressure, elevated cerebrospinal fluid pressure, sweating, convulsions, especially in children, chills, pallor, respiratory difficulty, collapse.

Identification

By common recognition (red hourglass on ventral side).

Treatment

Prevent secondary infection with antibiotics. Keep patient quiet and warm; morphine for pain, sedatives; Valium or short-acting barbiturates (with caution). Calcium gluconate (1–2 gm IV). Robaxin (injectable) for severe muscle spasm.

Fatalities are rare except in individuals with heart ailments or in children.

Apply paste of sodium bicarbonate over area. Adrenalin or antihistamine.

Artificial respiration and oxygen therapy if indicated.

Specific antivenin distributed by Merck, Sharp & Dohme in 2.5-ml ampules and should be given intramuscularly immediately.

Recovery usually within 48 hours, or convalescence may be prolonged for weeks with residual muscular weakness. Repeated calcium gluconate therapy intravenously may be of value to hasten convalescence. Corticosteroids have been helpful.

STRYCHNINE ($C_{21}H_{22}N_2O_2$)

Synonyms: Nux vomica; rat paste or powder.

Uses: Rodenticide; gopher, mice, and rat killer; Kilmice.

Properties: White crystalline; basic alkaloid; Mp 268°C; soluble in chloroform, less soluble in ether.

MLD: Approximately 30 mg/70 kg person.

APPROXIMATE BLOOD LEVEL: Lethal, 0.5 mg/dl in blood, (or less) ; half-life, about 5 hours.

Remarks: It is no longer used (dangerous) as a tonic to stimulate taste buds and appetite and gastric juices. Sensitivity to taste (very bitter) can be as low as 1:2000. It is readily absorbed from the GI tract and then rapidly metabolized by the liver. About 20 percent is eliminated in the urine and this can be detected within 30 minutes, up to about 12 hours later. Strychnine is not cumulative and is rapidly eliminated from the blood and tissues. Death may be within 15 minutes, or delayed up to 10 hours or more, during or following a massive convulsion with exhaustion of the phrenic and intercostal muscles, and resulting apnea.

Symptoms: The muscles of the neck and face become rigid, hypersensitivity to all senses (smell, vision, sound, taste, touch). Slightest stimulation may trigger a convulsion. Patient is conscious and extremely perceptive to all sensations; tingling of the skin and extremities. Body may be "arched" backwards. Convulsions may last a minute or more, then muscles relax and respiration is resumed. If convulsion is prolonged, this could lead to coma due to apnea and anoxia. Second convulsion usually follows in about 10 minutes. Two or three or more convulsions usually precede death, but can occur also with a very prolonged first convulsion. Respiratory muscles become exhausted. There may be foaming of the mouth, cyanotic skin and mucosa, increased blood pressure and dilated pupils. At death there is early rigor mortis.

Identification

Isolated by NH$_4$OH-chloroform extraction. Urine (or liver) is better than blood; blood may sometimes be negative even in fatal poisoning. Residue in container and fresh vomitus (if available) is best. Strychnine can still be reliably identified in putrefied and embalmed tissue. (Morano)

1. Ultra-violet spectrophotometry: Twenty (20) ml of urine is made alkaline with ammonium hydroxide and is then extracted with 40 ml of chloroform. Allow to separate. Filter the chloroform through course filter paper to eliminate water droplets, then re-extract the chloroform with 5 ml of 0.5 N H$_2$SO$_4$. Read (scan) in UV spectrophotometer (qualitative and quantitative) Maximum density, 254 nm (shoulder at 276–286 nm, very characteristic). E$_{1cm}^{1\%}$ 390, minimum density, 228 nm.

2. Alkaloidal precipitants: Extract a new sample or re-extract the 0.5N H$_2$SO$_4$ with NH$_4$OH-chloroform as described above. Evaporate (gently) the chloroform to dryness.

Dissolve an aliquot portion of this residue with 1 ml of 2% acetic acid. Mix and dissolve and transfer several 1 drop portions onto individual microscope slides. Then add to each singularly, 1 drop of an alkaloidal reagent such as Wagners reagent, Mayer's reagent, picric acid, platinic chloride, ferricyanide, chromate, or gold chloride. The absence of a precipitate *will rule out* strychnine. A positive alkaloid reaction is further studied microscopically for typical crystals by parallel comparison with known strychnine.

3. Color tests: Transfer small aliquot portions of residue to a porcelain spot plate (see under Alkaloids).
   a. Mandelin's reagent → blue → violet (red → (very sensitive) → orange after about 15 minutes)
   b. Marquis' reagent → colorless → greenish brown with heat
   c. Vitali's → violet
   d. Fading purple test: Dissolve a small aliquot of residue with 1 drop of H_2SO_4. Pass a single small crystal of potassium dichromate through this solution (very slowly). The track of the $K_2Cr_2O_7$ crystal will be → purple → changing to orange-red. This eventually in time → colorless (yellow).

4. Three (3) ml of the 0.5N H_2SO_4 (used in test 1) is converted to hydrostrychnine and then reacted with nitrous acid. Add 1 ml HCl and several small pieces of zinc; heat in a water bath for about 10 minutes.

   Remove the zinc and cool; add 1 drop of 10% sodium nitrite. A pink-red suggests strychnine.

5. Thin layer chromatography (TLC) : See Section I.
   a. methanol:acetone:triethanolamine (100:100:3).
      Spray: Dragendroff's reagent; Rf: 20 (Fiorese).
   b. chloroform:methanol (80:20) ; Rf 29. chloroform:methanol (60:20) ; Rf 34.
      Spray: Mandelin's reagent → blue-violet → red → orange
   c. methanol:ammonium hydroxide (100:1.5) ; Rf 15
   d. ethyl acetate:methanol:ammonium hydroxide (85:10:1); Rf 20

6. Gas Chromatography (GLC) : See Section I.

Treatment

First (immediate action) minimize increased reflex excitability (in spinal cord). Avoid all contact (quiet, free from all stimuli) until patient can be *sedated* to prevent onset of or continuing convulsion.

Succinyl choline (Anectine) or diazepam (Valium) may be useful in controlling convulsions. Rapid sedation has also been reported with ether or short-acting barbiturates. Convulsions *must be controlled;* maintain minimal contact or stimulation to patient (sound, light, touch, etc.).

Avoid morphine or long-acting barbiturates.

Supportive measures; maintain respiration; keep sedated. After hyperactivity (and convulsions) *are controlled,* gastric lavage may be attempted.

Prognosis is good if patient survives 24 hours.

SULFA DRUGS

Derivatives: Sulfanilamide; sulfathiazole; sulfapyridine; sulfamerazine; sulfaguanidine; etc.

Use: Bacteriostatic.

Properties: White crystalline, neutral. Sparingly soluble in water; soluble with mineral acids or as sodium salt.

MLD: Varies with agent.

Remarks: May produce crystals in kidney tubules.

Symptoms: Nausea, vomiting, vertigo, skin rash, cyanosis. mental confusion, light sensitivity, hemolytic anemia, acidosis, fatigue, psychoses, acidemia, fever, hematuria, albuminuria, kidney crystals, liver damage, agranulocytosis, nephrosis, oliguria, anuria, sulfhemoglobinemia.

Identification

1. Place 1 drop of urine on lignin (wood pulp) or on a piece of newspaper (good-quality paper is unsatisfactory) ; put 1 drop of concentrated hydrochloric acid onto urine. Normal urine stains paper yellow. Sulfa derivatives stain paper a definite orange. Diamox and Diuril also give reaction.

faint yellow   = about 0.01% or less
deep yellow   =   0.05
orange-yellow =   0.10
deep orange   =   0.25 and above

2. Above test is satisfactory to use directly with a small pulverized portion of a sulfa tablet.

3. Diazotization with Bratton-Marshall procedure. (Refer to any biochemistry or clinical pathology book.)

4. sulfanilamide: mp 165°C.
   sulfapyridine: mp 190–193°C.
   sulfaguanidine: mp 190–193°C.
   sulfamerazine: mp 234–238°C.
   sulfathiazole: mp 200–204°C.
   sulfadiazine: mp 252–256°C.

5. TLC (From Stahl by Waldi).
   a. chloroform:methanol (80:15).
   b. cyclohexane:acetone:acetic acid (40:50:10).
   c. acetone:methanol:diethylamine (90:10:10).

Treatment

Gastric lavage or emetics. Cathartics such as sodium sulfate (30 gm).

Maintain body heat, fluids, and electrolyte balance. Combat acidosis and stone formation with sodium bicarbonate orally and large intake of fluids.

Antibiotics for agranulocytosis (prevent infection). Blood transfusion if indicated for anemia.

For liver damage liberal administration of glucose, calcium salts, and B complex vitamins. Diet should be low in fat. Support against kidney damage. General supportive.

Hemodialysis to hasten elimination.

SULFIDES

Derivatives: Zinc sulfide, barium sulfide, sodium sulfide, selenium sulfide, ammonium sulfide, hydrogen sulfide; stink damp.

Uses: Paints, reagents, depilatory.

Properties: Hydrogen sulfide is a foul-smelling gas (odor like rotten eggs), irritating, penetrating odor even at 10 ppm, sense of smell is quickly dulled.

MLD: 200 ppm as H_2S gas, very rapid at 500 ppm.

Remarks: Is a very toxic poison. Found in sewers, tanneries, mines, refineries, animal manure.

Symptoms: Powerful odor of rotten eggs, sulfhemoglobinemia, eye irritation, nausea, vomiting, diarrhea, hypotension, pulmonary edema, dizziness, palpitation, headache, convulsions or more likely coma, apoplectic type of collapse, marked cyanosis, green discoloration of skin, respiratory failure. High concentrations produce *sudden* unconsciousness and death from respiratory failure (like cyanide produces tissue anoxia).

CHRONIC: Cough, lacrimation, irritation of mucous membranes, diarrhea, loss of weight, fatigue, anorexia, tachycardia. Disturbances of consciousness, memory, and intelligence. Polyneuritis is possible.

Identification

1. Hydrogen sulfide has a foul penetrating odor and can be detected in small traces (1 ppm).
2. Lead acetate paper, when exposed to traces of hydrogen sulfide gas, will turn black immediately (specific).
3. Salts of sulfides, when treated with dilute hydrochloric acid, will liberate gaseous hydrogen sulfide, which can be detected by characteristic odor or by treatment with lead acetate paper → PbS (black)
4. Conway microdiffusion: (See Section I).
   Outer chamber: 5 gm of homogenate + 1 ml 10% H_2SO_4.
   Inner chamber: 2 ml of 10% lead acetate.
   Reaction: Turns black in presence of sulfide.
   Time: 2 hours at room temperature; 1 hour at 37°C.
   Remarks: Cadmium acetate may be substituted for the lead. This produces a yellow sulfide.

Treatment

If salts were taken orally, use emetics and/or gastric lavage with activated charcoal.

Support respiration with artificial respiration and oxygen. Blood transfusion if needed. Keep patient warm and quiet; maintain body temperatures and fluid balance. Guard against pulmonary edema and secondary infection (if inhaled). Symptomatic and supportive measures. Amyl nitrite may help to minimize histotoxic anoxia at cell level. See Cyanide.

SULFURIC ACID (H_2SO_4)

Synonym: Oil of vitriol.

Derivative: $NaHSO_4$

Uses: Storage batteries, industry, cesspool cleaner, pipe and drain cleaner.

Properties: Oily, colorless, heavy liquid. Hygroscopic.

MLD: Approximately 3 ml.

Remarks: Very corrosive to skin and clothing; dehydrating agent. Sodium bisulfate ($NaHSO_4$) gives H_2SO_4 reactions.

Symptoms: Dehydration and carbonization of skin and tissue, brown eschars on lips and mouth. Severe corrosive gastrointestinal irritation; pain in mouth, throat, esophagus, and abdomen. Sour taste, nausea, vomiting, diarrhea, charred black stomach contents, intense thirst, difficult swallowing, acidemia, rapid and weak pulse, slow shallow breathing, convulsions, collapse.

Identification

In stomach contents:

1. Solution is oily, heavy; chars tissue surface or decomposes clothing (turns it black); chars paper, sugar, wood, etc.
2. Becomes hot when added to water.
3. Turns litmus paper pink.
4. Addition of barium chloride (10%) produces a heavy white precipitate, which is insoluble after adding 1 cc of nitric acid (specific).
5. One (1) ml of lead nitrate (10%) → white precipitate, which is insoluble in HNO_3.

Treatment

Do not use stomach tube or emetic if severe corrosion is evident. Dilute with water with caution. Neutralize with milk of magnesia, limewater, soap suds, Amphojel, Cremalin, or other mild antacid. Do not use sodium bicarbonate or other carbon dioxide forming compounds. Give milk, cream, or white of egg as demulcent.

Keep patient warm and quiet. Give morphine for pain. Give sedatives, antibiotics, and combat shock as necessary. Give crushed ice to relieve thirst. If there are signs of asphyxia, tracheotomy may be indicated. Protect against respiratory obstruction, perforation; or stricture formations with corticosteroids.

Guard against infection. Corticosteroid therapy has been recommended in persistent shock. Supportive.

If burns are *external,* wash with plenty of soap and water and then apply a paste of sodium bicarbonate.

SULFONAL ($C_7H_{16}O_4S_2$)

Derivatives: Trional; tetronal.

Uses: Hypnotic action, sedation.

Properties: White crystalline. Nearly tasteless, colorless, Almost insoluble in cold water. Mp 124–126°C.

MLD: Approximately 10 gm/70 kg person.

Remarks: Rarely used. Barbiturates have replaced it.

Symptoms: Nausea, vomiting, diarrhea, vertigo. May be cumulative. Often drowsiness, liver damage, cyanosis, formation of methemoglobin, ataxia, wine-colored urine, depression, coma, increased temperature, weak pulse, irregular breathing, gradual failure of respiration and circulation, collapse, coma.

Identification

Acid-ether extraction group. Test aliquot of residue.

1. If ether is allowed to evaporate spontaneously, characteristic Sulfonal crystals appear that are cubic (six sides equilateral) .
   Sulfonal: mp 125°C.
   Trional: mp 76°C.
   Tetronal: mp 87°C.

2. residue, plus pinch of charcoal, plus heat → mercaptan (foul) odor

3. residue plus pinch of powdered iron, plus heat → mercaptan (foul) odor

4. residue plus hydrochloric acid → hydrogen sulfide (rotten eggs odor)

5. Melt some crystals with potassium cyanide → mercaptan and potassium thiocyanate. Add 3 ml of water to dissolve salts. Test for thiocyanate with 1 ml of ferric chloric (5%) → red color.

Treatment

Activated charcoal and gastric lavage; or emetics. Cathartics (30 gm of sodium sulfate). Cardiac and respiratory support. Protect against liver damage. Treatment generally similar (for depression) as for barbiturates. Supportive.

TARACTAN (CHLORPROTHIXENE)

Properties: MW, 315; Mp 94°C.

Approximate Blood Levels: Single dose (50 mg) in adult: blood level 0.04 r/ml after 8 hours. 4 × 100 mg dose every 3 hours: blood levels 0.06–0.3 r/ml. Half-life is 17 to 24 hours. (Roche Laboratories).

Symptoms: Drowsiness, coma, respiratory depression, hypotension within 3 hours and may persist for about 3 days. Tachycardia, pyrexia, contracted pupils, convulsions (late).

Identification

Extract 4 ml of blood, 2 ml of water, 1 ml of 5N NaOH for 15 minutes with 15 ml of heptane-isoamyl alcohol mixture. Centrifuge and transfer 10 ml of extract and again shake with 1 ml of 10% acetic acid for about 10 minutes. Centrifuge; transfer 0.7 ml of acid extract to small tube. Cool in ice and add 0.1 ml of stannous chloride and 1.2 ml H_2SO_4; mix. Cool; transfer to quartz cuvette and read fluorescence within 1 hour in a spectrofluorometer at 560 nm activating at 390 nm.

Treatment

Charcoal and gastric lavage; or emetics. Guard against hypotension, maintain respiration. Valium or short-acting barbiturates for convulsions.

THALLIUM

Derivatives: Thallous sulfate, acetate, nitrate, carbonate.

Uses: Depilatory; rat and ant poison; glass and dye industry.

Properties: Inorganic white crystalline salts. Absorbed through all portals; accumulates in hair, skin, bones, and muscle.

MLD: Approximately 0.8 gm/70 kg person.

APPROXIMATE URINE LEVEL: Toxic, 0.3 mg/dl.

Remarks: Cumulative poison. Symptoms and signs very vague and not easily recognized; persists for many months; eliminated slowly by way of urinary and gastrointestinal tracts.

Symptoms

May be delayed several hours to several days. Usually begins with gastrointestinal upset within about 12 hours: nausea, vomiting, abdominal pain, diarrhea, hemorrhage, salivation, stomatitis. Vasomotor disturbances; puffiness of cheeks, eyelids, and lips. Chest pains, sore throat, fever, slate-gray complexion. Neurologic signs appear in about 3 days: ataxia, paresthesia (more frequent of lower limbs with severe pain in hands, legs, or soles of feet). Muscular tremors, weakness or atrophy, lethargy, delirium, stupor, psychic changes, cranial nerve effects with ptosis, facial paralysis, retrobulbar neuritis.

Symptoms may persist for a month or more. In about 10 days, scalp hair will start to fall out until completely bald, but there is no facial or axillary hair loss nor any loss of the inner one-third of the eyebrows. This alopecia is temporary, and new hair grows after about 1 month or so.

Congestion of viscera and cardiovascular signs with tachycardia, arrhythmias, hypertension, and EKG changes after about 2 weeks. Also there may be scaly dermatitis, dystrophy of the nails, and Mee's lines (white transverse bands of the nails).

Ataxia, blindness, paralysis of some special senses, peripheral neuritis and kidney damage. Recovery is slow.

Identification

Digest urine, blood, or gastric contents with HNO_3, H_2SO_4.

1. Atomic absorption (if available).
2. Dithizone (similar to lead), see Lead.
3. a. Dilute KI → white precipitate as iodide.
   b. Carefully neutralize with NH_4OH; then acidify with acetic acid and add potassium chromate solution → yellow precipitate as chromate. (Sensitive to 100 μg.) Lead also gives positive tests for a and b above.
   c. Carefully neutralize with NH_4OH and then add potassium ferricyanide solution → brown precipitate.
   Reference: Gettler and Weiss: *Am J Clin Path, 13*:322, 368, 422, 1943.
4. To 1 ml of urine (vomitus) add 2 drops of hydrochloric acid and 5 drops of (sat.) bromine water (use with great caution).
   Allow to stand 5 minutes and then add 5 drops of 20% sulfosalicylic acid, and 0.5 ml of benzene, and 5 drops of 0.1% aqueous methyl violet; shake → blue-green in the benzene layer is positive for thallium, which is sensitive to 1 μg/ml.
   Does not follow Beer-Lampert.
   Semiquantitation for matching visually with standards 1 μg to 6 μg.
   Must match quickly because colors fade.
   With high concentration, use smaller aliquot sample.
   Reference: Decker and Treuting: *Clin Tox, 4*:89, 1971.
5. a. Qualitative test: To 100 ml of freshly voided urine, add 2 ml of 2.5% cadmium sulfate solution. Dissolve 0.25 gm of sodium sulfide crystals in 10 ml of 4% sodium hydroxide solution and add this to the urine while stirring with a glass rod. Let stand for 1 hour or overnight. Draw off the supernatant and discard. Transfer the sediment with a little water to a graduated centrifuge tube. Centrifuge. Draw off the supernatant and discard. To the sediment, add 2 parts

of 6N hydrochloric acid.　Mix to *expel* hydrogen sulfide. Add bromine solution *drop* by *drop* until the solution *remains* a yellow color (5 minutes).　Add sulfosalicylic acid solution *drop* by *drop* until the yellow color fades.　*(Avoid overdose of bromine or sulfosalicylic acid.)*　Add 0.2 ml of rhodamine B solution.　Mix well.　Transfer to a separatory funnel; add 10 ml of benzene and shake.　Return the solution to the centrifuge tube and centrifuge.　The presence of thallium is indicated by a red fluorescent color in the benzene layer.　(Test is sensitive to approximately 2 μg and is positive even several weeks after exposure).

May be modified for quantitation and for serum.

Reagents

• Bromine solution:　Dissolve 10 gm of sodium bromide in 10 ml of water.　Add 20 ml of 6N hydrochloric acid followed by 2.5 ml of liquid bromine *(Caution)*.

• Sulfosalicylic acid: Mix 1 part saturated sulfosalicylic acid with 2 parts 6N hydrochloric acid.

• Rhodamine B (0.05% solution) in concentrated hydrochloric acid.

Reference:　Rappaport and Eichorn: *Clin Chim Acta, 2*:16, 1957.

b. Semiquantitative test.　Use 26 mg $TlNO_3$ in 1000 ml of water; 1 ml = 20 μg Tl.

Prepare standards of 2, 4, 8, 16, and 20 μg of Tl (0.1, 0.2, 0.4, 0.8 and 1.0 ml of standard stock), each in 5 ml of freshly voided urine.

Continue as under qualitative test above but eliminate the sulfosalicylic acid and remove the bromine excess with air bubbling in a water bath until the yellow color disappears.

Add 0.3 ml of rhodamine B solution, mix, and add 2 ml of benzene. Transfer to a separatory funnel and shake for about 2 minutes.　Transfer to a test tube and centrifuge. Collect benzene layer by aspiration and again repeat extraction with 2 ml of benzene.　Combine both benzene extracts. If color still remains, extract again with 2 ml of benzene (until all color is extracted).

The combined benzene-colored extracts are read in a spectrophotometer at 540 nm, with benzene as reference blank. Compare with standards.

If small amounts of thallium are expected, use 100 ml of urine; for larger amounts, use 5 ml of urine. Compare with standards similarly prepared.

If large amounts of albumin are present, first remove this by adding a few drops of acetic acid and boil in a water bath; cool and then filter.

Treatment

No specific therapy is available. Gastric lavage after giving activated charcoal or milk or dilute sodium thiosulfate (3%); or give emetics (syrup of ipecac); enema (high); saline cathartics (30 gm of sodium sulfate) may also help. Fluids (oral) plus 3 to 5 gm of potassium chloride daily for about 5 days to promote urine elimination (but this may be hazardous).

Morphine derivatives for severe muscular pain; Valium or short-acting barbiturates for severe tremors or convulsions; castor oil or soap enemas for constipation. Unfortunately, there is no consistent useful antidote; prognosis remains very poor.

Maintain body temperature, fluids, and electrolyte balance. Symptomatic and supportive.

THIOCYANATE (KSCN)

Synonyms: Potassium thiocyanate; sulfocyanate.

Uses: Medicinal, treatment for hypertension; herbicide.

Properties: White crystalline.

MLD: Approximately 15 gm/70 kg person.

Remarks: Relatively low toxicity. Some patients may show special intolerance to much smaller amounts. Blood levels should not be allowed to go above 10 mg%.

Symptoms: Nausea, vomiting, possible heart failure, anemia, agranulocytosis, blood dyscrasias, cerebral thrombosis, psychoses, renal shutdown, thyroxin formation with goiter formation during treatment. Toxic phenomenon occurs when blood levels are about 18 mg%. Skin rash, vertigo, slurring of speech, hallucinations, pain and weakness in legs and arms, lowered blood pressure, albuminuria, anuria.

Identification

5 ml of serum or plasma precipitate with 5 ml of trichloroacetic acid (10%). Stopper, shake well, allow to stand 15 minutes, filter. To 5 ml of filtrate, add 1 ml of ferric nitrate (5%). Intensity of deep red color is directly proportional to concentration of thiocyanate present (specific). Prepare thiocyanate standards by similar treatment. Small traces are normally found in blood and body fluids. Urine usually contains 0.03–0.06 mg per 100 ml. Smoking may slightly increase normal levels.

Treatment

Remove from exposure. Large fluid intake. Exchange blood transfusion, if indicated, or hemodialysis would hasten elimination in serious acute cases. Elimination is otherwise very slow (1 week or so). Supportive and symptomatic treatment.

ALIPHATIC THIOCYANATES (RHODANATES)

lauryl thiocyanate, less toxic.
Lethane-60, intermediate.
ethyl thiocyanate, most toxic.
methyl thiocyanate, most toxic.

All these compounds are much more toxic than inorganic thiocyanates. Organic thiocyanates probably convert to cyanide in the body.

Treat as for cyanide poisoning with immediate gastric lavage. Intravenous sodium nitrite and thiosulfate. Avoid fats and oils; use milk and egg white as demulcents. Symptomatic treatment for either depression or convulsions.

If compound contained kerosene or another petroleum solvent, this may dominate symptoms.

Antibiotics if needed; oxygen therapy with artificial respiration if in respiratory distress. Supportive measures for possible liver damage.

THIOUREA (CH₄N₂S)

Derivatives: Thiouracil and propyl thiouracil are similar in symptoms and treatment to thiourea.

Uses: Thiouracil and propyl thiouracil are used for thyrotoxicosis. Photography, manufacture of resins and rubber.

Properties: White crystalline. Mp 180–182°C. Neutral.

MLD: Approximately 10 gm/70 kg person.

Remarks: These drugs should be discontinued with first signs of sore throat, coryza, fever, malaise, change in blood count.

Symptoms: Nausea, headache, abdominal cramps, characteristic odor on breath, agranulocytosis, skin eruptions, jaundice, arthragia, hyperpyrexia.

Identification

Separated by acid-ether extraction.

1. ammoniacal silver nitrate → black precipitate
2. Nessler's reagent → black precipitate
3. Two drops of sodium hydroxide (10%) ; heat gently; add 2 ml of water plus 2 drops of sodium nitroprusside (10%) → purple color.
4. TLC. See Section I.

Treatment

Withdrawal of drugs. Guard against secondary infection. Supportive.

TOXALBUMINS

Members: Abrin *(Abrus precatorius)*, rosary pea, or precatory bean; jequirity croton *(Croton tiglium)*; ricin *(Ricinus communis, Castor bean)*; curin *(Jatropha curcas)*.

Origin: Seeds of above-mentioned plants.

MLD: Not known, but *very* toxic. May have a delayed action up to 10 hours before symptoms occur, with small doses.

Symptoms: Nausea, vomiting, diarrhea, general irritation, abdominal pain. Somewhat resembles bacterial toxins. Trembling, weakness, perspiration, hyperpyrexia followed by hypopyrexia, hematuria, albuminuria, agglutination of red blood cells, enlarged lymphatic glands, enlarged spleen, kidney damage.

Identification

1. Separated by dialysis. Toxalbumins are not dialyzed so that the residue is tested. Agglutination test: 1 drop of normal blood is diluted with normal saline and 1 drop of test material added. Examine microscopically for agglutination. pH should not be too acid or alkaline.

2. Black-eyed suzy beans (red small bean with black eye) used for necklace and bracelet and noise maker in "Maracas:" Aqueous extract is salted out with $(NH_4)_2SO_4$ (saturated). Centrifuge at 10,000 rpm for 10 minutes; retain precipitate but dialyze to remove excess $(NH_4)_2SO_4$. Pick up residue in normal saline and read in UV spectrophotometer
   Maximum density 243 nm; minimum density 267 nm.
   Same in H_2O; HCl; NH_4OH.
   Reference: Abrin (Niyogi: *J Foren Sci, 15:*529, 1970.

Treatment

Activated charcoal and gastric lavage; or emetics. Demulcents, cathartics. Blood transfusion of whole blood. Support against kidney damage. Symptomatic and supportive treatment.

TOXAPHENE ($C_{10}H_{10}Cl_8$)

Synonym: Chlorinated camphene.

Use: Insecticide—especially against cotton insects, grasshoppers.

Properties: White powder. Oil soluble; insoluble in water. Pleasant pine odor. Mp 65–90°C.

MLD: Approximately 3 gm/70 kg person.

Remarks: Moderately irritating to skin; can be absorbed through all portals including skin. Toxic effects within an hour; death may occur early or may be delayed 24 hours.

Symptoms: Gastric irritation, nausea, vomiting, diarrhea. Stimulation of central nervous system, effects within an hour, epileptiform convulsions associated with depression; these are aggravated by external stimuli; internal hemorrhages, high temperature. Respiratory failure. Similar in symptoms to camphor, which it resembles chemically. Liver and kidney damage.

Identification

1. Liver and kidney function tests are of presumptive value.
2. TLC and GLC: See Section I.
3. Toxaphene contains 67 to 69 percent chlorine. Determine chlorides similar to procedure given under DDT. Multiply results by 100/68.

Treatment

Gastric lavage with activated charcoal; or emetics; saline cathartics (sodium sulfate, 30 gm) .

Avoid oils. (Toxaphene is oil soluble.) Remove clothing. Thoroughly wash skin with soap and water.

Valium or short-acting barbiturates to combat convulsions: Support against liver and kidney damage. Symptomatic and supportive treatment.

TRICYCLIC ANTIDEPRESSANT TRANQUILIZERS

Members	Suggested therapeutic dose (mg) (PDR)	Approximate mg/dl* Blood Levels		
		Therapeutic	*Toxic*	*Lethal*
amitryptyline (Elavil) (Endep)	25 tid	0.02	0.04	1
desipramine (Norpramine) (Pertofrane)	50 tid	0.15	0.5	1
doxepin (Adapin) (Sinequan)	25 tid	0.002		1
imipramine (Tofranil) (Presamine)	25 tid	0.015	0.1	0.2
nortriptyline (Aventyl)	25 tid	0.015	0.5	1
opipramol (Ensidon)				
trimipramine (Surmontil)				
protriptyline (Vivactil)	10 tid			

*Winek, McBay, Clarke, others.

Uses: Antidepressant (endogenous depression); blocks pain arousal. Large doses may produce sedation. Mechanism of action is possibly to prevent the uptake of norepinephrine by the sympathetic nerves.

Properties: Soluble in ether (best), also soluble in *n*-heptane or hexane or chloroform. After a 10 minute hydrolysis with HCl make alkaline with NaOH and then chloroform extracts the metabolite (Clarke).

MLD: 1–2 gm/70 kg person. Desipramine less toxic; protriptyline more toxic.

Imipramine metabolizes → desipramine.

Serum half-life can be several days; in serious overdose, high levels may persist 4 to 5 days.

Remarks

Potentiation by amino oxidase inhibitors, and also with ethanol or the barbiturate group. Death can occur even 3 days after apparent recovery. There is cross tolerance within the group.

Absorption is fairly rapid from the GI tract and is deposited in select tissues; conjugates with glucuronides; Demethylation produces active metabolites. There may be some resecretion into the stomach cavity.

Symptoms: Generally similar to atropine; may appear early with greatest severity during the first 12 hours. In general, there is vomiting, thirst, drowsiness (or dizziness), hypo- or hyperthermia, stimulation, excitement, tachycardia, dilated pupils, hypo- or hypertension, tremors, agitation, convulsions, stupor, coma, bowel and bladder paralysis, respiratory depression, cardiac arrhythmias, death by cardiac arrest.

Doxepin: Gastric corrosion, pulmonary and cerebral edema.

Identification

1. 1 ml of urine + 1 ml reagent → green color, positive for desipramine, imipramine, trimipramine.

   Blue color may suggest Mellaril.

   Lilac color may suggest a phenothiazine compound.

   Reagent: Forrest & Forrest: 10 ml each of 0.2% $K_2Cr_2O_7$; 30% H_2SO_4; 20% $HClO_4$; 50% HNO_3.

2. 1 ml of urine + 1 ml Forrest & Forrest reagent → yellow-green if amitriplylin or blue-green if desipramine.

3. UV spectrophotometer
   a. 25 ml of urine is alkalinized with NaOH and is then extracted with 2 × 25 ml of ether. Combined ether is extracted with 5 ml of 0.5N H_2SO_4. Scan in UV spectrophotometer. Save extract for later confirmation.

| Member | 0.5N H$_2$SO$_4$ | | | 0.5N NaOH | |
	Max den nm	E$_{1cm}^{1\%}$	Min den nm	Max den nm	Min den nm
amitriptyline	238	550	228	238	
desipramine	251	340	231	251	340
doxepin	292	130	272		
	(shoulder at 250 nm)				
imipramine	250	270	231	253	231
nortriptyline	239	400	230	239	––

b. (Clarke) 25 ml of urine (or urine residual from test a above) is made neutral with 6N HCl + 0.2 ml in excess. Hydrolyze for 1 hour on a water bath; cool; make alkaline with 10% NaOH; extract with 50 ml of CHCl$_3$; re-extract CHCl$_3$ with 0.1N HCl and scan in UV spectrophotometer. Maximum density of the metabolite of amitriptyline and nortripyline is at 290 nm.

4. Thin Layer Chromatogrpahy (TLC)

a. To the 5 ml of H$_2$SO$_4$ extract in 3a above make definitely alkaline with 20% NaOH. Extract with 2 × 25 ml ether. Gently evaporate the combined ether. Pick up residue with minimal methanol and spot onto TLC plate. (See Section I.)

b. To a new 25 ml sample of urine (if available) extract with 2 × 25 ml ether and continue as above.

Plate: Silica gel G, 250 micron

Developing solvent systems:

- methanol:NH$_4$OH (100:1.5) (Clarke; Sunshine) —solvent 1
- acetone:methanol:isopropanolamine (85:15:1) (Sunshine)— solvent 2
- acetic acid:ethanol:H$_2$O (30:50:20) (Clarke) —solvent 3
- benzene:dioxane:NH$_4$OH (60:35:5) (Clarke) —solvent 4
- ethyl acetate:methanol:NH$_4$OH:H$_2$O (85:13.5:5:1.0) (Modified Davidow Assays) — solvent 5
- methanol:CHCl$_3$:NH$_4$OH (50:50:1)
- acetone:NH$_4$OH (100:1)

Spray:

• chloroiodoplatinate → purple
• FPN → blue → overspray with chloro-iodoplatinate for FPN

	Solvent				
	1	2	3	4	5
Amitriptyline	0.75	70	78	75	0.90
Desipramine	0.53				0.41
Doxepin	0.72				0.79
Imipramine	0.73	72	76	86	0.81
Nortriptyline	0.59				0.39
Protriptyline	0.38				0.17

Treatment

Control convulsions with inhalation anesthetics or diazepam (Valium) ; succinylcholine may also be useful. When convulsions are controlled, remove drug by gastric lavage and saline cathartics. Repetative lavage may be of some additional help. Symptomatic and supportive measures with particular attention to cardiac arrhythmias, convulsions, blood pressure, and respiration especially during the first 15 hours. Maintain good respiratory exchange, support against cardiac arrhythmias, maintain blood pressure (if possible without vasopressure agents) ; maintain electrolyte, water, and heat balance. Hemodialysis has been reported of little value.

During the recovery phase, a deep lethargy may alternate with tremors, agitation, delirium, hallucinations, mental confusion, and persistent insomnia. A sudden relapse and death can occur after apparent recovery.

Continuing cardiac monitoring may be advisable.

Physostigmine salicylate has been reported of some use for the atropine effects; but use with caution.

TURPENTINE

Synonyms: Oil of turpentine; oleoresin from Pinus; oil of pine.

Uses: In paints, polishes, paint or lacquer remover or thinner; rubefacient. Also see Essential Oils.

Properties: Oily liquid; volatile, odorous, colorless.

MLD: Approximately 15 ml/70 kg person.

Remarks: Absorbed through skin or by inhalation. Death may occur within a few hours; pine oil is less volatile and is less toxic; (See Essential oils).

Symptoms: Strong odor on the breath, severe gastrointestinal irritation producing nausea, vomiting, diarrhea, abdominal pain, dizziness, giddiness, general weakness, headache, insomnia, ataxia, central nervous system disturbances, restlessness, delirium, painful urination (urine has odor of violets), albuminuria, oliguria, dark urine, exposed skin is reddened, unconsciousness, shallow breathing, convulsions, pulmonary edema, bronchopneumonia, kidney involvement, collapse.

Identification

Separated by steam distillation; add sodium chloride to salt saturate distillate, extract with ether. Evaporate ether → turpentine.

1. Marquis reagent → pink-red.
2. 2 ml ethanol + 1 ml 1% vanillin in HCl + heat → green → blue
3. nitrosyl chloride → crystals (mp 103°C)
4. 1 drop on a piece of paper → translucent
5. Excreted in urine: odor of violets; reduces Benedict's or Fehling's reagents.
6. hydrochloric acid (1 drop) + ferric chloride (1 drop of 10%) + heat → pink → violet → blue
7. dilute solution + reagent → green-blue turbidity
   Reagent: 0.5 gm of potassium ferricyanide, 0.2 gm of ferric chloride dissolved in 250 ml of water.
8. Distill into carbon tetrachloride and examine with NIR spectrophotometry, see Section I.
9. Turpentine + H_2SO_4 → red — brown.

Treatment

Dilute with milk, then gastric lavage with great care to prevent aspiration. Saline cathartics (sodium sulfate, 30 gm); milk as demulcent; do not give fats or oils. Artificial respiration and oxygen as needed.

Keep patient warm and quiet. Support against kidney damage. Valium or short-acting barbiturates for restlessness or convulsions. Support against pulmonary edema. Guard against secondary infections, circulatory collapse. Supportive.

VACOR

Synonyms: DLP-787; *N*-3-pyridylmethyl-*N'p*-nitrophenylurea.
Uses: Rodenticide, single dose-quick kill.

Symptoms

INITIAL (4–48 hours) : Nausea, vomiting, abdominal pain, chills and mental confusion; pleasant odor of peanuts.

INTERMEDIATE: Anorexia, body aches especially in limbs, dilated pupils, dehydration, chest pain, glycosuria and elevated blood glucose, diabetic type of keto acidosis, dysphagia, leukocytosis, gastrointestinal dystonia, urinary retention (bladder dysfunction) , cardiovascular involvement with arrhythmias, postural hypotension, peripheral neuropathy, fine tremors of extremities, muscular weakness.

LATE: Severe autonomic dysfunction, cardiovascular collapse, respiratory failure, coma, death.

Identification

Thin Layer Chromatography (TLC) :

Adsorb 50 ml of urine onto Amberlite XAD-4 (50–80 mesh) Rohm and Haas; or the Brinkmann extraction kit; or Porapak Q (50-80 mesh) Waters Associates.

Elute the adsorbate with 3 ml acetone. Carefully evaporate below 70°C with a stream of air or N_2 gas. Reconstitute residue with minimal methanol and spot onto plate. Develop with acetone:benzene (60:40) .

Air dry and then spray with Erhlichs' reagent. After 5 minutes, heat the plate to develop color. Start at 70°C and gradually advance up to 200°C.

vacor → yellow brown at Rf 25
vacor amino → bright yellow at Rf 20

Sensitive to about 0.1 ppm in 50 ml urine. Vacor (*p*-nitrophenylurea) metabolizes → vacor (*p*-aminophenylurea), which is the principle compound found in urine; at higher levels, the parent compound vacor (nitrophenylurea) plus a second metabolite, vacor (acetamido) may be also detected in urine.

Reagent: Erhlich's: 1 gm *p*-dimethylaminobenzaldehdye in 30 ml methanol + 3 ml H_2SO_4 + 180 ml *n*-butanol.

Reference: W.C. Geyer of the Rohm-Haas Co.

Treatment

Gastric lavage or emesis as early as possible. Emesis or lavage is warranted up to 12 hours postingestion. This is followed by 30 ml of mineral oil plus a cathartic. It is recommended (Rohm & Haas) that 500 mg of niacinamide (nicotinamide) be given IM *immediately,* then follow with 100–200 mg every 4 hours up to 48 hours. If signs of toxicity develop (as noted above), increase frequency to every 2 hours. Do not exceed 3 gm per day per adult. When patient is able to take medication by mouth, continue to give 100 mg niacinamide p.o. 3 to 5 times daily for the next two weeks. Signs of diabetes mellitus may respond to insulin therapy.

Reference: Rohm & Haas Co., Philadelphia, Pennsylvania (11/30/76).

Telephone when human poisoning occurs: Medical Director, (215) 592-2912 (office hours), (215) 592-3000 (after hours).

VITAMINS AND SUPPLEMENTS

Vitamin A, 500 USP units: Symptoms come on 30–60 minutes later; nausea, vomiting, drowsiness, diplopia, severe gastroenteritis, diarrhea, dehydration, acidosis, collapse, coma.

Vitamin B_1 (thiamine), B_2 (riboflavin), B_6 (pyridoxine), niacinamide, and calcium pantothenate: All are water soluble with low toxicity.

Vitamin C (ascorbic acid): Dose 100–500 mg Tab; water soluble and essentially of low toxicity; possible mild GI irritation with massive doses.

Vitamin D: Possible chronic toxicity.

Vitamin E: 100–600 IU; capsules; oil soluble; low toxicity.

$FeSO_4$ (300 mg) may be fatal in children; see Ferrous sulfate.

WARFARIN ($C_{19}H_{16}O_4$)

Synonyms: 3 - α - phenyl - β - acetylethyl - 4 - hydroxycoumarin; WARF-42; Dethmore; d-Con; Rat powder; O-phenyl-β-acetylethylhydroxycoumarin; Chemrat; Meyerkil; Pival is warfarinlike.

SALTS: Warfarin: Coumadin; Marevan; Panwarfin; Prothromadin. Warfarin potassium: Athrombin K.

OTHER COUMARIN DERIVATIVES: Bishydroxycoumarin (dicumarol); acenocoumarin (Sintrom); phenprocoumon (Liquamar).

Uses: Therapeutically; sodium and potassium salts are used as anticoagulant; 12 to 18 hours to be effective and persists up to 6 days; absorption is rapid, but elimination in urine is slow (as metabolites). Used as a rodenticide (toxic to rats in small doses) it accumulates giving rise to internal hemorrhages (hypoprothrombinemia).

Properties: White crystalline; Mp 161°C; soluble in acetone, alcohol, and dioxane. Slightly soluble in chloroform and ether.

Coumadin (Na salt) is soluble in water; dicumarol is practically insoluble but is slightly soluble in chloroform, which can then be re-extracted into 0.5N NaOH.

MLD: Above 100 mg/70 kg person. It shows high toxicity for gray rats and low toxicity for man and dog.

Coumadin therapeutic blood levels: 2–8 ug/ml (Jatlow).

Remarks: Single dose shows maximum effects in 4 days. It prevents thrombus in therapeutic levels. Onset of action about 24–36 hrs.

Symptoms: Diminished prothrombin formation, capillary damage, increased clotting time of blood, bleeding upon slight trauma, visible external hematoma, internal hemorrhages; bloody sputum, nose, gums, gastrointestinal tract, stools, and urine. Back pain, abdominal pain, and vomiting.

Identification

SPECIMENS: Stomach content; metabolites found in urine upon acid-chloroform extraction.

1. Clotting time of blood increased; Measure Prothrombin Activity (1–2 days later).

2. UV-spectrophotometry: Re-extract with 0.5N NaOH. Maximum density, 307 nm; $E_{1cm}^{1\%} = 505$; minimum density. 257 nm; shoulder at 290–294 nm.
   dicoumarol: maximum density, 312 nm; minimum density, 260 nm.
3. Gas liquid chromatography: See Section I.
4. Thin layer chromatography: See Section I.
   Developing solvents:
   * cyclohexane:chloroform:acetone (40:50:10), Rf 45. Spray: Rhodamine B
   * benzene:acetic acid (20:3), Rf 25
   * ether:hexane:acetic acid (7:25:1), Rf 46 (Curry) (detect with UV at 254 nm).
   * ammonium hydroxide (3N):n-butanol (1:1). Saturate butanol then decant (discard the excess NH₄OH). Spray: Diazotized sulfonilic acid, dry, then spray with 3N HCl (Clarke).

	Rf	Color
Coumadin	63	White
dicoumarol	55	Yellow
salicylic acid	40	Orange
meprobamate	57	White
Darvon	50	Orange

Spray:
* rhodamine B
* 3% vanillin in H_2SO_4
* 20% H_2SO_4

Warfarin at very low concentrations gives good spots, but not for Coumadin or dicumarol. In contrast with larger amounts, Coumadin (Rf 54) and dicumarol (Rf 19) are now visible but not warfarin (Pinel de Rodríguez).

Try to elute all spots with ethyl acetate and scan in the UV spectrophotometer in isopropanol (1% acetic acid).

Maximum density, 305; $E_{1cm}^{1\%} = 361$ (Curry)

5. Fluorescence: The sodium salt of warfarin (Coumadin) does not emit fluorescence. In those warfarin compounds that do

emit, this will disappear by adding 0.1N NaOH (Cohn). Urine (normal) may emit some fluorescence that can interfere (does not disappear by adding NaOH).

To be able to see fluorescence in TLC: should not be the sodium salt; special fluorescent silica gel should be used; and short wave UV lamp at 254 nm should be used to identify spot.

Treatment

Induce vomiting with ipecac syrup (repeat in 20 minutes); or gastric lavage with normal saline. Vitamin K_1 emulsion can be used if prothrombin time is abnormal (phytonadione: Metphyton). However, prothrombin time is not usually effected unless repeated large ingestions occur.

Minimize chances for hemorrhage by limiting activity (if necessary).

Supportive measures. Symptoms and treatment are similar for overdose with Fumarin, Pival, or dicumerol.

Ferrous sulfate (hematinic) may help to replace iron loss; supportive measures for possible secondary anemia.

It is necessary to correct and maintain normal prothrombin activity. Laboratory monitoring is essential.

WARFARE POISONS

NERVE POISONS

Members: Parathion and related organic phosphate esters.

Remarks: Destroys cholinesterase and thereby builds up accumulated acetylcholine. Interferes with nerve function. Members of this group are *highly toxic* and readily absorbed through all portals including the eyes. Protective rubber gloves must be used during treatment; however, these agents will even penetrate rubber so periodic washings are necessary.

Symptoms: Rhinorrhea, bronchoconstriction, difficult breathing, pain and tightness in chest, convulsions, pinpoint pupils. See details under Parathion.

Treatment

Immediate use of atropine. See details under Parathion.

NOTE: This group may be dispersed as liquid or gas.

VESICANTS

Members: Nitrogen mustards and arsenical vesicants.

Remarks: These agents will cause systemic poisoning when absorbed.   Can be absorbed through all portals.   May be used in gas warfare or to contaminate food or drink.   Nitrogen mustards are very persistent; oily, colorless or pale yellow liquids; faint fish odor.

The arsenicals are organic chlor-vinyl dichloroarsines (lewisite).   These are colorless to brown liquids; fruity or geranium-like odor.   Will even penetrate rubber.

Symptoms: Erythema, itching, burning, multiple, large vesicant blisters, severe gastrointestinal irritation, nausea, vomiting, abdominal pain, diarrhea, cough, fever, dyspnea, moist rales, bronchopneumonia, hoarseness, conjunctivitis, corneal involvement, salivation, bradycardia, cardiac irregularities.

Treatment

Immediate action is necessary.   Decontaminate.   Remove patient's clothing.   Blisters treated; denuded areas treated as for burns.

Atropine to reduce gut motility.   Blood transfusions if indicated.   Guard against secondary infection.

For the arsenical exposure, give BAL immediately.   This is very important.   (For details, see under Arsenic.)

Convalescence may be slow.   Supportive and symptomatic treatment.

LUNG IRRITANTS

Members: Phosgene is most important; chlorine or chloropicrin.

Remarks: Phosgene is a colorless gas and smells like green silage.   It is nonpersistent.

Symptoms: Gastrointestinal irritation.   Especially irritating to lungs, possible bronchopneumonia, massive pulmonary edema, tightness in chest, cyanosis, collapse.

Treatment

Oxygen therapy; symptomatic and supportive. Guard against collapse and secondary infection.

Avoid barbiturates, atropine, *also avoid* alcohol, cardiac or respiratory stimulants, or vasopressors.

SYSTEMIC POISONS

Members: Hydrocyanic acid and cyanogen chloride are most important members. Arsine is no longer used.

Remarks: Both are gases and very volatile. Cyanogen chloride is similar in symptoms and treatment to cyanide.

Symptoms: See details under Cyanide.

Treatment

See details under Cyanide.

STERNUTATORS

Members: Adamsite, diphenylchloroarsine, diphenylcyanoarsine.

Remarks: These are crystalline solids; smell like fireworks. Irritant smoke; vomiting gases.

Symptoms: Gastrointestinal irritation, nausea, vomiting, abdominal pain, diarrhea, burning in throat, hoarseness, tightness and pain in chest, coughing, nasal secretions, increased salivation, mental depression, temporary prostration, pneumonia.

Tear gas: Chloroacetophenone (Mace) for riot control.

ZINC

Derivatives: Zinc salts (sulfate, chloride, oxide, phosphide, or stearate).

Uses: Solder flux, alloys, galvanized plating, rodenticide.

Properties: White crystallin soluble salt, acidic reaction, corrosive.

MLD: Approximately 15 gm as zinc sulfate for a 70/kg person; phosphide or chloride is more toxic; oxide is least toxic.

Remarks: Relatively nontoxic in small amounts. Small amounts normally found in the body: approximately 5 mg% in liver, 1 mg% in blood, 0.5 mg% in urine, cumulative; zinc chloride and phosphide are very caustic. Zinc stearate in talc, when inhaled, may produce chemical pneumonitis. Astringent.

Symptoms: Metallic taste, chills, nausea, vomiting, intense thirst, diarrhea, abdominal pain, leukocytosis, fever; if inhaled will produce above symptoms plus respiratory irritation, pulmonary edema, possible pneumonia.

Identification

1. Blood, urine, etc., can be digested with sulfuric-nitric-perchloric acid. See Section I (under Acid Digestion).
2. This digest is diluted (1:9) with water to give approximately 10% sulfuric acid. Remove a small aliquot and add 2 ml of 10% potassium ferrocyanide → white-yellow precipitate sensitive to approximately 0.020 mg per 10 ml of solution. Compare with standards. Cu, Cd, Ni, or Co interfere.
3. This digest or other solution specimen is treated dropwise with 20% sodium hydroxide until just slightly acid. Divide into 3 aliquot portions.
   a. Aliquot plus several drops of 10% sodium hydroxide until alkaline (or a precipitate appears). Add excess sodium hydroxide → precipitate dissolves.
   b. Aliquot plus dithizone → orange color at pH 5.5 (see Mercury).
      Reference: Gettler, A.O.: *Am J Clin Path, 17*:244, 1947.
   c. Aliquot plus ammonia until barely alkaline; then saturate with hydrogen sulfide gas → zinc sulfide (white precipitate).
4. Atomic absorption (if available) is best.

Treatment

Induce emesis (ipecac syrup is best), unless contraindicated (severe corrosion). Demulcents; morphine as needed for abdominal pain.

Maintain body heat and water and electrolyte balance. Guard against shock. Supportive measures.

Note: Inhalation of zinc metal fume may produce "metal fume fever" with pulmonary edema and powerful irritation to respiratory tract.

BIBLIOGRAPHY

Arena, Jay M: *Poisoning: Symptoms and Treatment,* 4th ed. Springfield, Thomas, 1979.

Arena, Jay M: Treatment of poisoning, *Clinical Symposia, 30(2):* 1978.

Clarke, E.G.C.: *Identification of Drugs.* Pharmaceutical Press, London, 1969.

Comstock, Eric: personal communications.

Curry, A.: *Advances in Forensic and Clinical Toxicology.* Cleveland, CRC Press, 1972.

Curry, A.: *Poison Detection in Human Organs,* 2nd ed. Springfield, Thomas, 1969.

Cutting, W.C.: *Handbook of Pharmacology,* 5th ed. New York, Appleton-Century-Croft, 1972.

Deichmann, W.B. and Gerarde, H.W.: *Signs, Symptoms, and Treatment of Certain Acute Intoxications.* 2nd ed. Springfield, Thomas, 1958.

Dreisbach, R.H.: *Handbook of Poisoning,* 7th ed. Los Altos, California, Lange Med Publ, 1977.

Stefanini, Mario (Ed.): *Clinical Pathology,* New York, Grune & Stratton, Vol. 11, 1969.

Gleason, M.N., Gosselin, R.F., Hodge, H.C., and Smith, R.P.: *Clinical Toxicology of Commercial Products,* 4th ed. Baltimore, Williams & Wilkins, 1976.

Goodman, L.S. and Gilman, A.: *Pharmacological Basis of Therapy,* 5th ed. New York, MacMillan, 1975.

Goth, A.: *Medical Pharmacology, Principles and Concepts,* 6th ed. St. Louis, Mosby, 1972.

Hayes, W.J.: *Clinical Handbook on Economic Poisons,* USPHS Publ. 476; 1963.

Handbook of Common Poisonings in Children, HEW Publication (FDA) 76-7004, 1976.

Kline, N.S., Alexander, S.F., and Chamberlain, A.: *Manual for Emergency Management of Psychotropic Drug Overdosage,* Orandell, N.J., Medical Economics Co., 1977.

Mathews, H. and Lawson, A.A.: *Treatment of Common Acute Poisoning,* 3rd ed. Longman, New York, 1975.

Mienscher, W.C.: *Poisonous Plants of the United States,* 2nd ed.   Mac-

Millan, New York, 1957.

Patty, F.A.: *Industrial Hygiene and Toxicology*. New York, Interscience, Vol. II, 1967.

Physician's Desk Reference (PDR) to Pharmaceutical Specialities, latest edition. Orandel, NJ, Medical Economics, Inc.

Spitz, W. and Fisher, R.S.: *Medico-Legal Investigation of Death*. Springfield, Thomas, 1973.

Sunshine, I. (Ed.): *Handbook of Analytical Toxicology,* Cleveland, CRC Press, 1969.

Sunshine, I. (Ed.): *Methodology for Analytical Toxicology.* Cleveland, CRC Press, 1975.

Thienes, C.H. and Haley, T.J.: *Clinical Toxicology,* 5th ed. Philadelphia, Lea & Febinger, 1972.

Winek, C.L.: *Blood and Chemistry Blood Level Data,* Fisher Co., Pittsburg.

Phone your nearest poison control center—See your local phone book. Look for name and location of drug manufacturer on the bottle and ask for telephone information; information is usually available.

National Clearinghouse for Poison Control Centers, Washington, D.C.

Center of Disease Control, Atlanta, Georgia.

INDEX

527

B